ADVANCES IN MOLECULAR AND CELLULAR ENDOCRINOLOGY

ADVANCES IN MOLECULAR AND CELLULAR ENDOCRINOLOGY

Series Editor
BORIS DRAZNIN

NEW TRANSCRIPTION FACTORS AND THEIR ROLE IN DIABETES AND ITS THERAPY

Editor

Jacob E. Friedman

Department of Pediatrics,
Biochemistry and Molecular Genetics
University of Colorado School of Medicine
Aurora, Co, USA

ELSEVIER

AMSTERDAM – BOSTON – HEIDELBERG – LONDON – NEW YORK – PARIS
SAN DIEGO – SAN FRANCISCO – SINGAPORE – SYDNEY – TOKYO

Elsevier
Radarweg 29, PO Box 211, 1000 AE Amsterdam, The Netherlands
The Boulevard, Langford Lane, Kidlington, Oxford OX5 1GB, UK

First edition 2006

Library of Congress Cataloguing-in-Publication Data
A catalogue record for this book is available from the British Library of Congress

British Library Cataloguing in Publication Data
A catalogue record for this book is available from the British Library

ISBN-13: 978-0-444-51158-4
ISBN-10: 0-444-51158-X

For information on all Elsevier publications
visit our website at books.elsevier.com

Printed and bound by CPI Antony Rowe, Eastbourne
Transferred to digital print 2007

Working together to grow
libraries in developing countries

www.elsevier.com | www.bookaid.org | www.sabre.org

ELSEVIER   BOOK AID
International   Sabre Foundation

Contents

Colour Plate Section can be found at the back of this book

Preface

The activation of nuclear receptors and DNA binding proteins serves as a final target for hormones and intracellular signaling pathways underlying many important physiological and biochemical pathways. Over the last 5–10 years, a new era of research has begun, arising from the application of molecular biology to the field of transcriptional regulation of metabolism and obesity. In addition, the application of transgenic and gene knockout technology to uncover the role of these transcription factors, and their potential application for therapeutic intervention, has led to new insights and broader understanding of the clinical relevance of these proteins in metabolic research.

Efforts to understand the mechanisms that underlie susceptibility to diabetes have primarily focused on structure–function of genes encoding receptors, enzymes, and transporters. More recently, the study of specific transcription factors has provided a new basis for understanding the integrated mechanisms of diabetes and metabolism. A powerful example of this integration is the discovery in 1996 of mutations in genes encoding transcription factors HNF-1α and HNF-4α (hepatic nuclear factor 4α/1α) as underlying causes of inherited MODY (maturity onset diabetes of youth). Another excellent example is the discovery of the thiazolidinedione (TZD) receptor class of drugs, which bind to PPARγ, a nuclear hormone receptor. The uncovering of associations between transcription factors and the pathophysiology of diabetes is an exciting new field with many recent new findings. Thus, understanding how transcription factors regulate fundamental metabolic processes should have broad appeal to an array of basic and clinical scientists.

Through specific examples, with broad applications, this book will provide a comprehensive look at several examples of how transcription factors may underlie the pathogenetic mechanisms of diabetes and obesity. We hope that this volume will provide a valuable overview of the status of the field, while also providing valuable information of practical utility to those who do not necessarily work in this field. The integration of basic biology with physiologically and clinically relevant proteins should provide the reader with a theoretical background to understanding the strategies for new potential therapeutic targets and their application to disease.

As the editor, I have asked several eminent experts in the fields of genetics, biochemistry, and pathophysiology of diabetes for their contributions, and they have graciously accepted. I am particularly grateful to these individuals for their efforts. The genetic approach for understanding obesity and diabetes ultimately relies upon a strong knowledge base of metabolism and metabolic pathways. Thus, I would particularly like to thank the two outstanding metabolic biochemists, my former mentors, Dr. Lynis Dohm (East Carolina University SOM) and Dr. Richard Hanson (Case Western Reserve University SOM). These individuals impressed upon me very early the importance of understanding organ-based metabolism together with molecular biology and its metabolic consequences. As Sir Issac Newton once remarked to fellow scientist Robert Hooke on February 5th, 1676, "my success has been built on the achievement of others: If I have seen further it is by standing on the shoulders of giants".

Jacob E. (Jed) Friedman, Ph.D.
Professor, Department of Pediatrics, Biochemistry & Molecular Genetics
University of Colorado School of Medicine

January 27, 2006

List of contributors

Michael N. Weedon

St. Lukes Laboratories
Peninsula Medical School
Exeter, United Kingdom

Andrew T. Hattersley

St. Lukes Laboratories
Peninsula Medical School
Exeter, United Kingdom

Timothy M. Frayling

St. Lukes Laboratories
Peninsula Medical School
Exeter, United Kingdom

Catherine S. Mitchell

Department of Medicine
University of Cambridge
Addenbrooke's Hospital
Cambridge, United Kingdom

Mark Gurnell

Department of Medicine
University of Cambridge
Addenbrooke's Hospital
Cambridge, United Kingdom

Uwe Dressel

Centre for Diabetes and Endocrine
Research (CDER)
The University of Queensland
Princess Alexandra Hospital
Brisbane, Australia

George E.O. Muscat

Institute for Molecular Bioscience (IMB)
The University of Queensland
Brisbane, Australia

Knut R. Steffensen

Receptor Biology Unit
Department of Biosciences at NOVUM
Karolinska Institute
Huddinge, Sweden

Pascal Ferré   INSERM U671
                         Université Pierre et Marie Curie
                         Paris Cedex, France

Delphine Eberlé   INSERM U671
                         Université Pierre et Marie Curie
                         Paris Cedex, France

Bronwyn Hegarty   INSERM U671
                         Université Pierre et Marie Curie
                         Paris Cedex, France

Fabienne Foufelle   INSERM U671
                         Université Pierre et Marie Curie
                         Paris Cedex, France

Robert R. Henry   VA San Diego Healthcare System
                         University of California, San Diego
                         San Diego, CA, USA

Susan A. Phillips   University of California, San Diego
                         San Diego, CA, USA

Sunder R. Mudaliar   VA San Diego Healthcare System
                         University of California, San Diego
                         San Diego, CA, USA

Theodore P. Ciaraldi   University of California, San Diego
                         San Diego, CA, USA

Sven Enerbäck   Medical Genetics
                         Department of Medical Biochemistry
                         Göteborg University
                         Göteborg, Sweden

Isabelle Gerin   Department of Molecular and
                         Integrative Physiology
                         University of Michigan Medical School
                         Ann Arbor, MI, USA

                         Laboratoire de Chimie Physiologique
                         Université Catholique de Louvain
                         Brussels, Belgium

Hyuk C. Cha

Department of Molecular and
Integrative Physiology
University of Michigan Medical School
Ann Arbor, MI, USA

Ormond A. MacDougald

Department of Molecular and
Integrative Physiology
University of Michigan Medical School
Ann Arbor, MI, USA

Judy Tsai

Department of Genetics and
Complex Diseases
Harvard School of Public Health
Boston, MA, USA

Qiang Tong

USDA/ARS Children's Nutrition Research Center
Baylor College of Medicine
Houston, TX, USA

Gökhan S. Hotamisligil

Department of Genetics and
Complex Diseases
Harvard School of Public Health
Boston, MA, USA

Andreas Barthel

Department of Medicine I
Kliniken Bergmannsheil
Ruhr-University Bochum
Bochum, Germany

Stephan Herzig

Department of Molecular
Metabolic Control
German Cancer Research Center
Heidelberg, Germany

Dieter Schmoll

DG Metabolic Diseases
Aventis Pharma Deutschland
Industriepark Höchst
Frankfurt, Germany

Jane E.B. Reusch

Division of Endocrinology
Veterans Affairs Medical Center
University of Colorado Health Sciences Center
Denver, CO, USA

Peter A. Watson

Division of Endocrinology
Veterans Affairs Medical Center
University of Colorado Health Sciences Center
Denver, CO, USA

Subbiah Pugazhenthi

Division of Endocrinology
Veterans Affairs Medical Center
University of Colorado Health Sciences Center
Denver, CO, USA

Jussi Pihlajamäki

Research Divison, Joslin Diabetes Center
Harvard Medical School
Boston, MA, USA

Mary Elizabeth Patti

Research Divison, Joslin Diabetes Center
Harvard Medical School
Boston, MA, USA

Jill M. Schroeder-Gloeckler

Medical University of Ohio at Toledo
Block Health Science Building
Toledo, OH, USA

Shaikh Mizanoor Rahman

Department of Pediatrics, Biochemistry and
Molecular Genetics
University of Colorado, Health Sciences Center
Aurora, CO, USA

Jacob E. Friedman

Department of Pediatrics, Biochemistry and
Molecular Genetics
University of Colorado, Health Sciences Center
Aurora, CO, USA

Bankim A. Bhatt

Department of Medicine
Division of Endocrinology/Metabolism
University of Pittsburgh, PA, USA

Robert M. O'Doherty

Department of Medicine, Divison of
Endocrinology/metabolism,
Department of Biochemistry and
Molecular Genetics
University of Pittsburg
Pittsburgh, PA, USA

Chapter 1

Transcription factor genes in type 2 diabetes

Michael N. Weedon, Andrew T. Hattersley, Timothy M. Frayling

Institute of Biomedical and Clinical Science, Peninsula Medical School, Exeter, UK

Abstract

Researchers in diabetes genetics first became aware of the importance of transcription factor genes in 1996, when two seminal papers described mutations in hepatocyte nuclear factor (HNF)1α and HNF4α as causes of the beta-cell disorder, maturity onset diabetes of the young (MODY). Since then, mutations in the HNF1β, insulin promoter factor (IPF)1 and NeuroD genes, have been described as causes of MODY. Rare mutations in the transcription factor peroxisome proliferative-activated receptor γ (PPARG) have been described as a cause of diabetes associated with severe insulin resistance. Recently researchers have described the importance of common variation in these genes in type 2 diabetes risk. Here, we review the evidence for common variants of transcription factor genes predisposing to type 2 diabetes. We briefly summarise the evidence for the role of the Pro12Ala variant of PPARG in type 2 diabetes and related disorders, as this has been the subject of extensive previous reviews. The evidence that subjects carrying at least one copy of the Ala allele are at reduced risk of type 2 diabetes has now gone beyond the stringent levels of significance required for genetic association studies. Of the MODY transcription factor genes that have been extensively analysed, there is strong evidence that variants of HNF1 α and HNF4 α predispose to type 2 diabetes. We conclude that further, comprehensive analyses are needed of all transcription factor genes where rare mutations cause a Mendelian disorder related to type 2 diabetes.

1. Introduction

Transcription factor genes play an important role in the aetiology of type 2 diabetes. Both rare, severe changes to transcription factor gene sequences (mutations) and more common, less severe changes (polymorphisms), contribute to different forms of diabetes. The role of transcription factor genes in type 2 diabetes can be split into

ADVANCES IN MOLECULAR AND CELLULAR ENDOCRINOLOGY
VOLUME 5 ISSN 1569-2566/DOI 10.1016/S1569-2566(06)05001-0

two groups:

(a) Peroxisome proliferative-activated receptor γ (PPARG) in monogenic severe insulin resistance-associated diabetes and type 2 diabetes risk
(b) Beta-cell transcription factors in Maturity onset diabetes of the young (MODY) and type 2 diabetes risk

We briefly summarise the evidence for the role of PPARG in type 2 diabetes and related disorders, as this has been the subject of extensive previous reviews [1–3]. We therefore focus on the role of the beta-cell transcription factors, mutations in which cause MODY. Many previous reviews have described how severe mutations in the MODY genes cause autosomal dominantly inherited beta-cell dysfunction and the clinical characteristics associated with this disorder [4–6]. In this chapter, we therefore concentrate on recent exciting findings, which suggest that common variation in some MODY transcription factor genes increases the risk of type 2 diabetes. We briefly describe MODY and why it is different from type 2 diabetes, before discussing each of the transcription factor genes and its role in type 2 diabetes.

2. The PPARG gene

Rare, severe mutations in the PPARG gene cause type 2 diabetes. Barroso et al. reported two heterozygous missense mutations that result in proteins that inhibit the action of the normal copy of the protein – a dominant-negative effect [7]. Patients with these mutations have other features of the metabolic syndrome in addition to type 2 diabetes, including severe insulin resistance, dyslipidaemia and hypertension [8]. Although these mutations have only been described in a handful of patients, these studies showed that PPARG is a critical molecule in the maintenance of normal glycaemia.

The role of the PPARG common, amino-acid changing variant, Pro12Ala in type 2 diabetes susceptibility is well-established. Since the study of Altshuler et al., which showed that the Pro allele increases the relative risk of type 2 diabetes by 25% [9], other studies have confirmed the findings so that the significance of the result ($p < 2 \times 10^{-8}$), in the latest meta-analysis [2], is beyond the stringent thresholds needed for genetic association studies [10]. The role of the Pro12Ala variant in intermediate and related traits such as, insulin resistance, obesity and cardiovascular disease is less clear. A recent meta-analysis of 19,136 subjects by Masud et al. showed that the Ala allele is associated with increased BMI, but, after showing there was significant heterogeneity among studies that this effect may be limited to subjects with $BMI > 27 \, kg \, m^2$ [11]. Further studies are needed to clarify the role of the Pro12Ala variant in type 2 diabetes intermediate traits.

3. Maturity onset diabetes of the young (MODY)

MODY is a type of non-insulin-dependent diabetes mellitus caused by rare autosomal-dominant mutations. MODY patients usually present before the age of 25 years and typically have a strong family history of diabetes [5]. Mutations in six different genes have been found to cause MODY: glucokinase [12–14]; hepatocyte nuclear factor 1α (HNF1α) [15]; HNF4α [16]; HNF1β [17]; insulin promoter factor-1 (IPF-1) [18] and NeuroD1 [19]. Others are likely to be described. Depending on the gene mutated, clinical course, extra-pancreatic features and response to drug treatment can vary widely [6,20]. MODY patients are often thought to have type 2 diabetes (T2DM, type 2 diabetes mellitus), especially if they are diagnosed late and/ or are obese (see Fig. 1); however, MODY, which accounts for 1–2% of diabetes mellitus cases, is not a subtype of T2DM as it has a defined monogenic basis. An understanding of MODY can aid our understanding of the molecular mechanisms involved in T2DM, the most common form of diabetes mellitus.

T2DM is a multifactorial disease. Twin, family, migration and admixture studies suggest that genetic differences explain a considerable proportion of the inter-individual variation in susceptibility to T2DM [21]. Unlike MODY, where a single mutation can cause the disease, the genetic component of T2DM predisposition is made up of multiple susceptibility variants, each with a small effect on disease risk (Table 1). Gene/gene and gene/environment interactions may also be important. Although the polygenic and heterogeneous nature of T2DM makes it a complicated task, identifying the genes involved in T2DM susceptibility will improve our understanding of the underlying pathophysiology. This should help improve treatment, as it is beginning to in MODY [20].

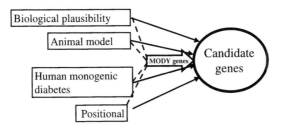

Fig. 1. MODY genes meet all the requirements for a good T2DM candidate gene.

Table 1
Contrasting the clinical presentation and genetic basis of transcription factor MODY and T2DM

	Transcription factor MODY	Type 2 diabetes mellitus
Age at diagnosis	Young onset, typically < 25 years	Older onset, usually > 45 years
BMI	Typically not overweight	Usually overweight or obese
Environmental factors	-	Obesity and inactivity
Genetic factors	HNF1α, HNF4α, HNF1β, NeuroD1, or IPF1 mutations	Polygenic – susceptibility due to large number of "minor" genetic variations
Diseaseaetiology	Severe, progressive, beta-cell failure	Progressive failure of beta-cell to compensate for insulin resistance
Treatment	OHA and insulin	Diet, OHA or insulin

Using DNA markers to perform a genome-wide scan (positional cloning) has been successful in identifying the mutations involved in many monogenic diseases [22]. Using positional cloning in large families, MODY3 was attributed to mutations of the HNF1α gene [15], and MODY1 to mutations of the HNF4α gene [16]. For monogenic diseases like MODY, where single mutations cause the disease and where large families are available, positional cloning is a valuable approach. A number of genome-wide scans have been performed for T2DM. In contrast to type 1 diabetes, where the HLA region has been identified as the major predisposing locus [23], no single large peaks showing increased sharing amongst affected relatives (linkage) have been demonstrated, and progress in positional cloning T2DM genes has been slow. Currently, calpain-10 is the only T2DM gene discovered through a genome-wide scan [24,25]. Consistent replication of relatively small linkage signals across genome scans implicate variation at a number of chromosomal regions [26], but the limited success of positional cloning suggests that candidate gene studies are also important in identifying T2DM susceptibility variants.

A gene may be considered a candidate gene for T2DM susceptibility for a variety of reasons (see Fig. 2). These include an understanding of the encoded proteins biological role; it may fall under a linkage peak, and so be a positional candidate; it may be implicated from transgenic animal studies; or because severe mutations result in human monogenic diabetes. MODY genes fall into all of these categories. Most importantly, mutations in the MODY genes result in autosomal dominant diabetes; this demonstrates that the protein they encode is a key biochemical factor and cannot be compensated for. Common variants of the MODY genes are strong candidates to play a role in human T2DM and related traits, because a small change in the activity or expression of one of these genes is likely to result in elevated blood glucose levels. This review looks at recent studies that suggest a comprehensive analysis of common variation in MODY genes is likely to be a particularly productive approach in identifying genetic susceptibility variants for T2DM.

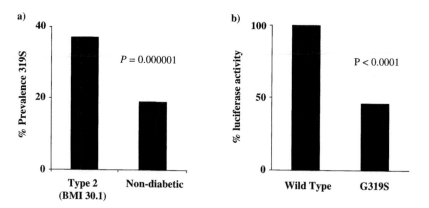

Fig. 2. The private S allele at G319S predisposes to T2DM in the Oji-Cree population. The S allele is not a MODY mutation as (a) it is present in the normal Oji-Cree population, and (b) the polymorphism causes only a moderate reduction in transactivation efficiency, with no evidence for a dominant-negative effect [35].

4. Transcription factor MODY genes

Five of the MODY genes are beta-cell transcription factors; the other one is the glycolytic enzyme glucokinase. Descriptions of each of the five transcription factor MODY genes are given in Table 2, along with a summary of the common variants of these genes that have been convincingly associated with T2DM or a related trait. The beta-cell transcription factor MODY genes are part of a regulatory network that is essential for the proper development, differentiation and survival of the beta-cell [27]. In contrast to mutations in glucokinase, mutations in HNF1α, HNF1β, HNF4α, IPF1 and NeuroD1 cause progressive, severe, beta-cell dysfunction [5].

4.1. *HNF1a*

Mutations in HNF1α are the commonest cause of MODY in the UK, accounting for approximately 63% of cases [28]. There is strong evidence that common variants of

Table 2
The MODY transcription factor genes, their function, clinical presentation and common variants of the genes reproducibly associated with T2DM or a related trait

MODY subtype	Gene	Monogenic phenotype	Strength of evidence for a role in t2dm predisposition	Common variants convincingly associated with t2dm or a related trait
MODY1	HNF4α	Severe, progressive beta-cell dysfunction	Strong	P2 promoter variation. MAF = 25%; RR = 1.3−1.5. References: [53,54]
MODY3	HNF1α(TCF1)	Severe, progressive beta-cell dysfunction	Strong	G319S. MAF = 9%; RR = 2−4. References: [32,35]
MODY4	IPF1 (PDX1)	Severe, progressive beta-cell dysfunction; pancreatic agenesis when homozygous mutant	Moderate	Multiple missense variants MAF ~1%; RR = 2−3 References: [59–61]
MODY5	HNF1β(TCF2)	Severe, progressive beta-cell dysfunction; renal and genital abnormalities (REF)	Mild, but no sufficiently large studies published	None as yet
MODY6	NeuroD1 (BETA2)	Severe, progressive beta-cell dysfunction	Mild, but no sufficiently large studies published	None as yet

MAF = minor allele frequency.

the HNF1α gene are also important in T2DM susceptibility. A genome-wide scan of Finnish insulin-deficient T2DM families identified the NIDDM2 linkage peak, which coincides with the MODY3 locus on chromosome 12q24 [29]. Some subsequent scans, in different populations, have also found evidence for linkage to this genomic region [26,30].

The most convincing evidence of a T2DM predisposition role for common variants of HNF1α comes from the Oji-Cree population of northwestern Ontario and Manitoba, Canada. This isolated native American population has one of the highest prevalences of type 2 diabetes in the world [31]. A common variant of the HNF1α gene, G319S, which is private to the Oji-Cree, has been shown to predispose to T2DM [32], and has a high diagnostic specificity for diabetes prediction [33]. The allele frequency of the S319 allele is around 9% in non-diabetic controls and 21% in type 2 diabetic subjects ($P = 0.000001$) (see Fig. 2a) [33]. The T2DM odds ratio (OR) for G319S heterozyotes is 1.97 (1.44–2.70) and for homozygous carriers of S319 is 4.00 (2.65–6.03) compared to G319 homozygotes. MODY3 mutations result in only residual activity of HNF1α, with haploinsufficiency the most common mutational mechanism [34]. This severe loss of function means that the mutation is sufficient to cause the disease. Importantly, *in vitro* functional studies have demonstrated that the S319 HNF1α allele product is ~50% transactivation deficient, with no evidence for a dominant-negative effect [35] (see Fig. 2b). As this variant leads to only a partial loss of HNF1α function, additional stresses such as obesity and insulin resistance are required for the onset of diabetes, and this explains why MODY3 patients and Oji-Cree type 2 diabetics have different clinical phenotypes [35].

Outside of the Oji-Cree population, no comparable HNF1α T2DM susceptibility variant has been identified. Within the Caucasian population there are three common missense polymorphisms: A98 V, I27L and S487N [36]. The A98 V variant was associated with a 20% reduction in 30 min plasma C-peptide and insulin response in OGTT (Oral Glucose Tolerance Test) studies on 240 middle-aged NGT (Normal Glucose Tolerant) Danish Caucasians [37]. In a further cohort of 377 young NGT subjects this association was only seen in homozygote V98 individuals (of which there were only 2, but who demonstrated a 39 and 44% reduction in acute C-peptide response in an OGTT). The study provided no evidence for a T2DM predisposing role (245 cases vs. 240 controls, OR = 0.83 [0.44–1.58], $P = 0.69$). The 30 min C-peptide result was replicated in a second study of 231 NGT first-degree relatives of T2DM probands [38]. In contrast, a study of 156 Chinese and 222 Finnish individuals [39] demonstrated a significant association of the *V* allele with T2DM (Chinese OR = 2.69 [0.32–infinity], Finnish OR = 2.20 [0.93–5.20], Combined $P = 0.01$), but found no evidence in 295 NGT and 38 IGT (Impaired Glucose Tolerant) subjects that it reduced beta-cell function (although they did not present C-peptide data). Replication of the A98 V result has been hindered by its low frequency (minor allele frequency (MAF) ~ 4% in European Caucasians), and its apparent absence in Chinese [40], Ashkenazi Jew [41] and the Pima Indian [42] populations. Confirmation of an association with beta-cell function and T2DM in a large-scale study is required.

While there is no evidence that the S487N (MAF 30–45%) variant influences beta-cell function or T2DM risk [36,37,39,41–44], there has been variable association of the I27L polymorphism (MAF 25–45%) [36,37,39,41–43,45]. No significant difference in the frequency of the variant was seen in an initial study of 245 NIDDM patients and 240 age-matched glucose-tolerant control subjects (OR = 1.29 [0.98, 1.70], $P = 0.09$) [36] and subsequent studies in Chinese (OR = 1.55 [0.96–2.51], $P = 0.09$) [39], Finnish (OR = 1.27 [0.86–1.87], $P = 0.27$) [39], Ashkenazi Jewish (OR = 1.09 [0.75–1.57], $P = 0.76$) [41], and Pima Indian (OR = 0.91 [0.54–1.53]) [42] populations also reported no association. Although these studies have not individually reported significant associations, overall the published literature appears to support a modest T2DM (OR ~ 1.2) predisposition effect for the Leucine allele. As all the studies so far have been underpowered to detect such an OR, confirmation by meta-analysis and a sufficiently powered replication study, consisting of > 2000 cases and > 2000 controls, is required.

There has also been some suggestion that the I27L variant affects beta-cell function. A study of 74 Danish Caucasian first-degree relatives of T2DM probands found a 32% reduction in 30 min serum C-peptide level ($P = 0.01$), and a 39% reduction in 30 min serum insulin ($P = 0.02$) during an OGTT [43]. However, in a larger cohort, of 230 NGT offspring of T2DM probands, these results were not replicated [43]. Although a subsequent study of 60 glucose-tolerant Caucasians found a significant effect of the I27L polymorphism on first and second phase insulin response [44], other larger studies have reported no association with beta-cell function [37,39].

It is becoming increasingly clear that well-designed, sufficiently powered, large-scale association studies are required to reproducibly detect small polygenic signals [9,46,47], and confirmation or refutation of an effect of these HNF1α variants is awaited. Even if A98 V and/or I27L are causal variants and play some role in the molecular pathology of T2DM, they probably do not explain the observed linkage signal at the HNF1α locus; other, silent or noncoding, HNF1α variants are likely to be important. As with all candidate genes, definitive answers about the role of common HNF1α variation in T2DM will only be achieved by a detailed analysis of the linkage disequilibrium and haplotype structure of the region. This should be followed by large association studies based on SNPs that capture a large proportion of all the variation across the gene.

4.2. *HNF4a*

Several T2DM genome-wide scans have provided evidence of linkage to 20q12-13.1, [26] where the HNF4α gene resides. Initial analysis of the coding regions and the P1 promoter did not identify any HNF4α variation significantly associated with T2DM that could explain the observed linkage [48,49]. However, the discovery and characterisation of an alternative promoter, P2, has led to a re-analysis of the role of the HNF4α gene in T2DM [50]. Figure 3 shows a schematic diagram of the HNF4α gene, with the P1 and P2 promoters. The P2 promoter occurs 46 kb upstream of the HNF4α transcription start site, and has been shown to be active in pancreatic beta-cells and hepatocytes [50]. Within hepatocytes, transcripts arising from the P1 promoter are more abundant; however, within beta-cells the HNF4α P2 splice variant predominates. The P2 promoter contains functional binding sites for the products of

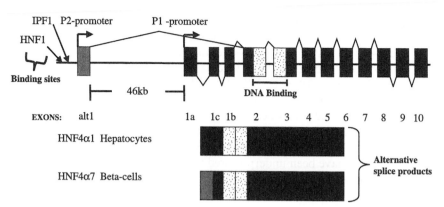

Fig. 3. Schematic representation of the HNF4alpha gene, with the alternate P2 promoter.

the other transcription factor MODY genes, and mutations in the IPF-1 and HNF1α sites have been shown to co-segregate with MODY1 [50,51]. The P2 promoter is therefore an important node in the complex beta-cell regulatory network that connects the MODY transcription factors. It has been suggested that this alternate 5' end of the HNF4α transcription unit may serve as a large target for transcriptional interference, and that variants in this region may explain the linkage of type 2 diabetes to this genomic area [50].

An initial screen of the P2 promoter and alternative first exon, in young-onset type 2 diabetic subjects and probands from families linked to chromosome 20, identified only rare variants that lacked biological significance [52]. However, two recent studies, in Finns [53] and Ashkenazi Jews [54], where there is evidence of linkage to 20q12-13.1 (current LODs of 2.48 and 2.05, respectively), have demonstrated that a P2 promoter haplotype is associated with T2DM. It can also explain the evidence of linkage in these two populations.

After finding the initial linkage, the two studies differed in their approach to identifying the causal gene/variants. The FUSION (Finland United States Investigation of Non-Insulin Dependent Diabetes) study used a DNA pooling approach to genotype 291 SNPs across a 10 Mb interval in a set of 793 cases and 413 controls [53]. The strongest association was with a variant of the HNF4α P2 promoter. They then went on to individually type 33 SNPs (that captured most of the genetic variation across the region) across a 247 kb region centred on HNF4α in a case/control study of 793 case and 413 controls. They identified a number of associated SNPs around the HNF4α P2 promoter. Most interestingly, a haplotype spanning the P2 promoter was associated with T2DM, with an OR of 1.34 [1.07,1.66], $P = 0.01$. This haplotype could also explain the evidence of linkage to 20q12-13.1 in this population (MLS = 1.86 vs. 0.28) [53].

The Ashkenazi Jewish study focused on HNF4α as the best candidate gene in the linked region [54]. They used a haplotype tagging SNP (htSNP) approach on a 78 kb region centred on HNF4α, and found association of two of the nine htSNPs with T2DM. One of these was a 3' intronic SNP (minor allele freq. 29.2% in cases vs.

21.7% in controls, $P = 0.0028$, OR 1.49 [1.15–1.90]). The second SNP (P2 SNP) was located ~3.9 kb upstream of P2 (minor allele freq. 26.9% cases vs. 20.3% controls, $P = 0.0078$, OR 1.46 [1.12–1.91]). The P2 SNP was shown to be part of a > 10 kb T2DM associated haplotype that extended 5' of the P2 promoter. In families where the proband carries at least one risk allele, the P2 SNP can account for the majority of the observed linkage signal on chromosome 20q in this population (MLS = 2.72 vs. 0.17). Importantly, this was the same P2 haplotype independently observed in the FUSION sample [53]. More recently we used 5256 subjects including 2004 cases, 1635 controls and 509 families, to show that the same haplotype is associated with T2DM risk in the UK [55]. The OR, 1.15 [1.02–1.29; P = 0.02], was smaller than that seen in the Finnish and Ashkenazi studies. This probably reflected the fact that we did not find any evidence for linkage to chromosome 20 in the UK genome-wide scan for T2DM [48]. Results from these three studies, two describing the initial association in populations with linkage to the region, and a large replication study, strongly suggest that common HNF4α regulatory element variants contribute to T2DM risk.

This HNF4α work also demonstrates the importance of a comprehensive linkage disequilibrium and haplotype analysis of a candidate gene region. The functionality of the region upstream of the P2 promoter was not obvious, and the P2 SNP association was missed by concentrating on "candidate SNPs" in and around the coding region of the gene.

4.3. *IPF-1*

IPF-1 (also known as PDX1) is key in the development of the pancreas and also in the mature islet, where it is involved in transcription of the insulin gene [56,57]. The importance of IPF-1 in human pancreatic function is demonstrated by the effect of rare mutations: homozygous mutation carriers present with pancreatic agenesis [58] and heterozygous mutants develop MODY [18]. A mutation in the IPF-1 binding site of the HNF4α P2 promoter has been shown to co-segregate with MODY [50]. An initial association study suggested that three coding polymorphisms, C18R, D76N and R197H, present in approximately 1% of the UK Caucasian population, predisposed subjects to type 2 diabetes with a relative risk of 3 [59]. *In vitro* work also suggested that these variants affect IPF-1 function [59]. Other studies from France and Sweden confirmed that functional missense mutations predisposed to type 2 diabetes, especially when subjects were diagnosed before 50 years [60,61]. The low frequency (in some populations these variants were absent) and the multiple variants detected, means that studies will have low statistical power; this may explain why other studies have not replicated these findings [62–64].

4.4. *NeuroD1 and HNF1β*

There has been limited analysis of the role of NeuroD1 and HNF1β in T2DM. In the populations screened so far, the only common (MAF > 5%) NeuroD1 coding variant identified is Ala45Thr. NeuroD1 occurs near the IDDM7 linkage peak and the majority of work has focused on the role of this variant in type 1 diabetes. As is typical of genetic association studies [47], the initial positive study suggested a major T1D predisposing role for the Thr45 allele [65], which subsequent studies have only variably replicated [66–70] although, the largest most recent, study shows no effect [71].

The evidence for a role of NeuroD1 variants in T2DM susceptibility is more limited [68,72], but a comprehensive analysis of this gene awaits. The same is true for HNF1β, on which few studies [73,74] have been performed.

5. Conclusion

The fact that heterozygous mutations of the PPARG and MODY transcription factor genes result in diabetes establishes that partial loss of function of these genes cannot be compensated for by other biochemical or cellular pathways. Therefore, common, less functionally severe, variants of these genes are among the best candidates to explain some of the population variation in T2DM risk or a related polygenic trait. This review has illustrated the same by showing that some common variation of MODY transcription factor genes, predisposes to T2DM. This is in addition to the well-established association of the PPARG Pro12 variant with type 2 diabetes risk. Further, comprehensive, large-scale analysis of the role of key transcription factor genes in the susceptibility to T2DM is required.

Acknowledgements

We thank all our colleagues in Exeter and the other centres who have contributed to our studies in MODY and type 2 diabetes genetics. We also acknowledge the kind financial support of Diabetes UK and the Wellcome Trust for the genetic work performed in Exeter reported in this study. A.T.H. is a Wellcome Trust Clinical Research Leave Fellow.

References

[1] M. Stumvoll, H. Haring, The peroxisome proliferator-activated receptor-gamma2 Pro12Ala polymorphism, Diabetes 51 (8) (2002) 2341–2347.

[2] J.C. Florez, J.N. Hirschhorn, D. Altshuler, The inherited basis of diabetes mellitus: implications for the genetic analysis of complex traits, Annu. Rev. Genomics. Hum. Genet. 4 (2003) 257–291.

[3] J.C. Florez, Phenotypic consequences of the peroxisome proliferator-activated receptor-gamma pro12ala polymorphism: the weight of the evidence in genetic association studies, J. Clin. Endocrinol. Metab. 89 (9) (2004) 4234–4237.

[4] S.S. Fajans, G.I. Bell, K.S. Polonsky, Molecular mechanisms and clinical pathophysiology of maturity-onset diabetes of the young, N. Engl. J. Med. 345 (13) (2001) 971–980.

[5] K. Owen, A.T. Hattersley, Maturity-onset diabetes of the young: from clinical description to molecular genetic characterization, Best Pract. Res. Clin. Endocrinol. Metab. 15 (3) (2001) 309–323.

[6] A. Stride, A.T. Hattersley, Different genes, different diabetes: lessons from maturity-onset diabetes of the young, Ann. Med. 34 (3) (2002) 207–216.

[7] I. Barroso, M. Gurnell, V.E. Crowley, M. Agostini, J.W. Schwabe, M.A. Soos, et al., Dominant negative mutations in human PPARgamma associated with severe insulin resistance, diabetes mellitus and hypertension, Nature 402 (6764) (1999) 880–883.

[8] D.B. Savage, G.D. Tan, C.L. Acerini, S.A. Jebb, M. Agostini, M. Gurnell, et al., Human metabolic syndrome resulting from dominant-negative mutations in the nuclear receptor peroxisome proliferator-activated receptor-gamma, Diabetes 52 (4) (2003) 910–917.

[9] D. Altshuler, J.N. Hirschhorn, M. Klannemark, C.M. Lindgren, M.-C. Vohl, J. Nemesh, et al., The common PPARγ Pro12Ala polymorphism is associated with decreased risk of type 2 diabetes, Nat. Genet. 26 (2000) 76–80.

[10] N. Risch, K. Merikangas, The future of genetic studies of complex human diseases, Science 273 (1996) 1516–1517.

[11] S. Masud, S. Ye, group S. Effect of the peroxisome proliferator activated receptor-gamma gene Pro12Ala variant on body mass index: a meta-analysis, J. Med. Genet. 40 (10) (2003) 773–780.

[12] A.T. Hattersley, R.C. Turner, M.A. Permutt, P. Patel, Y. Tanizawa, K.C. Chiu, et al., Linkage of type 2 diabetes to the glucokinase gene, Lancet 339 (1992) 1307–1310.

[13] N. Vionnet, M. Stoffel, J. Takeda, K. Yasuda, G.I. Bell, H. Zouali, et al., Nonsense mutation in the glucokinase gene causes early onset non-insulin-dependent diabetes mellitus, Nature 356 (6371) (1992) 721–722.

[14] P. Froguel, M. Vaxillaire, F. Sun, G. Velho, H. Zouali, M.O. Butel, et al., Close linkage of glucokinase locus on chromosome 7p to early onset non-insulin-dependent diabetes mellitus, Nature 356 (1992) 162–164.

[15] K. Yamagata, N. Oda, P.J. Kaisaki, S. Menzel, H. Furuta, M. Vaxillaire, et al., Mutations in the hepatic nuclear factor 1 alpha gene in maturity-onset diabetes of the young (MODY3), Nature 384 (1996) 455–458.

[16] K. Yamagata, H. Furuta, N. Oda, P.J. Kaisaki, S. Menzel, N.J. Cox, et al., Mutations in the hepatocyte nuclear factor 4 alpha gene in maturity-onset diabetes of the young (MODY1), Nature 384 (1996) 458–460.

[17] Y. Horikawa, N. Iwasaki, M. Hara, H. Furuta, Y. Hinokio, B. Cockburn, et al., Mutation in hepatocyte nuclear factor-1b gene (TCF2) associated with MODY, Nat. Genet. 17 (1997) 384–385.

[18] D.A. Stoffers, J. Ferrer, W.L. Clarke, J.F. Habener, Early onset type-II diabetes mellitus (MODY4) linked to IPF1, Nat. Genet. 17 (1997) 138–139.

[19] M.T. Malecki, U.S. Jhala, A. Antonellis, L. Fields, A. Doria, T. Orban, et al., Mutations in NEUROD1 are associated with the development of Type 2 diabetes mellitus, Nat. Genet. 23 (3) (1999) 323–328.

[20] E.R. Pearson, B.J. Starkey, R.J. Powell, F.M. Gribble, P.M. Clark, A.T. Hattersley, Genetic cause of hyperglycaemia and response to treatment in diabetes, Lancet 362 (9392) (2003) 1275–1281.

[21] A. Gloyn, M. McCarthy, The genetics of type 2 diabetes, Best practice and research clinical endocrinology and metabolism 15 (9) (2001) 293–308.

[22] Online Mendelian Inheritance in Man, OMIM (TM), in: McKusick-Nathans Institute for Genetic Medicine, John Hopkins University, Baltimore, MD and National Center for Biotechnology Information, National Library of Medicine, Bethesda, MD. 2000.

[23] F. Pociot, M.F. McDermott, Genetics of type 1 diabetes mellitus, Genes Immun 3 (5) (2002) 235–249.

[24] Y. Horikawa, N. Oda, N.J. Cox, X. Li, M. Orho-Melander, M. Hara, et al., Genetic variation in the gene encoding calpain-10 is associated with type 2 diabetes mellitus, Nat. Genet. 26 (2) (2000) 163–175.

[25] M.N. Weedon, P.E. Schwarz, Y. Horikawa, N. Iwasaki, T. Illig, R. Holle, et al., Meta-analysis and a large association study confirm a role for calpain-10 variation in type 2 diabetes susceptibility, Am. J. Hum. Genet. 73 (6) (2003) 1208–1212.

[26] M.I. McCarthy, Growing evidence for diabetes susceptibility genes from genome scan data, Curr. Diab. Rep. 3 (2) (2003) 159–167.

[27] J. Ferrer, A genetic switch in pancreatic beta-cells: implications for differentiation and haploinsufficiency, Diabetes 51 (8) (2002) 2355–2362.

[28] T.M. Frayling, J.C. Evans, M.P. Bulman, E. Pearson, L. Allen, K. Owen, et al., Beta-cell genes and diabetes: molecular and clinical characterization of mutations in transcription factors, Diabetes 50 (Suppl 1) (2001) S94–S100.

[29] M.M. Mahtani, E. Widen, M. Lehto, J. Thomas, M. McCarthy, J. Brayer, et al., Mapping of a gene for type 2 diabetes associated with an insulin secretion defect by a genome scan in Finnish families, Nat. Genet. 14 (1) (1996) 90–94.

[30] I. Reynisdottir, G. Thorleifsson, R. Benediktsson, G. Sigurdsson, V. Emilsson, A.S. Einarsdottir, et al., Localization of a susceptibility gene for type 2 diabetes to chromosome 5q34-q35.2, Am. J. Hum. Genet. 73 (2) (2003) 323–335.

[31] R.A. Hegele, B. Zinman, A.J. Hanley, S.B. Harris, P.H. Barrett, H. Cao, Genes environment and Oji-Cree type 2 diabetes, Clin. Biochem. 36 (3) (2003) 163–170.

[32] R.A. Hegele, H. Cao, S.B. Harris, A.J. Hanley, B. Zinman, The hepatic nuclear factor-1alpha G319S variant is associated with early onset type 2 diabetes in Canadian Oji-Cree, J. Clin. Endocrinol. Metab. 84 (3) (1999) 1077–1082.

[33] E. Abderrahim, F. Ben Moussa, T. Ben Abdallah, H. Hedri, R. Goucha, F. Ben Hamida, et al., Glomerulocystic kidney disease in an adult presenting as end-stage renal failure, Nephrol. Dial. Transplant. 14 (1999) 1276–1278.

[34] L.W. Harries, A.T. Hattersley, S. Ellard, Messenger RNA transcripts of the hepatocyte nuclear factor-1alpha gene containing premature termination codons are subject to nonsense-mediated decay, Diabetes 53 (2) (2004) 500–504.

[35] B.L. Triggs-Raine, R.D. Kirkpatrick, S.L. Kelly, L.D. Norquay, P.A. Cattini, K. Yamagata, et al., HNF-1alpha G319S, a transactivation-deficient mutant, is associated with altered dynamics of diabetes onset in an Oji-Cree community. Proc., Natl. Acad. Sci. USA. 99 (7) (2002) 4614–4619.

[36] S.A. Urhammer, S.K. Rasmussen, P.J. Kaisaki, N. Oda, K. Yamagata, A.M. Moller, et al., Genetic variation in the hepatocyte nuclear factor-1α gene in Danish Caucasians with late onset NIDDM, Daibetologia 40 (1997) 473–475.

[37] S.A. Urhammer, M. Fridberg, T. Hansen, S.K. Rasmussen, A.M. Moller, J.O. Clausen, et al., A prevalent amino acid polymorphism at codon 98 in the hepatocyte nuclear factor-1alpha gene is associated with reduced serum C-peptide and insulin responses to an oral glucose challenge, Diabetes 46 (5) (1997) 912–916.

[38] S.A. Urhammer, T. Hansen, C.T. Ekstrom, H. Eiberg, O. Pedersen, The Ala/Val98 polymorphism of the hepatocyte nuclear factor-1alpha gene contributes to the interindividual variation in serum C-peptide response during an oral glucose tolerance test: evidence from studies of 231 glucose-tolerant first degree relatives of type 2 diabetic probands, J. Clin. Endocrinol. Metab. 83 (12) (1998) 4506–4509.

[39] J. Rissanen, H. Wang, R. Miettinen, P. Karkkainen, P. Kekalainen, L. Mykkanen, et al., Variants in the hepatocyte nuclear factor-1alpha and -4alpha genes in Finnish and Chinese subjects with late-onset type 2 diabetes, Diabetes Care 23 (10) (2000) 1533–1538.

[40] H. Deng, W.L. Tang, Z. Liu, Relationship between Ala98Val variant of hepatocyte nuclear factor-1 alpha gene and late-onset type 2 diabetes in Han nationality, Hunan Yi Ke Da Xue Xue Bao 28 (2) (2003) 93–94.

[41] P.S. Behn, J. Wasson, S. Chayen, I. Smolovitch, J. Thomas, B. Glaser, et al., Hepatocyte nuclear factor 1alpha coding mutations are an uncommon contributor to early onset type 2 diabetes in Ashkenazi Jews, Diabetes 47 (6) (1998) 967–969.

[42] L.J. Baier, P.A. Permana, M. Traurig, A. Dobberfuhl, C. Wiedrich, J. Sutherland, et al., Mutations in the genes for hepatocyte nuclear factor (HNF)-1alpha, -4alpha, -1beta, and -3beta; the dimerization cofactor of HNF-1; and insulin promoter factor 1 are not common causes of early onset type 2 diabetes in Pima Indians, Diabetes Care 23 (3) (2000) 302–304.

[43] S.A. Urhammer, A.M. Moller, B. Nyholm, C.T. Ekstrom, H. Eiberg, J.O. Clausen, et al., The effect of two frequent amino acid variants of the hepatocyte nuclear factor-1alpha gene on estimates of the pancreatic beta-cell function in Caucasian glucose-tolerant first-degree relatives of type 2 diabetic patients, J Clin. Endocrinol. Metab. 83 (11) (1998) 3992–3995.

[44] K.C. Chiu, L.M. Chuang, A. Chu, M. Wang, Transcription factor 1 and beta-cell function in glucose-tolerant subjects, Diabet. Med. 20 (3) (2003) 225–230.

[45] K.C. Chiu, L.M. Chuang, A. Chu, C. Yoon, M. Wang, Comparison of the impact of the I27L polymorphism of the hepatocyte nuclear factor-1alpha on estimated and measured beta cell indices, Eur. J. Endocrinol. 148 (6) (2003) 641–647.

[46] A.L. Gloyn, M.N. Weedon, K.R. Owen, M.J. Turner, B.A. Knight, G. Hitman, et al., Large-scale association studies of variants in genes encoding the pancreatic beta-cell KATP channel subunits Kir6.2 (KCNJ11) and SUR1 (ABCC8) confirm that the KCNJ11 E23 K variant is associated with type 2 diabetes,, Diabetes 52 (2) (2003) 568–572.

[47] J.N. Hirschhorn, K. Lohmueller, E. Byrne, K. Hirschhorn, A comprehensive review of genetic association studies, Genet. Med. 4 (2) (2002) 45–61.

[48] S. Ghosh, R.M. Watanabe, E.R. Hauser, T. Valle, V.L. Magnuson, M.R. Erdos, et al., Type 2 diabetes: evidence for linkage on chromosome 20 in 716 Finnish affected sib pairs, Proc. Natl. Acad. Sci. USA. 96 (5) (1999) 2198–2203.

[49] M.A. Permutt, J. Wasson, L. Love-Gregory, J. Ma, G. Skolnick, B. Suarez, et al., Searching for type 2 diabetes genes on chromosome 20, Diabetes 51 (Suppl 3) (2002) S308–S315.

[50] H. Thomas, K. Jaschkowitz, M. Bulman, T.M. Frayling, S.M.S. Mitchell, S. Roosen, et al., A distant upstream promoter of the HNF-4alpha gene connects the transcription factors involved in maturity-onset diabetes of the young, Hum. Mol. Genet. 10 (19) (2001) 2089–2097.

[51] S.K. Hansen, M. Parrizas, M.L. Jensen, S. Pruhova, J. Ek, S.F. Boj, et al., Genetic evidence that HNF-1alpha-dependent transcriptional control of HNF-4alpha is essential for human pancreatic beta cell function, J. Clin. Invest. 110 (6) (2002) 827–833.

[52] S.M.S. Mitchell, M. Vaxillaire, H. Thomas, M. Parrizas, Y. Benmezroua, A. Costa, et al., Rare variants identified in the HNF-4α b-cell specific promoter and alternative exon 1 lack biological significance in maturity onset diabetes of the young and type 2 diabetes, Diabetelogia 45 (9) (2002) 1344–1348.

[53] K. Silander, K.L. Mohlke, L.J. Scott, E.C. Peck, P. Hollstein, A.D. Skol, et al., Genetic variation near the hepatocyte nuclear factor-4alpha gene predicts susceptibility to type 2 diabetes, Diabetes 53 (2004) 1141–1149.

[54] L.D. Love-Gregory, J. Wasson, J. Ma, C.H. Jin, B. Glaser, B.K. Suarez, et al., A common polymorphism in the upstream promoter region of the hepatocyte nuclear factor-4alpha gene on chromosome 20q is associated with type 2 diabetes and appears to contribute to the evidence for linkage in an Ashkenazi Jewish population, Diabetes 53 (2004) 1134–1140.

[55] M.N. Weedon, K.R. Owen, B. Shields, G. Hitman, M. Walker, M.I. McCarthy, et al., Common variants of the hepatocyte nuclear factor-4alpha P2 promoter are associated with type 2 diabetes in the UK population, Diabetes 53 (11) (2004) 3002–3006.

[56] W.M. Macfarlane, S.B. Smith, R.F.L. James, A.D. Clifton, Y.N. Doza, P. Cohen, et al., The p38/ reactiviating kinase mitogen activated protein kinase cascade mediates the activation of the transcription factor IUF1 and insulin gene transcription by high glucose in pancreatic beta-cells, J. Biol.Chem. 272 (1997) 20936–20944.

[57] W.M. Macfarlane, C.M. McKinnon, Z.A. Felton-Edkins, H. Cragg, R.F.L. James, K. Docherty, Glucose stimulates translocation of the homeodomain transcription factor PDX1 from the cytoplasm to the nucleus in pancreatic β-cells, J. Biol. Chem. 274 (1999) 1011–1016.

[58] D.A. Stoffers, N.T. Zinkin, V. Stanojevic, W.L. Clarke, J.F. Habener, Pancreatic agenesis attributable to a single nucleotide deletion in the human IPF1 gene coding sequence, Nat. Genet. 15 (1997) 106–110.

[59] W. Macfarlane, T. Frayling, S. Ellard, J. Evans, L. Allen, M. Bulman, et al., Missense mutations in the insulin promoter factor 1 (IPF-1) gene predispose to type 2 diabetes, J. Clin. Invest. 104 (1999) R33–R39.

[60] E.H. Hani, D.A. Stoffers, J.C. Chevre, E. Durand, V. Stanojevic, C. Dina, et al., Defective mutations in the insulin promoter factor-1 (IPF-1) gene in late-onset type 2 diabetes mellitus, J. Clin. Invest. 104 (9) (1999) R41–R48.

[61] J. Weng, W.M. Macfarlane, M. Lehto, H.F. Gu, L.M. Shepherd, S.A. Ivarsson, et al., Functional consequences of mutations in the MODY4 gene (IPF1) and coexistence with MODY3 mutations, Diabetologia 44 (2) (2001) 249–258.

[62] K. Silver, A. Shetty, IPF-1 gene variation and the development of type 2 diabetes, Mol. Genet. Metab. 75 (3) (2002) 287–289.

[63] A.F. Reis, W.Z. Ye, D. Dubois-Laforgue, C. Bellanne-Chantelot, J. Timsit, G. Velho, Mutations in the insulin promoter factor-1 gene in late-onset type 2 diabetes mellitus, Eur. J. Endocrinol. 143 (4) (2000) 511–513.

[64] L. Hansen, S. Urioste, H.V. Petersen, J.N. Jensen, H. Eiberg, F. Barbetti, et al., Missense mutations in the human insulin promoter factor-1 gene and their relation to maturity-onset diabetes of the young and late-onset type 2 diabetes mellitus in Caucasians, J. Clin. Endocrinol. Metab. 85 (3) (2000) 1323–1326.

[65] I. Iwata, S. Nagafuchi, H. Nakashima, S. Kondo, T. Koga, Y. Yokogawa, et al., Association of polymorphism in the NeuroD/BETA2 gene with type 1 diabetes in the Japanese, Diabetes 48 (2) (1999) 416–419.

[66] M.T. Malecki, T. Klupa, D.K. Moczulski, J.J. Rogus, The Ala45Thr polymorphism of BETA2/NeuroD1 gene and susceptibility to type 1 diabetes mellitus in Caucasians, Exp. Clin. Endocrinol. Diabetes 111 (5) (2003) 251–254.

[67] S. Yamada, Y. Motohashi, T. Yanagawa, T. Maruyama, A. Kasuga, H. Hirose, et al., NeuroD/beta2 gene G − > A polymorphism may affect onset pattern of type 1 diabetes in Japanese, Diabetes Care 24 (8) (2001) 1438–1441.

[68] L. Hansen, J.N. Jensen, S. Urioste, H.V. Petersen, F. Pociot, H. Eiberg, et al., NeuroD/BETA2 gene variability and diabetes: no associations to late-onset type 2 diabetes but an A45 allele may represent a susceptibility marker for type 1 diabetes among Danes. Danish Study Group of Diabetes in Childhood, and the Danish IDDM Epidemiology and Genetics Group, Diabetes 49 (5) (2000) 876–878.

[69] S. Dupont, C. Dina, E.H. Hani, P. Froguel, Absence of replication in the French population of the association between beta 2/NEUROD-A45T polymorphism and type 1 diabetes, Diabetes Metab 25 (6) (1999) 516–517.

[70] T. Awata, K. Inoue, I. Inoue, T. Abe, H. Takino, Y. Kanazawa, et al., Lack of association of the Ala45Thr variant in the BETA2/NEUROD1 with type 1 diabetes in Japanese, Diabetes Res. Clin. Pract. 49 (1) (2000) 61–63.

[71] A. Vella, J.M. Howson, B.J. Barratt, R.C. Twells, H.E. Rance, S. Nutland, et al., Lack of association of the Ala(45)Thr polymorphism and other common variants ot the NeuroD gene with type 2 diabetes, Diabetes 53 (4) (2004) 1158–1161.

[72] M.T. Malecki, K. Cyganek, T. Klupa, J. Sieradzki, The Ala45Thr polymorphism of BETA2/NeuroD1 gene and susceptibility to type 2 diabetes mellitus in a Polish population, Acta Diabetol 40 (2) (2003) 109–111.

[73] J. Ek, N. Grarup, S.A. Urhammer, P.H. Gaede, T. Drivsholm, K. Borch-Johnsen, et al., Studies of the variability of the hepatocyte nuclear factor-1beta (HNF-1beta/TCF2) and the dimerization cofactor of HNF-1 (DcoH/PCBD) genes in relation to type 2 diabetes mellitus and beta-cell function. Hum,, Mutat 18 (4) (2001) 356–357.

[74] N. Babaya, H. Ikegami, Y. Kawaguchi, T. Fujisawa, Y. Nakagawa, Y. Hamada, et al., Hepatocyte nuclear factor-1alpha gene and non-insulin-dependent diabetes mellitus in the Japanese population, Acta Diabetol 35 (3) (1998) 150–153.

Chapter 2

PPARγ, a key therapeutic target in the metabolic syndrome – unique insights derived from the study of human genetic variants

Catherine S. Mitchell, Mark Gurnell

Department of Medicine, University of Cambridge, Addenbrooke's Hospital, Cambridge, UK

Abstract

Diabetes is one of the most serious health issues facing developed countries today. In the UK it accounts for around 5% of all National Health Service (NHS) spending (~£10 million/day) and is a leading cause of heart disease, stroke, blindness, amputation and kidney failure. The majority (~90%) of these cases are type 2 in origin, reflecting a trend towards obesity and more sedentary lifestyles as the 'norm' rather than exception in western society. The development of insulin resistance is a critical step in the evolution of this disorder and, accordingly, improving insulin sensitivity, and thereby ameliorating excess vascular risk, is a primary goal for those concerned with its treatment. Recent interest has focussed on a novel class of antidiabetic agent, the thiazolidinediones which act as insulin sensitizers, thus targeting the underlying metabolic disturbance. These compounds are high affinity ligands for the nuclear receptor peroxisome proliferator-activated receptor γ (PPARγ), and a significant body of *in vitro* and *in vivo* data exists to support their increasing therapeutic use. Importantly, clinical and laboratory observations made in human subjects harbouring genetic variations in PPARγ have confirmed its pivotal role in the regulation of adipogenesis and glucose homeostasis, with evidence also emerging to indicate important contributions to lipid metabolism and control of blood pressure. It is not surprising then that this receptor has emerged as a key therapeutic target in the context of the metabolic syndrome. Indeed the 'race is on' to identify the next generation of PPARγ modulators, agents that will promote maximal therapeutic benefit by targeting specific facets of the metabolic syndrome (glucose intolerance/diabetes, dyslipidaemia and hypertension), while simultaneously avoiding undesirable side effects of PPARγ activation (e.g. weight gain and fluid retention).

ADVANCES IN MOLECULAR AND CELLULAR ENDOCRINOLOGY
VOLUME 5 ISSN 1569-2566/DOI 10.1016/S1569-2566(06)05002-2

1. Introduction

It has been predicted that by the end of this decade a staggering two to three hundred million people worldwide will meet World Health Organization (WHO) diagnostic criteria for diabetes mellitus [1] – worryingly, some sources consider this to be a conservative estimate. In the United Kingdom (UK) alone, there are nearly 1.8 million people already recognised to have this disorder, and the search is on to find the 'missing million' who are living with the condition, but in whom the diagnosis has yet to be made [2]. This 'explosion' of predominantly type 2 diabetes mellitus (T2DM) is inextricably linked to the increasing prevalence of obesity, which in turn reflects our shift towards 'unhealthy eating' and an increasingly sedentary lifestyle [3]. Obesity (and in particular excessive visceral adiposity) predisposes to the development of insulin resistance, which is a critical step in the evolution of both diabetic and 'pre-diabetic' (i.e. impaired glucose tolerance and possibly impaired fasting glucose) states. In the majority of subjects with T2DM, insulin resistance precedes overt hyperglycaemia, which only manifests once pancreatic β-cell function decompensates.

Atherosclerotic vascular events (ischaemic coronary, peripheral and cerebro-vascular disease) are more common in these populations [4,5], and in 1988 Reaven proposed the existence of a metabolic syndrome (also referred to as syndrome X) in which atherogenic risk factors cluster in the presence of insulin resistance [6]. Other workers have developed this concept to highlight key features of a disorder which includes: hyperinsulinaemia, abnormal glucose metabolism (impaired glucose tolerance or frank diabetes), hypertension, metabolic dyslipidaemia (typically high triglycerides and low levels of high density lipoprotein [HDL] cholesterol), obesity (especially visceral), hypercoagulability (with elevated levels of fibrinogen and plasminogen activator inhibitor-1), microalbuminuria and hyperuricaemia (Table 1). It has been estimated that 75% of individuals with T2DM fulfil WHO criteria [7] for the syndrome, which is associated with a three-fold excess risk of coronary heart disease and stroke [8]. The European Group for the Study of Insulin Resistance (EGIR) [9], the National Cholesterol Education Program (NCEP) expert panel (Adult Treatment Panel III -ATP III) [10] and, more latterly, a consensus statement issued under the auspices of the International Diabetes Federation (IDF) [11] have proposed further refinements to the diagnostic criteria (Table 1). Importantly, whilst all acknowledge insulin resistance as an integral component of the syndrome, each places particular emphasis on the role of central obesity (assessed by simple measurement of waist circumference) as a key factor in the development of insulin resistance.

Intriguingly, a similar pattern of metabolic disturbance is frequently found in subjects with lipodystrophy [12]. Together these findings suggest that there is an 'optimal range' for adipose tissue mass, above or below which metabolic dysfunction ensues. In lipodystrophy, a diminution in adipocyte storage capacity results in 'ectopic' fat deposition in liver and skeletal muscle, thus promoting insulin resistance. A similar end result occurs in obese individuals once normal adipocyte stores are 'saturated' and fat 'spills over' into ectopic sites. The inability to store triglycerides in

Table 1
Diagnostic criteria for the human metabolic syndrome

WHO, 1999	EGIR, 1999	NCEP ATP III, 2001	IDF, 2005
T2DM or IGT or IR	IR or hyperinsulinaemia, in non-diabetic subjects		*Central obesity:* WC≥ethnicity specific cut-offs with ≥2 of:
with ≥2 of:	with ≥2 of:	≥3 of:	
	Hyperglycaemia: fasting plasma glucose ≥ 6.1mmol/L, but non-diabetic	*Hyperglycaemia:* Fasting plasma glucose ≥ 6.1 mmol/L or treated with antidiabetic medication	*Hyperglycaemia:* Fasting plasma glucose ≥ 5.6 mmol/L or previously diagnosed T2DM
Dyslipidaemia: TG > 1.7 mmol/L and/or HDL < 0.9 mmol/L (M) HDL < 1.0 mmol/L (F)	*Dyslipidaemia:* TG > 2.0 mmol/L or HDL < 1.0 mmol/L or treated for dyslipidaemia	*Hypertriglyceridaemia:* TG ≥ 1.7 mmol/L	*Hypertriglyceridaemia:* TG > 1.7 mmol/L or treated for this lipid abnormality
		Low HDL cholesterol: HDL < 1.0 mmol/L (M) HDL < 1.3 mmol/L (F)	*Reduced HDL cholesterol:* HDL < 1.03 mmol/L (M) HDL < 1.29 mmol/L (F) or treated for this lipid abnormality
Hypertension: BP≥140/90 mmHg ± medication	*Hypertension:* BP ≥ 140/90 mmHg or treated for hypertension	*Hypertension:* BP ≥ 130/85 mmHg or treated for hypertension	*Hypertension:* BP ≥ 130/85 mmHg or treated for hypertension
Obesity: BMI ≥ 30 kg/m^2 or WHR > 0.9 (M) WHR > 0.85 (F)	*Central obesity:* WC ≥ 94 cm (M) WC ≥ 80 cm (F)	*Central obesity:* WC ≥ 102 cm (M) WC ≥ 88 cm (F)	*Central obesity:* See above – core requirement for diagnosis of syndrome
Microalbuminuria Urinary AER > 20 mcg/min			

Key: WHO, World Health Organization; EGIR, European Group for the Study of Insulin Resistance; NCEP ATP III, National Cholesterol Education Program Adult Treatment Panel III; IDF, International Diabetes Federation; T2DM, type 2 diabetes mellitus; IGT, impaired glucose tolerance; IR, insulin resistance; TG, triglycerides; HDL, high density lipoprotein cholesterol; BP, blood pressure; BMI, body mass index; WHR, waist hip ratio; WC, waist circumference; AER, albumin excretion rate; M, male; F, female.

adipose tissue, leading to accumulation in liver and muscle, and thus hepatic and muscle insulin resistance, glucose intolerance and overt diabetes, has been referred to as the 'overflow' hypothesis [13,14].

Accordingly, preventing/alleviating insulin resistance has become a key objective for those involved in the management of the human metabolic syndrome. At a population level, effective obesity prevention/treatment is likely to yield the greatest benefits in terms of improving insulin sensitivity. Unfortunately however, while this is a laudable goal, in practice it is very difficult to achieve, and hence attention has turned towards alternative therapeutic strategies. Over the past decade the nuclear receptor peroxisome proliferator-activated receptor γ (PPARγ) has emerged as a key molecular target for the pharmaceutical industry in this context. This receptor is a critical regulator of mammalian adipogenesis and glucose homeostasis, with evidence also accumulating to suggest important roles in the modulation of blood pressure and lipid status. While observations derived from the administration of both natural and synthetic PPARγ ligands *in vivo* and *in vitro* have contributed significantly to our understanding of the biology of this receptor, novel insights have also been derived from the study of naturally occurring human genetic variants, and their consequences for metabolic regulation. This article highlights the complementary nature of such studies, setting them in the wider context of existing pharmacological and animal data, and emphasises the unique contributions that they have made to our understanding of the pathogenesis of the human metabolic syndrome.

2. PPARγ – a 'metabolic' nuclear receptor

With the possible exception of biguanides (e.g. metformin), the majority of agents currently licensed for use in type 2 diabetes (e.g. sulphonylureas, prandial glucose regulators, alpha glucosidase inhibitors and insulin) confer little benefit in terms of ameliorating insulin resistance and it is not surprising therefore that diabetes is typically a progressive disease for most of those affected by it [15]. Recently, however, cautious optimism has been expressed that this situation might change with the introduction of the first of a group of novel agents – the thiazolidinediones (TZDs, e.g. rosiglitazone and pioglitazone) – which enhance insulin action in key target tissues, thereby specifically tackling the underlying metabolic defect [16]. Although originally synthesised as potentially hypolipidaemic derivatives of clofibrate, the TZDs were unexpectedly found to lower blood glucose, as a consequence of improving insulin sensitivity, in rodent models of T2DM and later in man. In the mid-1990s, Lehmann et al. [17] made the critical discovery that TZDs are selective high affinity ligands for the nuclear hormone receptor PPARγ, with their rank order of potency for receptor activation *in vitro* correlating closely with their glucose lowering activity *in vivo*. They were also able to demonstrate that these ligands could transactivate the receptor at nanomolar concentrations.

PPARγ belongs to a superfamily of nuclear receptors (which regulate target gene transcription in response to small lipophilic ligands) and is the third member of a subdivision within this broader family that also includes PPARα and PPARδ [18].

PPARα is principally expressed in tissues that exhibit a high rate of fatty acid metabolism (e.g. brown adipose tissue, liver, kidney and heart) and is the molecular target for the fibrate class of drugs. Less is known about the physiological roles of PPARδ, which is more ubiquitously expressed, although recent studies have implicated it in lipid trafficking in macrophages [19–21], blastocyst implantation [22] and wound healing [23].

Differential promoter usage, coupled with alternate splicing of the PPARγ gene, gives rise to a variety of mRNA isoforms, but just two receptors – PPARγ1 and PPARγ2 – which differ only in their extreme amino-terminal domains, with the latter containing an additional 28 amino acids. PPARγ1 exhibits widespread expression (e.g. adipose tissue, pancreatic beta cells, macrophages and vascular endothelium), albeit at low levels, while PPARγ2 is expressed almost exclusively in adipose tissue [24].

Like other nuclear receptors, PPARγ has a modular structure consisting of distinct functional domains (Fig. 1a). Many of its biological effects are mediated through direct regulation of target gene transcription in a ligand-dependent manner. Following binding to specific DNA response elements (PPAR response elements (PPREs) – located in the target gene promoter) as a heterodimer with the retinoid X receptor (RXR), binding of cognate or exogenous ligand(s) induces coactivator recruitment, which in turn promotes unfolding of the chromatin structure to permit greater levels of gene transcription (Fig. 1b). The identity(ies) of the endogenous ligand(s) for PPARγ remains a matter of debate (hence its original classification as an 'orphan receptor'), although several naturally occurring compounds, including polyunsaturated fatty acids (e.g. linoleic acid and arachidonic acid), 15-deoxy $\Delta^{12,14}$ prostaglandin J_2 (15d-PGJ$_2$) and eicosanoids (e.g. hydroxyoctadecadienoic acid (HODE) and hydroxyeicosatetraenoic acid (HETE)), have been shown to activate the receptor at concentrations comparable to physiological levels.

There is also evidence to suggest that PPARγ may exert regulatory effects in an 'off-DNA' manner, through interference with other transcriptional pathways – so called transrepression. This alternative mechanism has been suggested to account for some of the anti-inflammatory effects of PPARγ agonists such as the TZDs (Fig. 1c).

3. PPARγ – human genetic variants

To date, several different polymorphisms and mutations (both germline and somatic) have been identified in human PPARγ, each providing valuable insights into the diverse roles that this receptor plays in both normal physiology and in disease (Table 2). For example, a somatic gene rearrangement, which results in the generation of a mutant PAX8–PPARγ fusion protein, has been reported to occur in 20–60% of human thyroid follicular tumours [25], and intensive efforts are underway to exploit this finding for both diagnostic and therapeutic purposes. From the metabolic standpoint, several genetic variants have been described in association with phenotypes as diverse as lipodystrophy [26–28] and morbid obesity [29]. For the purpose of this article, we have chosen to focus on a small group of polymorphisms/mutations

Catherine S. Mitchell, Mark Gurnell

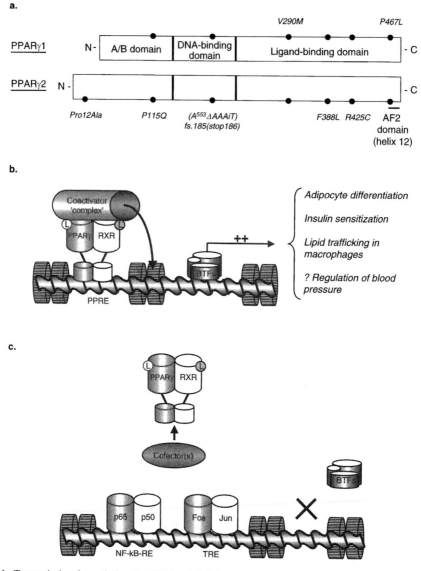

Fig. 1. Transcriptional regulation by PPARγ. (a) Schematic representation of the domain structure of PPARγ, denoting the location of several of the natural genetic variations, which have been identified in the human receptor. Note that mutations and polymorphisms have been depicted based on the nomenclature (γ1 or γ2) used in the primary publication [26,27,29,39,45,58]. (b) In transactivation, which is DNA dependent, addition of ligand (L) to the PPARγ–RXR heterodimer promotes recruitment of a 'coactivator' protein complex, which in turn modulates the transcription of target genes regulating different physiological processes. (c) In transrepression, which is DNA independent, PPARγ negatively interferes with other signal transduction pathways, e.g. nuclear factor-κB (NF-κB)- and Fos-Jun-mediated transcription, possibly through competition for limiting amounts of 'shared' transcriptional cofactors. PPRE, PPAR response element; BTFs, basal transcription factors; NF-κB-RE, NF-kB response element; TRE, TPA response element.

Table 2
Genetic variations in PPARγ and human disease

Germline PPARγ mutations	Molecular mechanism	Clinical Phenotype	Key references
Pro115Gln	Gain-of-function	? Obesity	29, 44
V290M	Loss-of-function, dominant negative	IR & partial lipodystrophy	28, 39, 40
P467L	Loss-of-function, dominant negative	IR & partial lipodystrophy	28, 39, 40
F388L	Loss-of-function	IR & partial lipodystrophy	27
R425C	Loss-of-function	IR & partial lipodystrophy	26
(A^{553}ΔAAAiT) fs.185 (stop 186)	Loss-of-function, ? haploinsufficiency	IR when combined with PPP1R3A loss-of -function mutation	58
-14A > G PPARγ4 promoter	Reduced promoter activity	IR & partial lipodystrophy	116

Somatic PPARγ variants	Molecular mechanism	Putative role	Key references
PAX8-PPARγ t(2;3) (q13;p25)	Fusion protein encompassing DBD of the thyroid transcription factor PAX8 and full length PPARγ1; ? functions as dominant negative oncogene	thyroid follicular carcinoma (25-63%); thyroid follicular adenoma (4-55%)	25, 111, 112, 113
Q286P, R288H, K319X, c.472delA	Loss-of-function	human colorectal adenocarcinoma (4/55)	114

PPARγ polymorphisms	Clinical Predisposition	Key references
Pro12Ala	Ala allele confers protection against risk of developing T2DM	45, 55, 56
C161T	? Reduced atherogenic risk	107
C1431T	? Reduced T2DM risk; ? Modulation of Pro12Ala effect	59, 60

Key: IR, insulin resistance; PPP1R3A, protein phosphatase 1 regulatory subunit 3A; DBD, DNA binding domain; T2DM, Type 2 diabetes mellitus.

which, in our opinion, have yielded particularly important findings in relation to the role of PPARγ in the human metabolic syndrome, either by virtue of their commonality in the population as a whole (e.g. the Pro12Ala polymorphism), or as a consequence of inducing an 'extreme' clinical phenotype (e.g. loss-of-function mutations within the ligand-binding domain).

4. PPARγ – a rational therapeutic target in the human metabolic syndrome

Patients with the metabolic syndrome frequently take a 'cocktail of drugs' to treat the individual manifestations of the disorder and its associated complications (e.g. antidiabetic agents, antihypertensives, 'statins' and/or fibrates and aspirin). This requirement for 'polypharmacy' places the patient at greater risk of side effects and can affect compliance. Moreover, the majority of drugs used in the treatment of this condition have little impact on the underlying metabolic disturbance, but rather deal with its consequences. In contrast, drugs that target PPARγ appear, at least in theory, to represent a unique resource with which to tackle the fundamental problem of insulin resistance. As evidence accrues of independent benefits of PPARγ modulation in terms of blood pressure regulation and lipid homeostasis, the move towards more widespread and earlier use of agents such as the TZDs gathers pace. The following sections highlight the human genetic evidence that supports such a strategy, with specific reference to each of the key components of the metabolic syndrome.

4.1. *Adipogenesis*

PPARγ is first and foremost a master-regulator of adipogenesis [30]. It is highly abundant in adipose tissue, with expression being induced early in preadipocyte differentiation [31]. Studies modulating PPARγ expression and/or action in rodent cell lines have established that the receptor is both essential and, in the presence of PPARγ agonists, sufficient for adipogenesis [32]. Although knocking out the murine PPARγ gene results in embryonic lethality, due to combined placental and cardiac defects [33,34], fusion of mutant and normal embryonic cells has enabled selective rescue of the placental pathology, thereby permitting the birth of a single live born runt, which exhibited no discernible adipose tissue [33]. Furthermore, heterozygous PPARγ null mice have reduced adipose tissue depots [35]. So, how do human studies corroborate and extend these findings?

As in rodents, human PPARγ (and in particular the γ2 isoform) is highly expressed in adipose tissue, and exposure of cultured primary human preadipocytes to PPARγ activators (e.g. TZDs) induces their differentiation [36]. Moreover, both chemical and biological receptor antagonists are capable of blocking this process [37]. In clinical practice, treatment with TZDs promotes weight gain in humans, thus suggesting an apparent conundrum, i.e. how can PPARγ activation improve insulin sensitivity while simultaneously promoting weight gain – the so-called 'TZD paradox'? One plausible explanation for this is that PPARγ agonists improve insulin sensitivity by promoting adipogenesis and postprandial fatty acid/triglyceride storage within adipocytes, both of which are likely to be associated with an increase in adipose tissue mass. In addition however, several studies have shown that the increase in body weight associated with TZD treatment is mediated principally by accumulation of subcutaneous fat, whereas visceral adipose tissue volume is reduced or unchanged (reviewed in detail in reference 14). These observations are consonant with *ex vivo* studies in which preadipocytes isolated from subcutaneous abdominal adipose tissue were found to differentiate more readily in response to TZDs than cells from visceral depots taken from the same subjects [36,38].

Recently, three groups have independently identified four heterozygous missense mutations within the ligand-binding domain of human PPARγ (Fig. 1a) [26–28,39], with functional studies confirming that these receptors are transcriptionally impaired [27,28,39]. In keeping with their dominant mode of inheritance, two of the mutants have been shown to inhibit the transcriptional activity of their wild type counterpart in a dominant negative manner, reflecting aberrant cofactor recruitment [39,40]. Together, these reports describe eight adult subjects, all of whom exhibit a stereo-typed pattern of partial lipodystrophy, in which subcutaneous fat is lost from the limbs and gluteal region, while being preserved in both the subcutaneous and visceral abdominal depots (Figs 2a, b). Some phenotypic differences were observed with facial adipose tissue, which was reported to be normal in those subjects harbouring the Pro467Leu and Val290Met mutations (PPARγ1 nomenclature), reduced in the single individual with the Arg425Cys mutation (corresponding to Arg397Cys in PPARγ1) and increased in the Phe388Leu kindred (corresponding to Phe360Leu in PPARγ1). The relative absence of gluteo-femoral fat, with preservation of visceral adipose tissue in these cases is again suggestive of a depot specific role for PPARγ in adipogenesis, and complements the observations made in subjects receiving TZD treatment. Clearly, one challenge is to understand why visceral adipose tissue appears relatively refractory to PPARγ regulation despite expressing comparable levels of receptor to its subcutaneous counterpart. Interestingly, a transgenic knockin mouse model based on the human Pro467Leu mutation (Pro465Leu) has recently been reported [41]. Heterozygous $Pparg^{P465L/+}$ mice have normal total adipose tissue weight, but exhibit reduced intra-abdominal fat mass and increased extra-abdominal subcutaneous fat compared to wild type (WT) animals, i.e. altered body fat distribution, but in a manner which is quite distinct from that observed in human subjects. The reason for this discordance currently remains unclear.

With loss-of-function mutations resulting in lipodystrophy, and PPARγ agonists promoting adipogenesis, it would seem reasonable to speculate that gain-of-function PPARγ mutations might increase body fat mass. Ristow et al. [29] have provided support for this hypothesis, with the identification of four morbidly obese (body mass index (BMI) 37.9–47.2 kg m^{-2}) German subjects, all of whom harboured a gain-of-function mutation (Pro115Gln) within the N-terminal domain of PPARγ2. The transcriptional activity of PPARγ is subject to inhibition through phosphorylation of a serine residue at codon 114 [42,43], and mutation of the adjacent proline was shown to interfere with this process, thus resulting in a receptor with constitutive transcriptional activity and enhanced adipogenic potential [29]. Recently however, a fifth subject harbouring the same amino acid substitution was reported to have only a mildly elevated BMI (28.5 kg m^{-2}), which is in marked contrast to the findings of the original study [44]. Clearly, the identification of other mutation carriers will be required to clarify the significance of this particular genetic variation.

The loss- and gain-of-function receptor mutations described hitherto are rare, having been identified in only a small number of individuals. In contrast, by far the most prevalent human PPARγ genetic variant reported to date is a polymorphism,

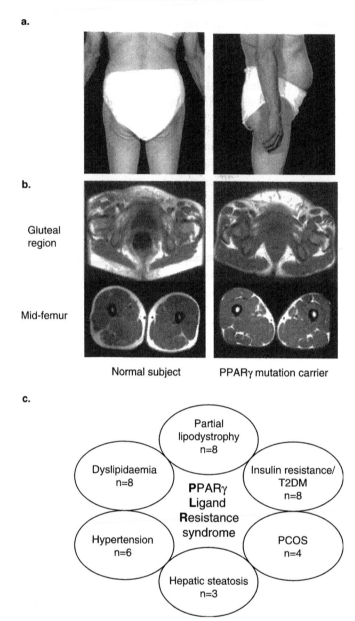

Fig. 2. Partial lipodystrophy in a female subject harbouring a loss-of-function mutation in PPARγ. (a) Note the prominent forearm veins and musculature and diminished gluteal fat depots, but with preservation of abdominal adiposity. (b) T1-weighted MRI images at the levels of the gluteal fat pad and mid-femur in a normal control (a lean healthy female) and in the subject shown in (a). Note the striking loss of gluteal and lower limb subcutaneous fat in the affected individual when compared with the control subject. (c) Schematic representation of the recognised components of the human PPARγ ligand resistance (PLR) syndrome, showing the number of affected individuals manifesting each clinical feature. In all instances the common denominator is 8 (the number of affected adults reported to date), except the polycystic ovarian syndrome (PCOS) where the denominator is 5 females.

substituting alanine for proline at codon 12 (Pro12Ala) in the unique PPARγ2 amino-terminal domain [45]. The allelic frequency of the Ala variant differs depending on the study population, e.g. approximately 12% in Caucasians, 10% in native Americans, 4% in Japanese and just 1% in Chinese [46]. Unlike PPARγ1, which is ubiquitously expressed at relatively low levels, the γ2 isoform is almost exclusively expressed in adipose tissue. In functional assays, Ala12-PPARγ exhibits reduced binding to DNA and modest impairment in target gene transactivation [45]. An association with lower BMI in an early study appeared to suggest a corresponding genotype–phenotype correlation [45]. However, numerous subsequent cross-sectional studies have yielded conflicting results by demonstrating either no difference [47,48] or a modestly greater BMI [49] in carriers of the Ala allele. It can be argued of course that the latter is also compatible with the *in vitro* properties of Ala12-PPARγ, given that carriers of this allele exhibit enhanced insulin sensitivity (see below) when compared with their Pro/Pro counterparts, and greater insulin sensitivity *per se* has been shown to predict future weight gain. In an attempt to resolve this issue, Masud et al. [50] have recently published a meta-analysis using data from 30 independent studies with a total of 19,136 subjects. They concluded that in the samples with a mean BMI value $\geqslant 27 \, \mathrm{kg \, m^{-2}}$, Ala12 allele carriers had a significantly higher BMI than non-carriers ($p = 0.0006$), whereas no difference was detected in the samples with a BMI value $< 27 \, \mathrm{kg \, m^{-2}}$. A further analysis using data from publications in which BMI for the three genotype groups (i.e. Pro/Pro, Pro/Ala and Ala/Ala) were presented separately revealed that the Ala12 homozygotes had significantly higher BMI than heterozygotes and Pro12 homozygotes [50]. It is important to bear in mind however, that the effects of the Ala allele are likely to be subject to modification by other genetic and environmental factors. For example, variations in dietary polyunsaturated fat versus saturated fat intake may influence BMI in carriers of the Ala variant, suggesting gene–nutrient interaction at the PPARγ locus [51]. Taken together, these genetic observations strongly support the notion that PPARγ is a critical regulator of human adipose tissue mass.

4.2. *Insulin sensitivity*

4.2.1. *Evidence for a link*
Given the associations of both obesity and lipodystrophy with insulin resistance, it is not surprising that PPARγ, a critical regulator of adipogenesis, should also be involved in the regulation of insulin sensitivity. In fact, several lines of evidence point to such a link: firstly, the *in vitro* binding affinities of TZD and non-TZD PPARγ ligands correlate closely with their *in vivo* potencies as insulin sensitizers [17,52]; secondly, RXR ligands, which can activate the PPARγ–RXR heterodimer, also exhibit insulin-sensitizing effects in rodents [53]; thirdly, mice harbouring a mutation at serine 112 (corresponding to serine 114 in human PPARγ2), which leads to a constitutively more active receptor (through inhibition of phosphorylation), are protected from obesity-associated insulin resistance [54].

Studies of human PPARγ genetic variants have proved complementary to this body of pharmacological and animal data. For example, severe insulin resistance (with or without overt T2DM) has proved to be a remarkably consistent finding in subjects with loss-of-function PPARγ mutations, being evident even in early childhood in affected individuals (Fig. 2c) [26–28,39]. At a population level, there is now a substantial body of evidence to implicate 'Pro12Ala' as a major T2DM susceptibility locus. Thus, while earlier studies provided conflicting views on the possible association between this polymorphism and diabetes risk, subsequent reports, including a meta-analysis encompassing more than 3000 individuals, have confirmed a modest (1.25-fold), but significant ($p = 0.002$), increase in diabetes risk with the Pro allele [55]. It has been suggested that if these findings held true in the population as a whole, then the global prevalence of T2DM would be ~25% lower simply by virtue of everybody carrying one or more copies of the Ala allele [46]. A recently published prospective study, arising from within the Nurses' Health Study, has provided additional support for such an assertion [56]. Using a nested case control study of 387 incident cases of T2DM and 771 matched controls (with corrections for age, alcohol consumption, physical activity, smoking and BMI), the authors reported an inverse relationship between the presence of the Ala12 variant and T2DM risk (OR = 0.74 [0.55–1.00]).

The finding that a transcriptionally less active human receptor polymorphism predisposes to increased insulin sensitivity appears, at first glance, to accord with observations derived from transgenic mouse models of PPARγ action. Thus, two groups have shown that heterozygous PPARγ null mice ($+/-$) exhibit increased insulin sensitivity when compared with their wild type littermates [34,57]. These animals have reduced fat depots, populated by smaller adipocytes, with lower levels of triglyceride accumulation and lipogenesis in white adipose tissue, skeletal muscle and liver [35]. However, it is worth noting that in a unique human pedigree, with perhaps greater similarities to the heterozygous null mice than the Pro12Ala polymorphism, evidence of improved insulin sensitivity was not observed [58]. In this kindred, two subjects harbouring a heterozygous frameshift/premature stop mutation in PPARγ, which results in a truncated receptor with no discernible dominant negative activity, exhibited normal rather than enhanced insulin sensitivity. Moreover, when combined with a second heterozygous 'genetic hit' in an unrelated molecule – a regulatory subunit of protein phosphatase 1 (PPP1R3A) – the double heterozygotes within this same kindred exhibited severe insulin resistance, suggesting that the presence of the dysfunctional PPARG allele served to predispose to, rather than protect against, the risk of developing insulin resistance.

In light of the findings with Pro12Ala, several groups have sought to determine whether other single nucleotide polymorphisms (SNPs) within PPARγ might also influence T2DM risk at a population level. In one study of ~ 4000 Asian subjects, a link with a second polymorphism C1431T (for which the presence of a T allele conferred a reduced diabetes risk when compared with CC homozygotes [OR 0.73, $p = 0.011$]), was reported [59]. Doney et al. [60] have taken analysis of this genetic variant further, establishing it to be in tight allelic disequilibrium with the Ala12 variant in their study population (70% of all Ala carriers also carried the C1431T polymorphism). Having genotyped individuals from three separate cohorts (1,997 subjects with T2DM, 2,444 non-diabetic children and 1061 middle-aged controls – all from a similar area in Tayside, Scotland) for the PPARG Pro12Ala and C1431 T polymorphisms, they concluded that the Ala12 variant was under-represented in the T2DM population when compared with similarly aged non-diabetic adults (OR 0.74, $p = 0.0006$). The 1431 T variant was also under-represented in the T2DM versus adult population. Intriguingly however, when the Ala12 variant was on a haplotype not bearing the 1431 T variant, it conferred greater protection (OR $= 0.66$, $p = 0.003$); in contrast, when it was present in haplotypes containing the 1431 T variant (70% of Ala12 carriers), this protection was absent (OR $= 0.99$, $p = 0.94$). Further studies are awaited with interest. Moreover, it remains to be seen how a silent polymorphism such as C1431 T could influence PPARγ function at a molecular level.

Thus, it is clear that the relationship between PPARγ activity and insulin sensitivity in humans is complex, with evidence for a gene dosage effect, which is subject to modification by other genetic and environmental factors.

4.2.2. Potential mechanisms

Maintenance of normal glucose homeostasis is dependent on retention of insulin sensitivity in key target tissues including liver and skeletal muscle. TZDs promote insulin sensitization in both of these sites, while muscle-specific knockout of the murine *Pparg* gene has been linked to muscle and/or hepatic insulin resistance [61,62]. It remains unclear however, as to whether TZDs are able to ameliorate insulin resistance in this setting, with two separate groups reporting conflicting findings [61,62]. Nevertheless, these observations raise the possibility that direct activation of PPARγ in skeletal muscle might account for at least some of the beneficial effects that are observed with TZD therapy.

In contrast to muscle, PPARγ expression is markedly higher in adipose tissue, and thus it seems likely that receptor activation in adipocytes contributes significantly to the clinical efficacy of PPARγ ligands in ameliorating insulin resistance. In keeping with this, mice lacking adipose tissue have been shown to be refractory to the anti-diabetic effects of TZDs [63], while adipose-specific deletion of PPARγ (which is associated with progressive lipodystrophy) predisposes mice to hepatic steatosis, and high fat feeding-induced skeletal muscle insulin resistance [64]. Moreover, because PPARγ2 is virtually exclusively expressed in fat cells, any metabolic effects of the Pro12Ala polymorphism, including those on glucose homeostasis, are likely to be secondary to alterations in adipose tissue metabolism. So how does PPARγ activity in fat impact on whole body insulin sensitivity?

4.2.2.1. Regulation of free fatty acid flux in adipocytes. It has long been recognised that circulating levels of free fatty acids (FFAs) are a major determinant of insulin sensitivity. Both lean and obese type 2 diabetics experience day-long elevations in plasma FFA concentrations, which fail to suppress normally in response to a glucose load or insulin [14]. Several studies have shown that the antidiabetic efficacy of TZDs correlates with their ability to lower circulating FFA levels [14]. Emerging evidence indicates that PPARγ activation in adipose tissue exerts coordinated effects on FFA flux (promoting uptake/trapping, while simultaneously impairing FFA release – the

Catherine S. Mitchell, Mark Gurnell

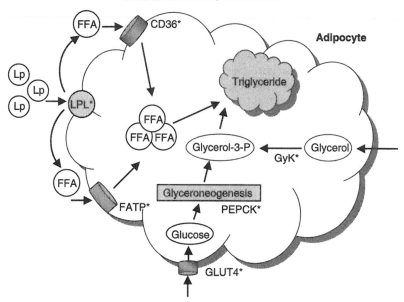

Fig. 3. PPARγ regulation of FFA flux in adipocytes. PPARγ ligands enhance the expression of lipoprotein lipase and the FFA transporters FATP and CD36, thereby promoting uptake of FFAs released from circulating lipoproteins. Inside the adipocyte, FFAs are esterified into triglyceride through combination with glycerol-3-phosphate. The latter is generated through two pathways: (i) phosphorylation of exogenous glycerol under the influence of glycerol kinase and (ii) glyceroneogenesis, which is subject to regulation by PEPCK. Lp, lipoprotein; LPL, lipoprotein lipase; FATP, fatty acid transport protein; CD36, fatty acid translocase; FFA, free fatty acids; GyK, glycerol kinase; PEPCK, phosphoenolpyruvate carboxykinase; glycerol-3-P, glycerol-3-phosphate; GLUT4, glucose transporter 4. * denotes potential sites of regulation by PPARγ.

so-called 'fatty acid steal' hypothesis), through the regulation of a panel of genes involved in FFA metabolism (Fig. 3). Adipocyte lipoprotein lipase (LPL) expression is up regulated in response to TZD treatment, thereby potentially enhancing release of FFAs from circulating lipoproteins [65]. Simultaneous up regulation of FFA transporters such as CD36 and fatty acid transport protein (FATP) on the adipocyte surface facilitates their uptake [66]. TZDs may also reduce FFA efflux from adipocytes through enhanced expression of genes that promote their storage in the form of triglycerides (e.g. glycerol kinase – directs the synthesis of glycerol-3-phosphate directly from glycerol; phosphoenolpyruvate carboxykinase (PEPCK) – permits the utilisation of pyruvate to form the glycerol backbone for triglyceride synthesis) [67,68]. Together these actions ensure that fatty acids are stored appropriately in adipose tissue, and not 'ectopically' in other sites such as liver and skeletal muscle, where they are capable of inducing 'lipotoxicity'. It is worth pointing out that this concept is far from novel, with Randle et al. [69] first postulating that increased FFA oxidation could restrain glucose oxidation and hence uptake into skeletal muscle more than 40 years ago.

Observations in human subjects with genetic variations in PPARγ may be consistent with this hypothesis. For example, it appears that even the existing residual adipose tissue depots in individuals with loss-of-function mutations in PPARγ are dysfunctional, resulting in exposure of skeletal muscle and liver to unregulated fatty acid fluxes, with consequent impairment of insulin action at these sites [28]. In addition, there is evidence that the Pro12Ala polymorphism facilitates insulin-mediated suppression of lipolysis, and hence FFA release, possibly by shifting the balance from large to small adipocytes, which are more insulin sensitive [46]. However, others have failed to detect any relationship between circulating FFA levels and Pro12Ala status [70].

4.2.2.2. *Regulation of genes governing glucose uptake.* Promotion of glucose uptake into skeletal muscle and adipose tissue, coupled with suppression of hepatic glucose production, are critical steps in the insulin-mediated response to a glucose load. The glucose transporter 4 (GLUT4) (insulin-dependent) transporter, which translocates to the plasma membrane from intracellular storage sites, is a key modulator of glucose disposal in both muscle and fat (Fig. 4). Binding of insulin to its tyrosine kinase receptor engages a cascade of intracellular phosphorylation events, including activation of phosphatidylinositol-3-OH kinase [PI(3)K] and other downstream kinases,

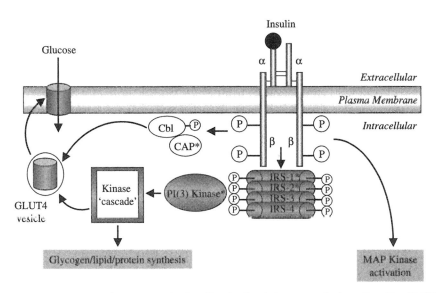

Fig. 4. PPARγ regulation of glucose uptake. Insulin stimulated glucose uptake is mediated by GLUT4, a specific glucose transporter. Activation of PI(3)K promotes trafficking of GLUT4 containing vesicles from intracellular sites to the plasma membrane. In addition phosphorylation of Cbl, which associates with CAP, provides a second signal that acts in parallel with the PI(3)K pathway to augment this process. IRS-1 to 4, insulin receptor substrates-1 to 4; PI(3)K, phosphatidylinositol-3-OH kinase; Cbl, c-Cbl protooncogene; CAP, c-Cbl-associated protein. * denotes potential sites of regulation by PPARγ. Reproduced with permission from reference 115.

which promote trafficking of GLUT4 containing vesicles to the plasma membrane. A second pathway, which involves a distinct group of signalling molecules including the c-Cbl protooncogene product and c-Cbl-associated protein (CAP), augments this process (Fig. 4). Evidence is accumulating to suggest that PPARγ activation in adipose tissue can influence insulin signalling at various points in these pathways, e.g. through up regulation of insulin receptor substrates-1 and -2 (IRS-1, IRS-2) [71,72], the p85 subunit of PI(3)K [73], and CAP [74,75] – all of which might be predicted to enhance GLUT4 activity. Increased glucose uptake into adipocytes contributes to whole body glucose disposal, and provides important substrate for triglyceride synthesis (see above). However, it remains to be seen whether similar direct effects on glucose uptake are also operational in skeletal muscle, where much lower levels of PPARγ expression are observed, but where the majority (∼80%) of glucose disposal occurs. Unfortunately, conflicting findings in the two existing mouse models of muscle-specific *Pparg* deletion have so far failed to resolve this issue [61,62].

4.2.2.3. *Regulation of adipokine release.*   As already alluded to in the context of FFA metabolism, it is of course possible that PPARγ 'stimulated' glucose uptake into skeletal muscle is dependent in significant part on receptor activation in adipose tissue. This hypothesis is supported not only by the findings in adipose-specific *Pparg* knockout mice fed a high fat diet [64], but also those arising from the study of mice with adipose tissue-specific knockout of the *Glut4* gene, which develop insulin resistance in muscle and liver, manifesting as hyperinsulinaemia and glucose intolerance, despite normal GLUT4 expression in these tissues [76]. Importantly, when studied *ex vivo*, basal and insulin-stimulated glucose transport in skeletal muscle from the transgenic mice did not differ from that observed with their wild type littermates, leading the authors to conclude that one or more factors secreted from adipose tissue *in vivo*, as a consequence of impaired glucose uptake in adipocytes, must be acting to impair insulin sensitivity in other target tissues.

In light of these and other similar findings, there is now a general consensus that adipose tissue should no longer be viewed simply as a reservoir for energy storage during 'times of plenty' and energy release during 'times of need', but also as a true endocrine organ in its own right [77]. Indeed, adipocytes are not only critical regulators of circulating FFAs, but they also act as a rich source of hormones, collectively referred to as adipokines (e.g. leptin, adiponectin, tumour necrosis factor-α (TNFα), interleukin-6 (IL-6), resistin), many of which are capable of exerting profound effects on insulin-mediated glucose disposal and/or hepatic glucose output. For example, circulating adiponectin levels have been shown to correlate closely with insulin sensitivity, and inversely with fat mass (especially visceral adiposity) [78–80]. Adiponectin is produced exclusively by adipose tissue and exerts both insulin sensitizing and anti-atherogenic properties in mice. TZDs increase adiponectin gene expression, suggesting that this adipokine may represent a critical link between PPARγ activation and insulin sensitization [81]. Consonant with this, circulating adiponectin levels were found to be dramatically lower in three individuals harbouring loss-of-function PPARγ mutations when compared with healthy controls or subjects with non-PPARγ-mediated severe insulin resistance, suggesting a direct correlation between PPARγ activity and adiponectin expression [82]. In contrast resistin, a novel protein expressed in preadipocytes undergoing differentiation into mature adipocytes [83], induces severe hepatic insulin resistance, correlating with the finding that circulating levels and resistin expression in fat cells are increased in humans with T2DM and obesity [84].

In general, PPARγ activation in adipocytes appears to enhance the expression of 'factors' that facilitate insulin action (e.g. adiponectin), while simultaneously suppressing those which are antagonistic (e.g. resistin, TNFα and IL-6), thereby altering the profile of adipocyte gene expression in a manner that is likely to promote insulin sensitization (Fig. 5).

4.2.2.4. *Modulation of other adipocyte genes.* Prolonged exposure to hypercortisolaemia, as observed in subjects with Cushing's syndrome, is associated with

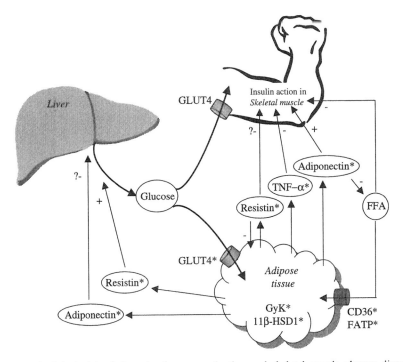

Fig. 5. At a physiological level, hepatic glucose production and skeletal muscle glucose disposal are subject to regulation by a number of adipocyte derived factors (adipokines). Ambient blood glucose levels reflect, at least in part, the balance that exists between factors which impair insulin action (e.g. TNFα, FFA and resistin) and those with insulin sensitizing effects (e.g. Adiponectin). GyK acts to reduce FFA release through promotion of triglyceride synthesis. 11β-HSD1 serves to regenerate active cortisol from inactive cortisone. GLUT4, CD36, adiponectin and GyK gene expression are enhanced following treatment with PPARγ ligands, while TNFα and resistin are negatively regulated. '+' stimulation, '−' inhibition. TNFα, tumour necrosis factor-α; FFA, free fatty acids; FATP, fatty acid transport protein; CD36, fatty acid translocase; GyK, glycerol kinase; 11β-HSD1, 11β-hydroxysteroid dehydrogenase type 1. * denotes potential sites of regulation by PPARγ. Reproduced and adapted with permission from reference 115.

many features of the metabolic syndrome (visceral obesity, glucose intolerance, hypertension and dyslipidaemia). While circulating cortisol levels in ordinary obese non-Cushingoid individuals are normal, there is evidence to suggest that local regeneration of cortisol within adipose tissue could contribute to the development of insulin resistance in the setting of visceral obesity [85]. 11β-hydroxysteroid dehydrogenase type 1 (11β-HSD1) directs the production of active cortisol from inactive cortisone in liver and fat, thereby facilitating cortisol-induced adipocyte differentiation. In keeping with this, adipose-specific over-expression of 11β-HSD1 in transgenic mice induced a phenotype of insulin resistance and central obesity [86]. PPARγ ligands have been shown to down-regulate adipocyte 11β-HSD1 expression and activity [87], and the subsequent modulation of glucocorticoid-induced gene expression may conceivably contribute to their insulin sensitizing actions.

4.3. Dyslipidaemia

PPARγ agonists, which improve insulin sensitivity, would be predicted to lower circulating triglycerides and raise HDL levels. Indeed the latter has been a consistent finding in several clinical studies with both rosiglitazone and pioglitazone. Intriguingly however, while pioglitazone also reduces serum triglycerides, this is not the case with rosiglitazone – the mechanisms underlying these divergent responses remain to be elucidated [16]. One possible explanation is that pioglitazone may also be acting as a partial PPARα agonist (akin to a fibrate), while at the doses used in clinical practice rosiglitazone retains pure γ-agonist activity [88]. Rosiglitazone has also been noted to elevate low density lipoprotein (LDL) cholesterol, possibly through increasing levels of large buoyant LDL particles [16]. It has been suggested that this beneficial effect on particle size will translate into delayed progression of atheromatous disease, although ongoing long-term studies designed to assess cardiovascular endpoints will yield more conclusive data on this.

To date, the majority of subjects with loss-of-function mutations in the ligand binding domain of PPARγ have exhibited hypertriglyceridaemia and low HDL levels, with unremarkable LDL cholesterols [26–28]. It remains unclear however, as to whether these abnormalities are simply a 'metabolic consequence' of severe insulin resistance *per se*, or whether they indicate an additive and independent effect of dysfunctional PPARγ signalling in relation to lipoprotein metabolism.

Although there is now an extensive body of data concerning the potential effects of the Pro12Ala polymorphism on glycaemic control, there are relatively few studies focusing on its consequences for lipid homeostasis. Moreover, given the potential confounding effects of insulin resistance, cohort selection (particularly with respect to diabetic status and/or BMI) is critical when trying to identify a specific independent link between PPARγ action and lipid handling. Accepting these limitations, there is some evidence to suggest that the Ala allele may confer additional benefits with respect to circulating lipid levels. For example, in the original study of Deeb et al. [45], higher HDL cholesterol ($p = 0.001$) and lower triglyceride ($p = 0.002$) levels were also observed among elderly subjects with the Ala/Ala genotype compared with Pro/Ala and Pro/Pro genotypes. A similar association was described in over 4000

Singapore Asians whose genotype was analysed as a dichotomous variable (i.e. presence or absence of the Ala variant), and in whom Ala allele carriers had significantly higher HDL cholesterol levels compared with Pro/Pro homozygotes ($p < 0.05$) [59]. However, other groups have reported conflicting results. For example, in a study of 663 Caucasian subjects from Western Australian, obese (BMI > 30 kg m^{-2}) carriers of the Ala allele exhibited significantly lower HDL cholesterol levels, and non-significantly higher triglycerides [48]. No such association was found within a group of lean subjects (BMI < 25 kg m^{-2}). While the obese cohort was significantly older and had a greater prevalence of diabetes, these associations remained significant after adjusting for these as co-variants [48].

4.4. *Hypertension*

The prevalence of hypertension has been estimated to be 1.5- to 2-fold higher in subjects with T2DM compared with the general population. Insulin resistance *per se* is also associated with hypertension, which may in part reflect effects on the renin–angiotensin system. It is not surprising then that early onset (and in some cases severe) hypertension has been a notable finding in the majority of human subjects with PPARγ loss-of-function mutations [26–28]. In contrast, TZD therapy is associated with a modest reduction in blood pressure in a variety of clinical settings including (i) patients with type 2 diabetes and hypertension (ii) non-hypertensive type 2 diabetics (iii) obese subjects without diabetes and (iv) non-diabetic hypertensives [88]. The latter might suggest possible additional effects on blood pressure regulation, independent of insulin sensitization, and indeed several lines of evidence suggest that PPARγ may directly regulate vascular tone, e.g. through blockade of calcium channel activity in smooth muscle [89], inhibition of release of endothelin-1 [90] and enhancement of C-type natriuretic peptide release [91]. While no studies of vascular tone or endothelial function have as yet been reported in human subjects with PPARγ mutations, mice heterozygous for the equivalent Pro465Leu mutation were found to be hypertensive in the absence of insulin resistance, exhibiting enhanced expression of the angiotensinogen gene in their subcutaneous adipose tissue [41]. These findings lend strong support to the hypothesis that specifically targeting PPARγ function in the metabolic syndrome is likely to confer additional benefits over and above those derived simply from improving insulin sensitivity.

Data relating to differences in blood pressure and Pro12Ala status have proved less informative, again reflecting in part the confounding variable of insulin resistance. In a small cross-sectional observation study limited to subjects with T2DM, an association between the Pro12Ala polymorphism and lower diastolic blood pressure (of the order of 3–7 mmHg) was observed [92]. However, it is important to note that the link with blood pressure in this study was restricted to male subjects. While this may represent a novel gender difference, no plausible biological explanation has been offered, and the possibility remains therefore, that this was a chance finding. In contrast, in an American study of 619 individuals from 52 familial T2DM kindreds no link between Pro12Ala genotype and blood pressure was noted [93], while in a large Finnish cohort the only significant association was in the morbidly obese subgroup ($BMI > 40 \, kg \, m^{-2}$), where the Ala allele was actually linked with higher diastolic blood pressure [94]. Rodriguez-Esparragon et al. [95] examined the relationship between polymorphic markers in two genes – PPARγ and endothelial nitric oxide synthase (eNOS) – in 235 hypertensive patients and 223 normotensive matched controls [95]. They observed that the Pro-Pro genotype of PPARγ was associated with hypertension and was particularly influential in patients who were normohomocysteinaemic. Moreover, when analysed together the 'unfavourable' alleles of PPARγ and eNOS increased the risk of hypertension in a synergistic manner with the authors proposing that nitric oxide is the common denominator. However, it remains unclear as to whether PPARγ is capable of regulating eNOS expression and, moreover, the proposed hypothesis would depend on an upregulation of eNOS by PPARγ, whereas previous work has demonstrated that the apparently 'favourable' Ala allele exhibits reduced transcriptional activity [45]. These results are also potentially at odds with the observation that PPARγ activators such as TZDs exert beneficial effects on blood pressure. It is clear that further epidemiological studies will be required to explore the potential influences of polymorphisms such as Pro12Ala on the regulation of blood pressure.

4.5. *PPARγ and atherosclerotic vascular disease*

Collectively, the individual components of the metabolic syndrome conspire to dramatically increase the risk of cardiovascular disease in affected individuals [8]. PPARγ activation with exogenous ligands such as the TZDs would be predicted to confer significant benefits in this setting, through the amelioration of insulin resistance, dyslipidaemia and possibly hypertension, albeit at a potential 'cost' of mild weight gain (as a consequence of enhanced adipogenesis). Although it is too early to know whether these theoretical benefits will translate into a genuine risk reduction in the longer term, early studies of carotid arterial intima-media thickness (IMT), a surrogate marker of atherosclerosis, have proved reassuring, reporting a significant reduction in subjects with T2DM treated with troglitazone, rosiglitazone and pioglitazone [96].

It was therefore surprising and of potential therapeutic concern when Tontonoz et al. [97] reported that PPARγ activation in a pre-macrophage cell line induced expression of CD36 (also known as fatty acid translocase (FAT)), a cellular 'scavenger' receptor for atherogenic LDL. Enhanced CD36 expression might be predicted to increase intracellular accumulation of oxidised LDL cholesterol, which could then be catabolized to generate PPARγ ligands (e.g. 9-hydroxyoctadecadienoic acid [9-HODE] and 13-HODE) capable of further receptor activation, thereby creating a 'vicious' feed-forward cycle of increasing lipid uptake, and ultimately driving conversion of the macrophage into an atherogenic foam cell [97]. The finding that PPARγ is expressed at relatively high levels in human atherosclerotic plaques, further served to fuel concerns [98,99].

However, almost coincident with these observations, several groups reported that PPARγ ligands reduce the release of inflammatory cytokines (e.g. TNF-α and IL-6) from macrophages, an effect that might be predicted to be anti-atherogenic [100,101].

Subsequent studies have further redressed the balance, with the demonstration that PPARγ ligands exert an opposing effect on SR-A, a second LDL scavenger receptor, down regulating its expression in mouse macrophages [102]. In addition, the nuclear receptor liver X receptor α (LXRα), which enhances expression of ABCA1 (ATP-binding cassette transporter A1), a protein which mediates cellular cholesterol efflux [103], has also been shown to be a PPARγ target gene in human and mouse macrophages [104,105]. Taken together, these data suggest a broader spectrum of PPARγ effects within the macrophage with the overall balance favouring cholesterol efflux and an anti-atherogenic effect.

Circulating adiponectin levels are typically low in patients with insulin resistance and have also been shown to be reduced in the setting of coronary artery disease. The ability to raise adiponectin levels would also speak therefore, to a cardioprotective effect of treatment with PPARγ activators such as the TZDs.

In light of these findings, one might predict a predisposition to atheromatous vascular disease in subjects harbouring loss-of-function mutations within PPARγ. In the eight affected adult subjects reported to date, only one vascular event has been described (a myocardial infarct in a male member of the Phe388Leu kindred, occurring at 56 years of age in a non-smoker). In addition however, we have recently identified five novel mutations in PPARγ (Gurnell, O'Rahilly, Chatterjee - manuscript in preparation) with three affected female subjects from these kindreds exhibiting premature ischaemic coronary disease.

There is also an emerging body of epidemiological evidence to suggest an association between the naturally occurring PPARγ polymorphisms and IMT and thus, indirectly, cardiovascular risk. A study of 154 Japanese T2DM patients found those carrying the Ala12 allele to have a significantly lower carotid IMT than their Pro/Pro counterparts, despite no observed differences in gender, age, fasting blood glucose, lipid profile or HbA1c [106]. However, differences in BMI and the degree of insulin resistance between the two groups were not reported. Yan et al. [107] used IMT as a secondary outcome measure to investigate the prevalence of the C161T PPARγ polymorphism within four different Chinese cohorts; 248 subjects with insulin resistance syndrome (IRS), 163 with essential hypertension, 115 with T2DM and 121 normal controls. They observed that the CC genotype (prevalence 75%) was significantly associated with increased IMT compared to CT and TT genotypes (prevalence 22 and 4% respectively) within 248 'metabolic syndrome' patients. However interestingly, the Pro12Ala and C161T polymorphisms within PPARγ were neither over- nor under-represented in a large Caucasian cohort (1170 individuals) with angiographically proven coronary heart disease [50], and it is clear further large-scale studies are needed.

5. Conclusions and future directions

While there is genuine excitement that the introduction of TZDs has at last provided clinicians with an appropriate therapeutic agent with which to target insulin resistance and its sequelae, it is also apparent that these drugs are not without their problems. Indeed, the initial wave of enthusiasm that accompanied their introduction into clinical practice was tempered by the withdrawal of troglitazone, the first TZD in widespread use, on the grounds of hepatotoxicity; subsequent studies have suggested that this potentially fatal idiosyncratic adverse event is unlikely to be a class effect, but rather reflects the generation of a toxic metabolite unique to troglitazone. Close surveillance for hepatic dysfunction following the introduction of rosiglitazone and pioglitazone has provided added reassurance, but other potentially troublesome side effects have been reported, e.g. weight gain and peripheral oedema.

With the major metabolic effects of PPARγ being promotion of fat cell formation (adipogenesis) and enhancement of tissue sensitivity to insulin, this raises the intriguing possibility that it might be possible to uncouple these biological responses, by developing selective receptor modulators (the so-called SPPARMs), which preferentially affect glucose metabolism. Precedent for such an approach is provided by raloxifene, a selective estrogen receptor (ER) modulator (SERM), which is an ER antagonist in breast and endometrium but an agonist in bone. Promisingly, several groups have independently identified PPARγ ligands with either partial agonist or antagonist activity, which exhibit divergent biological responses: GW0072 and LG100641 are compounds which inhibit adipocyte differentiation yet stimulate cellular glucose uptake [108,109]; FMOC-L-leucine, a chemically distinct receptor ligand, has been shown to improve insulin sensitivity yet exert relatively weak adipogenic effects in rodent diabetic models [110]. Similarly, enhancing the ability of TZDs to further alter the dyslipidaemic profile of insulin resistance, would clearly offer added therapeutic benefit, in a high-risk diabetic population. A greater understanding of the PPARγ target genes which mediate these effects, in conjunction with studies of patterns of cofactor recruitment and gene activation in response to novel receptor ligands, may lead to the development of newer agents which promote desirable PPARγ responses with greater selectivity.

Accordingly, it seems likely that PPARγ will continue to be a focus of attention for those interested in exploring the pathogenesis of the human metabolic syndrome, with the anticipation that improved understanding will bring with it more effective therapeutic agents for its treatment. Given the apparent inexorable rise in the prevalence of obesity, insulin resistance and T2DM, the need for such novel therapies could not be more urgent.

References

[1] A.F. Amos, et al., The rising global burden of diabetes and its complications: estimates and projections to the year 2010, Diabetes Med. 14 (suppl 5) (1997) 81–85.

[2] Diabetes in the UK, Diabetes UK Report.(2004).

[3] A.H. Mokdad, et al., Prevalence of obesity, diabetes, and obesity-related health risk factors, 2001, Am. Med. Assoc. 289 (2003) 76–79.

[4] S.H. Saydah, et al., Subclinical states of glucose intolerance and risk of death in the US, Diabetes Care 24 (2001) 447–453.

[5] N. Unwin, et al., Impaired glucose tolerance and impaired fasting glycaemia: the current status on definition and intervention, Diabetes Med. 19 (2002) 708–723.

[6] G. Reaven, Banting lecture: role of insulin resistance in human disease, Diabetes 37 (1988) 1595–1607.

[7] World Health Organization, Definition, Diagnosis and Classification of Diabetes Mellitus and its Complications. Part 1. Diagnosis and Classification of Diabetes Mellitus, WHO, Geneva, 1999.

[8] B. Isomaa, et al., Cardiovascular morbidity and mortality associated with the metabolic syndrome, Diabetes Care 24 (2001) 683–689.

[9] European Group for the Study of Insulin Resistance (EGIR), Diabetic Med. 16 (1999) 442–443.

[10] Executive summary of the third report of the National Cholesterol Education Program (NCEP) expert panel on detection, evaluation and treatment of high blood cholesterol in adults (Adult treatment Panel III), JAMA 285 (2001) 2486–2497.

[11] International Diabetes Federation. The IDF consensus worldwide definition of the metabolic syndrome. April 14, (2005). http://www.idf.org/webdata/docs/Metac_syndrome_def.pdf

[12] A. Garg, Acquired and inherited lipodystrophies, New Engl. J. Med. 350 (2004) 1220–1234.

[13] J.D. McGarry, et al., Fatty acids, lipotoxicity and insulin secretion, Diabetologia 42 (2) (1999) 128–138.

[14] H. Bays, et al., Role of the adipocyte, free fatty acids and ectopic fat in pathogenesis of type 2 diabetes mellitus: peroxisomal proliferator-activated receptor agonists provide a rational therapeutic approach, J. Clin. Endocrinol. Metab. 89 (2004) 463–478.

[15] United Kingdom Prospective Diabetes Study (UKPDS) Group, Intensive blood glucose control with sulphonylureas or insulin compared with conventional treatment and risk of complications in patients with type 2 diabetes (UKPDS 33), Lancet 352 (1998) 837–853.

[16] H. Yki-Jarvinen, Thiazolidinediones, New Engl. J. Med. 351 (2004) 1106–1118.

[17] J.M. Lehmann, et al., An antidiabetic thiazolidinedione is a high affinity ligand for peroxisome proliferator-activated receptor γ (PPARγ), J. Biol. Chem. 270 (1995) 12953–12956.

[18] T.M. Willson, et al., The PPARs: from orphan receptors to drug discovery, J. Med. Chem. 43 (2000) 527–550.

[19] W.R. Oliver Jr., et al., A selective peroxisome proliferator-activated receptor delta agonist promotes reverse cholesterol transport, Proc Natl. Acad. Sci. USA 98 (2001) 5306–5311.

[20] H. Vosper, et al., The peroxisome proliferator-activated receptor delta promotes lipid accumulation in human macrophages, J. Biol. Chem. 276 (2001) 44258–44265.

[21] A. Chawla, et al., PPARδ is a very low-density lipoprotein sensor in macrophages, Proc. Natl. Acad. Sci. USA 100 (2003) 1268–1273.

[22] H. Lim, et al., PPAR delta functions as a prostacyclin receptor in blastocyst implantation, Trends Endocrinol. Metab. 11 (2000) 137–142.

[23] N.S. Tan, et al., Critical roles of PPAR β/δ in keratinocyte response to inflammation, Genes Dev. 15 (2001) 3263–3277.

[24] L. Fajas, et al., The organization, promoter analysis, and expression of the human PPARgamma gene, J. Biol. Chem. 272 (1997) 18779–18789.

[25] T.G. Kroll, et al., PAX8-PPARγ1 fusion oncogene in human thyroid carcinoma, Science 289 (2000) 1357–1360.

[26] A.K. Agarwal, A. Garg, A novel heterozygous mutation in peroxisome proliferator-activated receptor-γ gene in a patient with familial partial lipodystrophy, J. Clin. Endocrinol. Metab. 87 (2002) 408–411.

[27] R.A. Hegele, et al., PPARG F388L, a transactivation-deficient mutant, in familial partial lipodystrophy, Diabetes 51 (2002) 3586–3590.

[28] D.B. Savage, et al., Human metabolic syndrome resulting from dominant-negative mutations in the nuclear receptor PPARγ, Diabetes 52 (2003) 910–917.

[29] M. Ristow, et al., Obesity associated with a mutation in a genetic regulator of adipocyte differentiation, New Engl. J. Med. 339 (1998) 953–959.

[30] E.D. Rosen, et al., Transcriptional regulation of adipogenesis, Genes Dev 14 (2000) 1293–1307.

[31] R. Saladin, et al., Differential regulation of peroxisome proliferator activated receptor gamma1 (PPARgamma1) and PPARgamma2 messenger RNA expression in the early stages of adipogenesis, Cell Growth Differ. 10 (1999) 43–48.

[32] E.D. Rosen, et al., C/EBPalpha induces adipogenesis through PPAR-gamma: a unified pathway, Genes Dev. 16 (2002) 22–26.

[33] Y. Barak, et al., PPARγ is required for placental, cardiac and adipose tissue development, Mol. Cell 4 (1999) 585–595.

[34] N.T. Kubota, et al., PPARγ mediates high-fat diet-induced adipocyte hypertrophy and insulin resistance, Mol. Cell 4 (1999) 597–609.

[35] T. Yamauchi, et al., The mechanisms by which both heterozygous peroxisome proliferator-activated receptor gamma (PPARgamma) deficiency and PPARgamma agonist improve insulin resistance, J. Biol. Chem. 276 (2001) 41245–41254.

[36] M. Adams, et al., Activators of PPARγ have depot-specific effects on human preadipocyte differentiation, J. Clin. Invest. 100 (1997) 3149–3153.

[37] M. Gurnell, et al., A dominant negative peroxisome proliferator-activated receptor γ (PPARγ) mutant is a constitutive repressor and inhibits PPARγ-mediated adipogenesis, J. Biol. Chem. 275 (2000) 5754–5759.

[38] C.P. Sewter, et al., Regional differences in the response of human pre-adipocytes to PPARgamma and RXRalpha agonists, Diabetes 51 (2002) 718–723.

[39] I. Barroso, et al., Dominant negative mutations in human PPARγ associated with severe insulin resistance, diabetes mellitus and hypertension, Nature 402 (1999) 880–883.

[40] M. Agostini, et al., Tyrosine agonists reverse the molecular defects associated with dominant negative mutations in human peroxisome proliferator-activated receptor γ, Endocrinology 145 (2004) 1527–1538.

[41] Y.S. Tsai, et al., Hypertension and abnormal fat distribution but not insulin resistance in mice with P465L PPARgamma, J. Clin. Invest. 114 (2004) 240–249.

[42] E. Hu, et al., Inhibition of adipogenesis through MAP kinase-mediated phosphorylation of PPARγ, Science 274 (1996) 2100–2103.

[43] M. Adams, et al., Transcriptional activation by peroxisome proliferators-activated receptor gamma is inhibited by phosphorylation at a consensus mitogen-activated protein kinase site, J. Biol. Chem. 272 (1997) 5128–5132.

[44] M. Bluher, R. Paschke, Analysis of the relationship between PPARγ2 gene variants and severe insulin resistance in obese patients with impaired glucose tolerance, Exp. Clin. Endocrinol. Diabetes 111 (2003) 85–90.

[45] S.S. Deeb, et al., A Pro12Ala substitution in PPARγ2 associated with decreased receptor activity, lower body mass index and improved insulin sensitivity, Nat. Genet. 20 (1998) 284–287.

[46] M. Stumvoll, H. Haring. The peroxisome proliferator-activated receptor-gamma2 Pro12Ala polymorphism,, Diabetes 51 (2002) 2341–2347.

[47] K. Clement, et al., The Pro115Gln and Pro12Ala PPARγ gene mutations in obesity and type 2 diabetes, Int. J. Obes. Relat. Metab. Disord. 24 (2000) 391–393.

[48] M.M. Swarbrick, et al., A Pro12Ala polymorphism in the human peroxisome proliferator-activated receptor-gamma 2 is associated with combined hyperlipidaemia in obesity, Eur. J. Endocrinol. 144 (2001) 277–282.

[49] B.A. Beamer, et al., Association of the Pro12Ala variant in peroxisome proliferators-activated receptor-γ2 gene with obesity in two Caucasian populations, Diabetes 47 (1998) 1806–1808.

[50] S. Masud, et al., Effect of the peroxisome proliferators activated receptor-γ gene Pro12Ala variant on body mass index: a meta-analysis, J. Med. Genet. 40 (2003) 773–780.

[51] J. Luan, et al., Evidence for gene-nutrient interaction at the PPARgamma locus, Diabetes 50 (2001) 686–689.

[52] T.M. Willson, et al., The structure-activity relationship between peroxisome proliferator-activated receptor γ agonism and the anti-hyperglycemic activity of thiazolidinediones, J. Med. Chem. 39 (1996) 665–668.

[53] R. Mukherjee, et al., Sensitization of diabetic and obese mice to insulin by retinoid X receptor agonists, Nature 386 (1997) 407–410.

[54] S.M. Rangwala, et al., Genetic modulation of PPARgamma phosphorylation regulates insulin sensitivity, Dev. Cell 5 (2003) 657–663.

[55] D. Altshuler, et al., The common PPARγ Pro12Ala polymorphism is associated with decreased risk of type 2 diabetes, Nat. Genet. 26 (2000) 76–80.

[56] A. Memisoglu, et al., Prospective study of the association between the proline to alanine codon 12 polymorphism in the PPARγ gene and type 2 diabetes, Diabetes Care 26 (2003) 2915–2917.

[57] P.D. Miles, et al., Improved insulin-sensitivity in mice heterogeneous for PPAR-gamma deficiency, J. Clin. Invest. 105 (2000) 287–292.

[58] D.B. Savage, et al., Digenic inheritance of severe insulin resistance in a human pedigree, Nat. Genet. 31 (2002) 379–384.

[59] E.S. Tai, et al., Differential effects of the C1431T and Pro12Ala PPARgamma gene variants on plasma lipids and diabetes risk in an Asian population, J. Lipid Res. 45 (2004) 674–685.

[60] A.S. Doney, et al., Association of the Pro12Ala and C1431T variants of PPARG and their haplotypes with susceptibility to Type 2 diabetes, Diabetologica 47 (2004) 555–558.

[61] A.W. Norris, et al., Muscle-specific PPARgamma-deficient mice develop increased adiposity and insulin resistance but respond to thiazolidinediones, J. Clin. Invest. 112 (2003) 608–618.

[62] A.L. Hevener, et al., Muscle-specific PPARg deletion causes insulin resistance, Nat. Med. 9 (2003) 1491–1497.

[63] L. Chao, et al., Adipose tissue is required for the antidiabetic, but not for the hypolipidamic, effect of thiazolidinediones, J. Clin. Invest. 106 (2000) 1221–1228.

[64] W. He, et al., Adipose-specific peroxisome proliferator-activated receptor gamma knockout causes insulin resistance in fat and liver but not in muscle, Proc. Natl. Acad. Sci. USA 100 (2003) 15712–15717.

[65] K. Schoonjans, et al., PPARalpha and PPARgamma activators direct a distinct tissue-specific transcriptional response via a PPRE in the lipoprotein lipase gene, EMBO J. 15 (1996) 5336–5348.

[66] B.I. Frohnert, et al., Identification of a functional peroxisome proliferator-responsive element in the murine fatty acid transport protein gene, J. Biol. Chem. 274 (1999) 3970–3977.

[67] H.P. Guan, et al., A futile metabolic cycle activated in adipocytes by antidiabetic agents, Nat. Med. 8 (2003) 1122–1128.

[68] J. Tordjman, et al., Thiazolidinediones block fatty acid release by inducing glyceroneogenesis in fat cells, J. Biol. Chem. 278 (2003) 18785–18790.

[69] P.J. Randle, et al., The glucose fatty acid cycle: its role in insulin sensitivity and the metabolic disturbances of diabetes mellitus, Lancet 1 (1963) 785–789.

[70] O. Vaccaro, et al., Fasting plasma free fatty acid concentrations and Pro12Ala polymorphism of the peroxisome proliferator-activated receptor (PPAR) gamma2 gene in healthy individuals, Clin. Endocrinol. 57 (2002) 481–486.

[71] M. Iwata, et al., Pioglitazone ameliorates tumour necrosis factor-α-induced insulin resistance by a mechanism independent of adipogenic activity of peroxisome proliferator-activated receptor gamma, Diabetes 50 (2001) 1083–1092.

[72] U. Smith, et al., Thiazolidinediones (PPARγ agonists) but not PPARα agonists increase IRS-2 gene expression in 3T3-L1 and human adipocytes, FASEB J. 15 (2001) 215–220.

[73] J. Rieusset, et al., Regulation of gene expression by activation of the peroxisome proliferator-activated receptor γ with rosiglitazone (BRL49653) in human adipocytes, Biochem. Biophys. Res. Commun. 265 (1999) 265–271.

[74] V. Ribbon, et al., Thiazolidinediones and insulin resistance: peroxisome proliferator-activated receptor γ activation stimulates expression of the CAP gene, Proc. Natl. Acad. Sci. USA 95 (1998) 14751–14756.

[75] C.A. Baumann, et al., Cloning and characterization of a functional peroxisome proliferator activated receptor-γ -responsive element in the promoter of the CAP gene, J. Biol. Chem. 275 (2000) 9131–9135.

[76] E.D. Abel, et al., Adipose-selective targeting of the GLUT4 gene impairs insulin action in muscle and liver, Nature 409 (2001) 729–733.

[77] R.S. Ahima, et al., Adipose tissue as an endocrine organ, Trends Endocrinol. Metab. 11 (2000) 327–332.

[78] T. Yamauchi, et al., The fat-derived hormone adiponectin reverses insulin resistance associated with both lipoatrophy and obesity, Nat. Med. 7 (2001) 941–946.

[79] K. Hotta, et al., Circulating concentrations of the adipocyte protein adiponectin are decreased in parallel with reduced insulin sensitivity during the progression to type 2 diabetes in rhesus monkeys, Diabetes 50 (2001) 1126–1133.

[80] A.H. Berg, et al., The adipocyte-secreted protein Acrp30 enhances hepatic insulin action, Nat. Med. 7 (2001) 947–953.

[81] N. Maeda, et al., PPARgamma ligands increase expression and plasma concentrations of adiponectin, an adipose-derived protein, Diabetes 50 (2001) 2094–2099.

[82] T.P. Combs, et al., Induction of adipocyte complement-related protein of 30 kilodaltons by PPARgamma agonists: a potential mechanism of insulin sensitization, Endocrinology 143 (2002) 998–1007.

[83] C.M. Steppan, et al., The hormone resistin links obesity to diabetes, Nature 409 (2001) 307–312.

[84] P.G. McTernan, et al., Increased resistin gene and protein expression in human abdominal adipose tissue, J. Clin. Endocrinol. Metab. 87 (2002) 2407.

[85] I.J. Bujalska, et al., Does central obesity reflect 'cushings disease of the ommentum'? Lancet 349 (1997) 1210–1213.

[86] H. Masuzaki, et al., A transgenic model of visceral obesity and the metabolic syndrome, Science 294 (2001) 2166–2170.

[87] J. Berger, et al., Peroxisome proliferator-activated receptor-gamma ligands inhibit adipocyte 11beta-hydroxysteroid dehydrogenase type 1 expression and activity, J. Biol. Chem. 276 (2001) 12629–12635.

[88] A.A. Parulkar, et al., Nonhypoglycaemic effects of thiazolidinediones, Ann. Intern. Med. 134 (2001) 61–71.

[89] Y. Nakamura, Inhibitory action of insulin-sensitizing agents on calcium channels in smooth muscle cells from resistance arteries of guinea-pig, Br. J. Pharmacol. 123 (1998) 675–682.

[90] H. Satoh, et al., Thiazolidinediones suppress endothelin-1 secretion from bovine vascular endothelial cells: a new possible role of PPARγ on vascular endothelial function, Biochem. Biophys. Res. Commun. 254 (1999) 757–763.

[91] H. Itoh, et al., Hypertension and insulin resistance: role of peroxisome proliferator-activated receptor γ, Clin. Exp. Pharmacol. Physiol. 26 (1999) 558–560.

[92] C.J. Ostgren, et al., Peroxisome proliferator-activated receptor-γ Pro12Ala polymorphism and the association with blood pressure in type 2 diabetes, J. Hypertens. 21 (2003) 1657–1662.

[93] S.J. Hasstedt, et al., Effect of the peroxisome proliferator-activated receptor-gamma 2 pro(12)ala variant on obesity, glucose homeostasis, and blood pressure in members of familial type 2 diabetic kindreds, J. Clin. Endocrinol. Metab. 86 (2001) 536–541.

[94] J.A. Douglas, et al., The peroxisome proliferator-activated receptor-gamma2 Pro12Ala variant: association with type 2 diabetes and trait differences, Diabetes 50 (2001) 886–890.

[95] F.J. Rodriguez-Esparragon, et al., Peroxisome proliferator-activated receptor-gamma2 Pro12Ala and endothelial nitric oxide synthase-4 a/b gene polymorphisms are associated with essential hypertension, J. Hypertens. 21 (2003) 1649–1655.

[96] J. Minamikawa, et al., Potent inhibitory effect of troglitazone on carotid arterial wall thickness in type 2 diabetes, J. Clin. Endocrinol. Metab. 83 (1998) 1818–1820.

[97] P. Tontonoz, et al., PPARgamma promotes monocyte/macrophage differentiation and uptake of oxidized LDL, Cell 93 (1998) 241–252.

[98] M. Ricote, et al., Expression of the peroxisome proliferator-activated receptor γ (PPARγ) in human atherosclerosis and regulation in macrophages by colony stimulating factors and oxidized low density lipoprotein, Proc. Natl. Acad. Sci. USA 95 (1998) 7614–7619.

[99] N. Marx, et al., Macrophages in human atheroma contain PPARgamma: differentiation-dependent peroxisomal proliferator-activated receptor gamma(PPARgamma) expression and reduction of MMP-9 activity through PPARgamma activation in mononuclear phagocytes *in vitro*, Am. J. Pathol. 153 (1998) 17–23.

[100] C. Jiang, et al., PPAR-gamma agonists inhibit production of monocyte inflammatory cytokines, Nature 391 (1998) 82–86.

[101] M. Ricote, et al., The peroxisome proliferator-activated receptor-γ is a negative regulator of macrophage activation, Nature 391 (1998) 79–86.

[102] K.J. Moore, et al., The role of PPAR-gamma in macrophage differentiation and cholesterol uptake, Nat. Med. 7 (2001) 41–47.

[103] A.R. Tall, et al., Regulation and mechanisms of macrophage cholesterol efflux, J. Clin. Invest. 110 (2002) 899–904.

[104] G. Chinetti, et al., PPAR-alpha and PPAR-gamma activators induce cholesterol removal from human macrophage foam cells through stimulation of the ABCA1 pathway, Nat. Med. 7 (2001) 53–58.

[105] A. Chawla, et al., PPAR-gamma dependent and independent effects on macrophage-gene expression in lipid metabolism and inflammation, Nat. Med. 7 (2001) 48–52.

[106] M. Iwata, et al., The association of Pro12Ala polymorphism in PPARgamma2 with lower carotid artery IMT in Japanese, Diabetes Res. Clin. Pract. 62 (2003) 55–59.

[107] Z.C. Yan, et al., Peroxisome proliferator-activated receptor gamma C-161T polymorphism and carotid artery atherosclerosis in metabolic syndrome, Zhonghua Yi Xue Za Zhi 84 (2004) 543–547 (article in Chinese).

[108] R. Mukherjee, et al., A selective peroxisome proliferator-activated receptor-gamma (PPARgamma) modulator blocks adipocyte differentiation but stimulates glucose uptake in 3T3-L1 adipocytes, Mol. Endocrinol. 14 (2000) 1425–1433.

[109] J.L. Oberfield, et al., A peroxisome proliferator-activated receptor γ ligand inhibits adipocyte differentiation, Proc. Natl. Acad. Sci. USA 96 (1999) 6102–6106.

[110] S. Rocchi, et al., A unique PPARgamma ligand with potent insulin-sensitizing yet weak adipogenic activity, Mol. Cell. 8 (2001) 737–747.

[111] M.N. Nikiforova, et al., RAS point mutations and PAX8-PPARγ rearrangement in thyroid tumours; evidence for distinct molecular pathways in thyroid follicular carcinoma, J. Clin. Endocrinol. Metab. 88 (2003) 2318–2326.

[112] L. Cheung, et al., Detection of the PAX8-PPARγ fusion oncogene in both follicular thyroid carcinomas and adenomas, J. Clin. Endocrinol. Metab. 88 (1) (2003) 354–357.

[113] A.R. Marques, et al., Expression of PAX8-PPARγ1 rearrangements in both follicular thyroid carcinomas and adenomas, J. Clin. Endocrinol. Metab. 87 (8) (2002) 3947–3952.

[114] P. Sarraf, et al., Loss-of-function mutations in PPARγ associated with human colon cancer, Mol. Cell 3 (1999) 799–804.

[115] M. Gurnell, PPARγ and metabolism – insights from the study of human genetic variants, Clin. Endocrinol. 59 (2003) 267–277.

[116] K. Al-Shali, et al., A single-base mutation in the peroxisome proliferator-activated receptor γ4 promoter associated with altered *in vitro* expression and partial lipodystrophy, J. Clin. Endocrinol. Metab. 89 (2004) 5655–5660.

Chapter 3

PPARδ: Emerging therapeutic potential of novel agonists in lipid and glucose homeostasis

Uwe Dressel*, George E.O. Muscat

Institute for Molecular Bioscience, The University of Queensland, St. Lucia QLD 4072, Australia

1. Introduction

1.1. *Cardiovascular and metabolic disease*

Cardiovascular disease (CVD) is the most serious public health burden in western societies. For example, CVD is the leading cause of death and disability in the USA, accounting for nearly 40% of all deaths [1]. CVD includes heart disease, vascular disease, atherosclerosis, myocardial infarction, stroke, and hypertension. Major independent risk factors for CVD include hypertension, chronic inflammation, sedentary lifestyle, and smoking. Other risk factors include obesity, diabetes, and dyslipidemia. Dyslipidemia is associated with anomalous levels of the lipid triad: elevated levels of triglycerides and low-density lipoprotein (LDL, the "bad" cholesterol) and decreased levels of high-density lipoprotein (HDL, the "good" cholesterol).

It is now acknowledged that the worldwide escalation in the incidence of obesity is likely to have adverse effects on human health. The "obesity epidemic" is recognized by the World Health Organization as one of the top 10 global health problems. It is the leading cause of heart disease, cancer, and stroke – the top three causes of death in the USA. It also triggers hypertension, high cholesterol, and diabetes. Obesity leads to metabolic syndrome; a disorder that includes elevated levels of triglycerides and LDL cholesterol, low levels of HDL cholesterol, impaired fasting glucose, and hypertension. These are cardiovascular risk factors for diseases such as atherosclerosis and type II diabetes. In the USA, 65% of adults, aged 20 years and older are overweight and more than 30% are obese [2], meaning their health is at risk and representing a significant public health burden. One billion adults worldwide are now overweight, and at least 300 million are clinically obese. Among these, about half a

*Corresponding author. Present address: Centre for Diabetes and Endocrine Research (CDER), The University of Queensland, Princess Alexandra Hospital, Ipswich Rd, Buranda QLD 4102, Australia

ADVANCES IN MOLECULAR AND CELLULAR ENDOCRINOLOGY
VOLUME 5 ISSN 1569-2566/DOI 10.1016/S1569-2566(06)05003-4

million people in North America and Western Europe die from obesity-related diseases every year [3].

Western lifestyle of the later 20th and early 21st century have led to a shocking prediction that more than 33% of American children born in 2000 will develop type-II diabetes [4]. Similar predictions probably apply for other westernized countries. Currently, more than 170 million people worldwide suffer from diabetes. This figure is more than likely to exceed 360 million by 2030. Diabetes is a growing and massive silent epidemic that has the potential to cripple the health services worldwide. Currently, diabetes consumes 5–10% of the healthcare budget in many countries. More than 50% of that cost is due to diabetic complications [5]. At least 1 in 10 deaths among adults between 35 and 64 years old is attributable to diabetes worldwide, mainly through the increased risk of CVD.

Weight gain and physical inactivity lead to insulin resistance, making obesity and diabetes intrinsically linked. The risk factors for CVD; high cholesterol, high blood pressure, obesity, and diabetes are directly influenced by life-style patterns, particularly food consumption. Trials have consistently demonstrated that sustained changes in lifestyle, physical activity and diet substantially reduce the levels of overweight and obesity and the risk of developing type-II diabetes, dyslipidemia, and hypertension. Despite the efficacy of behavioural changes, compliance is often an issue. This lays behind the drive to the development of novel therapeutic interventions that target metabolism. Contemporary therapies that target obesity perform modestly, and are aimed at central appetite suppression or reduced fat absorption. Recent research suggests novel strategies that target lipid catabolism accompanied by increased energy expenditure (i.e. thermogenesis). This emerging evidence provides exciting new hope in the quest for novel anti-obesity drugs.

1.2. *Nuclear hormone receptors regulate lipid and carbohydrate metabolism*

Nuclear receptors (NRs) regulate the expression of genes involved in metabolism, reproduction, and development. NRs are hormone regulated transcription factors that bind specific regulatory sequences. Essentially, NRs function as an interface between environmental stimuli and gene expression. The ever-growing number of drugs that have been created to combat disorders associated with dysfunctional hormone signaling emphasizes the importance of NRs in human physiology. NRs are one of the largest families of transcription factors. They can be regulated by specific ligands (activated or blocked), which makes them a straightforward target for drug-mediated approaches. A number of NRs regulate all critical aspects of CVD such as energy homeostasis, lipid metabolism, glucose disposal, and inflammation. Therefore, the therapeutic utility of NRs has been exploited by the pharmaceutical industry: 12 of the top-selling drugs in the USA target NRs.

NRs are evolutionary highly conserved. Research demonstrates the development of a multi-layered autoregulated system that involves NRs for sensing and metabolizing biologically active lipids. NRs involved in control of lipid and cholesterol homeostasis, include the thyroid hormone receptors (TRs), liver X receptors (LXRs), farnesoid X receptor (FXR), RORα1, liver receptor homologue-1, the small heterodimeric partner and the peroxisome proliferator-activated receptors (PPARs), [6–8].

PPARs regulate the transcription of genes involved in lipid homeostasis, carbohydrate metabolism, energy expenditure and reverse cholesterol transport in a subtype and tissue-specific manner. Endogenously, a wide range of dietary factors activate PPARs, including saturated and unsaturated fatty acids (FAs), as well as oxidized FA metabolites derived through the lipoxygenase and cyclo-oxygenase pathways. Hence, PPARs act as dietary lipid sensors that regulate a variety of biological functions, including development, inflammation and metabolism. Three PPAR subtypes, designated PPARα (NR1C1), PPARγ (NR1C3) and PPARδ (NR1C2) have been identified in mammals. Selective synthetic compounds that activate PPARα or PPARγ (i.e. hypolipidemic fibrates and anti-diabetic thiazolidinediones (TZDs), respectively) have been employed successfully to treat metabolic dysfunctions. PPARδ was first cloned in *Xenopus* and termed PPARβ [9]. However, when first cloned in mammals [10], it was not obviously homologous to the *Xenopus* gene and given the name PPARδ. Other synonyms for PPARδ are NUC1 [11], or FAAR [12]. It is now accepted that they are bona fide orthologues, but the most agreed upon name for this receptor is PPARδ and therefore will be used in this review.

PPARs have demonstrated therapeutic utility in the treatment of dyslipidemia, diabetes, and obesity. For example, hypolipidemic compounds known as fibrates are agonists for PPARα and used in the treatment of dyslipidemia, while TZDs are agonists for PPARγ and established as hypoglycemic insulin sensitizing anti-diabetic drugs. Until recently, no specific agonists for the PPARδ subtype were available. The first comprehensive study presenting a potent, selective and efficacious agonist was published in 2001 by Oliver et al. [13]. This review gives an overview on the function of PPARδ in metabolism and focuses on the molecular regulation of lipid and energy homeostasis modulated by agonists for this receptor and their therapeutic potentials.

1.3. *Peroxisome proliferator activated receptors (PPARs): an overview*

All three PPARs bind to specific PPAR-responsive elements (PPREs) as heterodimers with the 9-*cis*-retinoic acid receptor (RXR), another member of the NR superfamily. As a consequence, genes under the control of a PPRE can be activated by ligands for RXR or PPAR-specific ligands. The endogenous ligand for RXR is 9-*cis*-retinoic acid, which is a vitamin-D derivative.

PPARα is preferentially expressed in metabolically demanding tissues such as liver and heart, and mediates high FA catabolism (β- and ω-oxidation). Regarding ligand specificity, PPARα is the most promiscuous subtype. Endogenous ligands for PPARα include saturated and polyunsaturated fatty acids (PUFAs), and their metabolites [10,14]. Another endogenous ligand for PPARα is leukotriene-B4, a mediator of inflammatory response [15]. Synthetic ligands for PPARα are hypolipidemic fibrates, drugs that are widely used for reducing blood triglyceride levels.

In contrast to the catabolic role of PPARα, the PPARγ isoform regulates lipid storage. The distribution of PPARγ is more restricted than that of PPARα. It is highly expressed in brown and white adipose tissue, but also found to a lesser extent in skeletal muscle, the retina, the intestinal endothelium, and lymphoid tissue. PPARγ expression is crucial for the differentiation of adipocytes [16] and plays a pivotal role in lipid metabolism. Unlike PPARα, PPARγ has a clear preference for PUFAs. Another endogenous ligand for PPARγ is 15-deoxyΔ12,14-prostaglandin J2 which is the terminal metabolite of the prostaglandin-J2 family. Synthetic ligands of PPARγ are the anti-diabetic TZDs or "glitazones" that are a class of insulin sensitizers used in the treatment of type-II diabetes.

The third member of the PPAR family, PPARδ, is expressed ubiquitously but often at a higher level than PPARα or PPARγ [14]. The binding profile of PPARδ to FAs is intermediate between that of PPARα and PPARγ. PPARδ was found to bind both saturated and unsaturated FAs [17], but not as promiscuous as PPARα. Numerous studies have suggested a role for PPARδ in a variety of biological functions such as embryonic development [18], cholesterol efflux and FA metabolism [13,19,20], inflammation [21], and wound healing [22,23]. Recent investigations also indicate a role for PPARδ in tumor development, particularly in colorectal cancers [24,25].

2. PPARδ: the rise of an abandoned orphan

2.1. *The neglected orphan*

PPARδ initially received much less attention than the other PPARs, partially because of its ubiquitous expression profile and the lack of a potent, selective agonist [26]. First, it was observed that PPARδ (then termed "NUC1") acts as a repressor for PPARα and the TR when ectopically expressed in HepG2 cells [27]. A more recent study supports this role for PPARδ in modulating PPARα and PPARγ activity, not only by competing for PPAR response elements (PPREs), but also by recruiting corepressors [28]. A study undertaken in preadipose cells, which lack PPARδ, suggested a role for PPARδ in the transcriptional activation of the uncoupling protein-2 (UCP2) gene [29]. Later, a transcriptional activation of another uncoupling protein (UCP3) was also described in L6 myotubes [30]. Together, these observations provide a potential link between FA metabolism, thermogenesis and energy expenditure in PPAR-expressing tissue that, as we will discuss later, is one of the key functions of PPARδ.

Early investigations into the specific function of PPARδ utilized the ectopically expressed receptor. Amri et al. [12] showed that overexpressing PPARδ in fibroblasts induced FA responsive gene expression, yet another study showed that PPARγ is predominantly responsible for adipogenesis and that overexpression of human PPARδ does not act adipogenic [31]. Grimaldi and co-workers [32] later provided evidence that the expression of the PPARγ gene is under the control of PPARδ in 3T3C2 preadipocytes and that activation of PPARδ by FAs induces PPARγ, thereby promoting adipogenesis. PPARδ is also involved in hormonal regulation of gene transcription in brown adipose tissue (BAT) during cold acclimatization. Levels of

PPARδ–mRNA progressively increase during cold induction, while levels for PPARα and PPARγ decrease within hours of cold exposure [33]. A recent study by Gonzalez and co-workers [34] further established a role for PPARδ in adipogenesis and lipid storage in adipocytes. Addition of the PPARδ ligand L165041 [13] (see below) enhanced adipocyte differentiation and this effect is diminished in adipocytes lacking the PPARδ gene.

2.2. *Ligands for PPARδ: an orphan becomes adopted*

As described above, natural ligands for PPARs are FAs and their metabolites. Thereby, PPARs act as dietary lipid sensors that regulate a variety of biological functions, including development, inflammation, and metabolism.

Stimulatory agents for PPARδ were first found in the pancreas and identified as methyl-palmitate, known to be enriched in pancreatic lipids and esters of palmitic and oleic acids [35]. These compounds also activate the other PPAR-subtypes. A subset of ligands for PPARα, endogenous PUFAs and synthetic hypolipidemic drugs such as bezafibrate and the eicosanoid carbaprostacyclin (cPGI) were found to be also ligands for PPARδ but not PPARγ [36,37]. This suggests that the overall balance between FA catabolism and storage may be determined by the relative levels of endogenous ligands for PPARα and PPARδ on the one side, and those for PPARγ on the other. Among these dual agonists, bezafibrate shows a stronger affinity for PPARδ than for PPARα, therefore representing the first antilipidemic drug with a preference for PPARδ [37]. Prior to this, PPARδ was given synonyms such as "lonesome orphan among the PPARs" [38], which was somehow appropriate until the synthesis of the first real specific agonist GW501516 ([13] see below). A number of other dual agonists for PPARδ and PPARα have been described, mainly L631033 [39,40], GW2433 [17,41], and linoleic acid [42,43]. Bezafibrate was used to investigate the function of PPARδ in PPARα-null mice and vice versa [44].

Dual agonists for PPARδ and PPARγ that do not activate PPARα have also been described [45]. Of these, L165041 acts more strongly on PPARδ than on PPARγ and has been used in a number of studies investigating the function of PPARδ. For example, in reaggregated brain cells that lack PPARγ, treatment with L165041 leads to transcriptional activation of the acyl-CoA synthetase-2 (ACS2) gene, demonstrating that PPARδ has a role in brain lipid metabolism [46]. A role for PPARδ in cholesterol metabolism was established by using L165041 in obese Lepr$^{db/db}$ mice [47]. As a result of a defective leptin receptor, Lepr$^{db/db}$ mice are obese, hyperglycemic and hypertriglyceridemic. Treatment of these mice with L165041 at low doses (where it presumably shows only weak PPARγ activation) significantly increased the number of HDL particles, with little change in the LDL fraction. In contrast, treatment with a specific agonist for PPARγ reduced HDL cholesterol and dramatically increased LDL levels. At these low doses, the dual agonist did not change PPARγ-specific effects on plasma glucose or triglyceride levels, as it did when used in higher doses, presumably due to on its affinity for PPARγ.

In 2001, GlaxoSmithKline published the potent, synthetic and selective PPARδ agonist, GW501516, a phenoxyacetic acid derivative [13]. GW501516 corrects hyperinsulinemia in insulin-resistant and obese primates. Furthermore, it raises mRNA expression of ABCA1 (reverse cholesterol transporter ATP-binding cassette-A1) and serum HDL cholesterol, while lowering triglycerides. Moreover, serum apoCIII levels and total cholesterol were raised. Since then, GW501516 has become the most exploited synthetic agonist for PPARδ [20,25,48–53]. Some outcome of this research will be discussed below. Another highly selective agonist for PPARδ synthesized by the same research group is GW0742, a derivative of GW501516 [54]. GW0742 is now also used to investigate the function of PPARδ [55–58]. A short and efficient synthesis of GW501516 is also reported by Wei et al. [51]. Other selective agonist for PPARδ, termed Compound F and Compound 1, have also been reported [48,59–62].

3. PPARδ in lipid and carbohydrate metabolism: a potential phoenix from the ashes

In recent times, a great deal of evidence showed that, among the other PPAR subtypes, PPARδ plays an important role in lipid and energy homeostasis. Potent and selective agonists for this receptor have demonstrated therapeutic utility in the treatment of hyperinsulinemia, insulin resistance, dyslipidemia, obesity, and inflammation.

3.1. *Ligands for PPARδ regulate cholesterol homeostasis*

The first comprehensive study using a highly selective agonist for PPARδ (GW501516, [13]) showed that induction of PPARδ by this agonist increased the expression of ABCA1 in macrophages, fibroblasts, and intestinal cells. This transcriptional activation of ABCA1 was accompanied by an induction of apolipoprotein A1-specific cholesterol efflux to an even greater extent than agonists for PPARα or PPARγ. When administered to insulin-resistant middle-aged obese rhesus monkeys, GW501516 dose-dependently increased serum levels of HDL cholesterol. The levels of small-dense LDL cholesterol, fasting triglycerides and fasting insulin were lowered.

Whether the reported dramatic increases in HDL cholesterol observed *in vivo*, could be accounted by the GW501516 induction of ABCA1 mediated increases in apoA1-specific cholesterol efflux in macrophages remains obscure. This issue was further addressed in our laboratory [20]. We investigated the contribution of skeletal muscle to the consequences of PPARδ activation. GW501516 induced ABCA1 mRNA expression, and apoA1-specific efflux of intracellular cholesterol in skeletal muscle cells. These effects in cells from a major mass peripheral tissue accounting for 30–40% of the total body mass are entirely consistent with the profound effects of this drug on HDL cholesterol.

After hydrolysis by lipoprotein lipase (LPL), triglycerides of very low-density lipoprotein (VLDL) particles strongly activate the expression of genes that are associated with lipid storage. These triglycerides are reported to act via PPARδ [63], establishing a role for PPARδ in response to atherosclerotic lesions. Moreover, PPARδ-KO mice show elevated levels of triglycerides and VLDL with no difference in total cholesterol or phospholipids [64]. In concordance to that PPARδ-KO mice on a high-fat diet showed an increased rate of hepatic VLDL production as well as lowered LPL activity. It is conceivable that in the absence of PPARδ, extrahepatic cells such as macrophages, are unable to detect and uptake VLDL–triglycerides and that the increased hepatic VLDL production presents a compensatory response (Fig. 1).

3.2. *PPARδ and fatty acid catabolism*

3.2.1. *Skeletal muscle*
Grimaldi and colleagues suggested that modulation of PPARδ expression or action mediated the adaptation of white adipose tissue to dietary changes [65]. Subsequently, PPARδ was implicated in FA catabolism and homeostasis from the observation that skeletal muscle from PPARα-knockout (KO) mice has similar oxidative capacity to muscle derived from wild-type animals [58]. Skeletal muscle is one of the major sites of FA catabolism and the earliest sign of developing type-II diabetes is the accumulation of intramuscular fat and insulin resistance in this tissue [66].

Muoio et al. reported that PPARα-KO mice showed greater rates of glycogen depletion in liver but not skeletal muscle during exercise [58]. Unlike in the liver and heart, PPARδ is severalfold more abundant in skeletal muscle of wild-type mice than either PPARα or PPARγ. It was postulated that this high abundance of PPARδ compensates for the lack of PPARα in the KO-mice. This assumption is supported

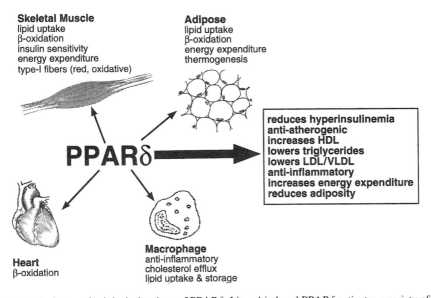

Fig. 1. Model of some physiological actions of PPARδ. Ligand-induced PPARδ activates a variety of key metabolic pathways (indicated by arrows) in muscle, heart, adipose tissue, and macrophages (blue background). The resulting anti-atherogenic effects in the vascular system (red background) include improved blood lipid profile (raised level of HDL, lowered levels of LDL, VLDL, and triglycerides), accompanied by increased energy expenditure, reduced adiposity and hyperinsulinemia, and anti-inflammatory effects.

by two observations: (i) exercise induces the classical PPARα target genes, pyruvate-dehydrogenase kinase 4 (PDHK4) and uncoupling protein-3 (UCP3) in skeletal (but not cardiac) muscle from the wild type (WT) and KO mice, and (ii) PPARδ agonists increase FA oxidation and induce the expression of lipid regulatory genes, such as PDHK4 and UCP3. These findings strongly support a redundancy in the functions of PPARα and PPARδ as regulators of FA metabolism in skeletal muscle. Holst et al. [66] previously showed that another uncoupling protein (UCP2) is also activated by PPARδ agonists in skeletal muscle cells, but not by agonists for the other PPARs. This observation indicates a more distinctive role for PPARδ in skeletal muscle.

A unique role of PPARδ in skeletal muscle was finally established by Holst et al. [68] who demonstrated that starvation induces PPARδ mRNA expression in murine gastrocnemius muscle. Moreover, fatty acid translocase (FAT/CD36) and heart fatty acid-binding protein (FABP) are concomitantly activated. However, expression levels are restored to control levels after refeeding. The authors went on to demonstrate that the PPARδ agonist GW1514 (a GW501516 analogue) induced CD36, FABP, and muscle carnitine palmitoyl transferase (M-CPT1 or CPT-1b) mRNA expression, and FA oxidation in skeletal muscle cells. Furthermore, they showed ectopic expression of PPARδ enhanced the expression of these genes in response to the selective agonist, and that ectopic expression of a dominant-negative PPARδ attenuated the response to agonist, and ablated the expression of these transcripts. These data suggested a role for PPARδ in skeletal muscle lipid homeostasis. PPARδ was also shown to be partially responsible for the dual effect of long-chain FAs as inhibitors of myogenesis and inducers of transdifferentiation of myoblasts into preadipose-like cells [69]. Ectopic expression of PPARδ in C2C12 myoblasts potentiates the FA induced expression of adipogenic markers, while expression of a dominant-negative PPARδ mutant exert the opposite effect.

Gilde et al. [53] similarly demonstrated in rodent neonatal cardiomyocytes that the PPARδ agonist induced the expression of the mRNAs encoding acyl-CoA synthetase (ACS), CPT1, UCP2, and UCP3. In concordance with these observations, they demonstrated an activation of the CPT1 promoter by PPARδ agonists, and an increase in FA oxidation.

In 2003, numerous publications collectively helped to clarify the role of PPARδ in this major mass tissue simultaneously. Dressel et al. [20] demonstrated that the selective PPARδ agonist GW501516 induces the expression of genes involved in lipid absorption, preferential lipid-utilization, lipid catabolism/β-oxidation, and energy expenditure in differentiated C2C12 myotubes (Fig. 2). For instance, a specific induction of FABP3, ACS4, LPL, CPT1, PDK4, UCP2, and UCP3 was observed. Furthermore, treatment of myotubes with the PPARδ agonist increased apo A1-specific cholesterol efflux. Promoter studies demonstrated that PPARδ (not PPARα) directly regulates the CPT-1 promoter in mouse skeletal muscle cells. Interestingly, an induction of genes involved in carbohydrate (glycogenin, GYG1) and lipid storage (adipocyte-related protein, ADRP, and stearoyl-CoA desaturase 1 and 2, SCD1&2) was also found.

To address the specific function of PPARδ, relative to PPARα and PPARγ, the authors treated differentiated C2C12 myotubes with selective and specific agonists

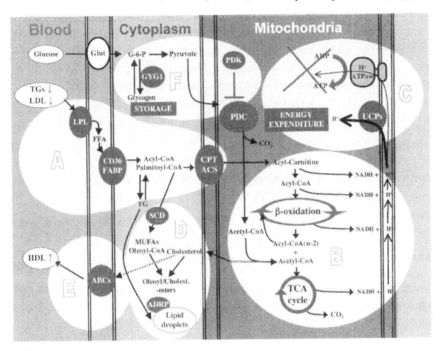

Fig. 2. Schematic overview of metabolic PPARδ action in skeletal muscle. Activation of PPARδ in skeletal muscle results in a number of metabolic effects (highlighted by the light-blue fields): Lipid uptake (A) which in turn facilitates increased lipid utilization (B), energy expenditure (C), increased lipid storage and cholesterol efflux (E), and inhibition of carbohydrate catabolism (F). These effects result in decreased blood levels of glucose, tri-glycerides (TGs), LDL-cholesterol, and increased levels of HDL-cholesterol. Enzymes and functions found to be activated by PPARδ agonists are marked in green. Red indicates inhibition of pathways. Modified after Dressel et al. 2003 [20].

for the other PPAR subtypes. It was found that fenofibrate, a PPARα agonist, induces genes involved in fructose uptake and glycogen formation, while the PPARγ agonist rosiglitazone induces genes associated with glucose uptake, FA synthesis and lipid storage. This clearly demonstrated the distinct roles for different PPARs in skeletal muscle cells. However, this specificity of PPAR function can vary in other tissues. In cardiomyocytes for example, PPARδ and PPARα increase FA oxidation [53]. We surmised that activation of PPARδ increases FA catabolism, cholesterol efflux, and energy expenditure in skeletal muscle, a major tissue that accounts for 30–40% of the total body mass, and that agonists for PPARδ would consequently have therapeutic utility in the treatment of hyperlipidemia, atherosclerosis, and obesity.

In agreement with the results discussed above, microarray expression profiling in GW501516-treated rat skeletal muscle cells (L6 myotubes) identified a large panel of genes involved in FA transport, β-oxidation and mitochondrial respiration [50]. Similar PPARδ-mediated gene activation was observed in skeletal muscle of GW501516-treated mice. The abundance of data by the end of 2003 underscored the role of PPARδ mediated regulation of gene expression involved in lipid absorption, FA oxidation, and energy expenditure. The authors went on to demonstrate that GW501516 treatment of mice stimulates FA oxidation in skeletal muscle. In contrast, β-oxidation was not induced in the liver. This was consistent with the activation of gene expression in muscle, including long-chain acyl-coenzyme-A dehydrogenase (LCAD), CPT1, UCP2, and UCP3.

Luquet et al. [70] developed an animal model that overexpresses PPARδ in skeletal muscle tissue. Staining for succinate dehydroxygenase (SDH) activity, which is a mitochondrial complex II marker revealed an increase in fiber number and an increase in fibers with high mitochondrial complex content (i.e. oxidative capacity). Concordantly, the activity of enzymes involved in oxidative (not glycolytic) metabolism and the expression of UCP2 increased.

3.2.2. Adipose tissue

PPARδ is expressed at similar levels in fat and skeletal muscle [71]. As discussed earlier, it is the PPARγ isoform that regulates lipid storage and adipogenesis, and that overexpression of human PPARδ does not act adipogenic [31]. There is, however, evidence from exogenous expression in 3T3C2 preadipocyte cells, that PPARδ activates the expression of the PPARγ gene in a FA-dependent manner (e.g. bromopalmitate and linolenate), thereby promoting adipogenesis [32]. Consistent with this, treatment with the PPARδ ligand L165041 enhances primary preadipocyte differentiation and this effect is not observed in preadipocytes lacking the PPARδ gene [34].

PPARδ was rigorously implicated in lipid homeostasis and having a critical role in omental tissue from studies using the KO animals. Most PPARδ-KO embryos die at an early stage due to a placental defect. However, survivors exhibit a reduction in fat mass and adiposity [72]. Curiously, this phenotype is absent in an adipocyte specific PPARδ KO-mouse, suggesting a complex autonomous action regulating systemic lipid metabolism rather than adipocyte functions [73]. This concept was strengthened by the observation that treatment with the synthetic compound GW501516 in insulin-resistant primates dramatically improves the serum lipid profile, and improves hyper insulinemia [13].

To pinpoint the *in vivo* function of PPARδ in brown and white adipose tissue, Evans and co-workers [19] fused the VP16 transcriptional activation domain of the herpes simplex virus to the N-terminal end of PPARδ and expressed this constitutive active fusion protein in mice under the control of an adipocyte-specific promoter. This gain-of-function approach led to animals that displayed reduced body weight and adiposity. Remarkably, these mice showed severe reduced amount of white fat tissue, resembling the phenotype of lipoatrophy that is caused by defects in adipogenesis. However, they do not exhibit hypertriglyceridemia, enlarged viscera, or fatty liver. These attributes do not indicate a defect in adipogenesis. Rather, these transgenic mice exhibit increased FA catabolization and energy dissipation, resulting in decreased triglyceride storage. The investigators hypothesized increased fat consumption by omental tissue, which is consistent with the observation that adipocytes from the transgenic inguinal and retroperitoneal fat depots were small and heterogeneous. This hypothesis is supported by induction of a panel of genes involved in FA oxidation and energy expenditure (including UCP1, UCP3, LCAS, VLCAS, AOX, and CPT-1) predominantly in BAT and to a significantly lesser extent in white fat. This is consistent with the observed selective accumulation of lipids in brown fat in PPARδ-KO mice [72].

Furthermore, these mice were also resistant to high-fat diet-induced obesity and hyperlipidemia. Expressing the constitutive active VP16–PPARδ transgene in adipocytes also protects from genetically induced obesity. Lepr$^{db/db}$ mice normally exhibit increased adiposity due to hyperphagia caused by mutation in the leptin receptor gene [74,75]. Lepr$^{db/db}$ mice harboring the VP16–PPARδ transgene do not develop an obese phenotype, indicating that the anti-obese function of PPARδ does not require the presence of the leptin signaling pathway. Treatment of obese Lepr$^{db/db}$ mice with the PPARδ agonist GW501516 also reversed the accumulation of fat in liver and brown, but not white adipose tissue.

Luquet et al. [70] demonstrated that muscle specific PPARδ overexpression promoted a decrease in body fat and in adipose cell size (from periovarian pads) with no change in cell number. In this context, Tanaka et al. [50] demonstrated that GW501516 treatment of mice ameliorated diet induced obesity accompanied by an enhanced metabolic rate, lipid oxidation, and increased mitochondria in skeletal muscle. Interestingly, lipid droplets were markedly reduced. However, very small increases in β-oxidation in intrascapular BAT were reported. Curiously, the GW501516 significantly reduced weight gain on a high-fat diet. Anatomical analysis revealed the resistance to increased body weight was largely due to reduced mass of visceral and epidermal fat depots. The drug treatment ameliorated the diet induced (i) hypertrophy in epidermal white adipose, and brown fat, (ii) hepatic steatosis, and (iii) accumulation of intramuscular lipid droplets. This was consistent with the GW5011516 treatment of Lepr$^{db/db}$ mice, with the absence of white adipose-specific effects [19].

3.3. *PPARδ and energy expenditure: implications for obesity and diabetes, and the creation of the 'Marathon Mouse'*

Several cell culture studies have identified induction of the mRNAs for uncoupling proteins (UCP1-3) and genes responsible for preferential lipid utilization in skeletal muscle and adipogenic cells by PPARδ [20,29,30,50,67].

PPARδ is significantly more highly expressed in oxidative slow twitch (type I) than in glycolytic fast twitch (type-II) skeletal muscle fibers. Endurance training leads to conversion into more type-I fibers. This fiber-type switch is accompanied by an increased expression of PPARδ [69]. The two fiber types display marked differences with respect to contraction, metabolism, and vulnerability to fatigue. Type-I fibers are richer in mitochondria and mainly use oxidative metabolism for ATP synthesis. Type-II fibers contain less mitochondria and rely preferentially on glycolytic metabolism as energy resource.

To elucidate the *in vivo* function of PPARδ in skeletal muscle, Evans and co-workers expressed the VP16–PPARδ construct under the control of the muscle-specific α-actin promoter [76]. Mice expressing the constitutive active VP16–PPARδ construct in skeletal muscle showed a higher content in type-I muscle fibers. The transgenic mice showed increases in succinate dehydrogenase, elevated citrate synthase, and β-hydroxyacyl-CoA activity. The authors also showed an induction of the myoglobin gene and other genes involved in increased oxidative metabolism, preferential lipid utilization, and increased energy expenditure (i.e. troponin-I-slow, cytochrome-C, UCP2, UCP3, and CPT1). This supports data from mice that over-express the wild-type PPARδ transgene in skeletal muscle [70]. These mice also showed the activation of certain oxidation enzymes in muscle, even though an actual muscle fiber switch did not occur. This observation indicates that activation of PPARδ, not just an increase of the receptor, is essential for functional manifestations such as fiber-type switching and prevention of obesity.

Constitutive expression of the VP16-activated form of PPARδ in skeletal muscle also profoundly increased the endurance capabilities and resistance to fatigue relative to their wild-type littermates. Hence the term "marathon mouse" was used in the press.

The studies of Tanaka et al. [50], and Wang et al. [76] demonstrated that GW501516 treated mice and the mice expressing activated PPARδ in skeletal muscle were resistance to high-fat diet-induced obesity, with improved metabolic profiles and reductions in intramuscular triglycerides. Furthermore, these studies plus the work from Luquet et al. [70] demonstrated a reduction in adipose cell size and decreased body fat content. These phenotypic effects were consistent with increased FA oxidation and elevated expression of the UCPs. Transgenic muscle specific expression of UCPs similarly leads to resistance to diet-induced obesity [77].

3.4. *PPARδ and carbohydrate homeostasis*

PPARδ seems to be prominently active in the regulation of genes involved in lipid metabolism and energy homeostasis. Until recently, there was not much evidence for a direct involvement in glucose metabolism. However, there is some evidence that PPARδ is involved in glycogen synthesis, the principal storage form of glucose in skeletal muscle. During exercise PPARα-KO mice exhaust earlier than wild-type mice and exhibit lesser rates of glycogen depletion in skeletal muscle, where PPARδ is able to compensate for the loss of PPARα, then in the liver [58]. Furthermore, it has been reported that glycogenin (GYG1), the enzyme that initiates the synthesis of glycogen, is activated by the PPARδ agonist GW501516 in skeletal muscle [20]. Under hypoglycemic and hyperinsulinemic conditions, muscle glycogen synthesis is the major pathway for glucose metabolism in both normal and diabetic individuals. Defective muscle glycogen synthesis plays a major part in causing insulin resistance [78].

Studies involving pharmacological treatment with PPARδ agonists in primates and rodents, and/or genetic manipulation, clearly demonstrate the utility of this receptor in the treatment of diabetes. For example, the primate study [13] reported a dose dependent decrease in serum insulin levels (~50%) whereas no changes in fasting glucose were reported. The study of Tanaka et al. [50] reported improved glucose tolerance, and lower fasting glucose levels after treatment of obese insulin-resistant *ob/ob* mice. Postprandial levels of plasma insulin and glucose were much lower in

GW501516 treated mice, relative to vehicle-treated animals. Concomitant with these observations was the reduction in intramuscular lipid droplets, and the normalization of *ob/ob* mouse islet hypertrophy due to increased insulin sensitivity. The study from Evans and colleagues [76] utilizing genetic manipulation of PPARδ activity in skeletal muscle demonstrated a profound reduction in blood glucose and improved glucose tolerance. In addition, another recent study from Evans and co-workers showed that treatment of diabetic *ob/ob* mice with a PPARδ agonist improves insulin sensitivity by increasing glycolysis and FA synthesis in the liver, thereby reducing hepatic glucose output [79].

It appears that carbohydrate and fat metabolism cross-react with each other and are inherently related. Insulin, usually recognized for its role in promoting cellular glucose uptake, also regulates triglyceride catabolism through its inhibition of hormone-sensitive lipase. Vice versa, dyslipidemia have effect on glucose homeostasis. Lipid infusion has been shown to cause insulin resistance in human skeletal muscle by reducing insulin-stimulated glucose transport activity [80] and intramyocellular triglyceride content was found to be an indicator for insulin resistance in subjects with an inherited high risk of developing type-II diabetes [81]. Depletion of intramuscular triglyceride accumulation is associated with an improvement of insulin sensitivity [82]. Analysis of polymorphisms of the PPARδ gene showed no significant association with the risk of type-II diabetes [83]. However, some association with fasting plasma glucose levels and body mass index were found in non-diabetic subjects. In conclusion, even though PPARδ directly doesn't regulate most enzymes involved in glucose homeostasis, it is likely that improvement of lipid metabolism through treatment with agonists for PPARδ, will in the long term also improve glucose homeostasis.

3.5. *PPARδ and inflammation: complex functions in complex tissues*

Lipid-laden macrophages are the major component of atherogenic lesions. A role for PPARδ in lipid homeostasis of macrophages has been documented, but its exact function is the subject of controversy [84]. On the one hand, it has been shown that PPARδ acts as a VLDL sensor and promotes ADRP mRNA expression, and lipid accumulation in macrophages [61,63]. On the other, it has also been shown that activation of PPARδ increases ABCA1 expression and apoA1 mediated cholesterol efflux. In strong contrast to these observations, mice that have been transplanted with PPARδ-KO-bone marrow (PPARδ$^{-/-}$BMT) show no significant difference in levels of VLDL, LDL, or HDL. This suggests that PPARδ does not modulate either cholesterol uptake or efflux [23]. Despite this, the average aortic lesion area was more than 50% reduced, compared to control mice.

PPARδ controls the inflammatory status of the macrophage cell. Gain or loss of function PPARδ analysis in macrophages suggests a pro-inflammatory role for PPARδ in the absence of an agonist [23]. In contrast, treatment with GW501516, a strong and selective PPARδ agonist, resulted in decrease of inflammatory cytokines. This was accompanied by the regulation of the expression and activity of BCL-6 and the monocyte chemoattractant protein (MCP-1). GW501516 treatment suppresses the expression of

MCP-1, and interleukin- (IL)-1b, clearly demonstrating an anti-inflammatory role of PPARδ in the presence of ligand. This process involves the selective association of BCL-6 with PPARδ (but not PPARα or PPARγ) in macrophages in the absence of ligand. Presence of PPARδ ligands result in the dissociation of BCL-6 that subsequently represses the expression of MCP-1. A recent study by Evans and colleagues [85] also demonstrated that activation of PPARδ by VLDL-derived FAs induces lipid catabolism in macrophages. Interestingly they provide evidence that the unliganded PPARδ is also able to repress basal β-oxidation, indicating a firm regulation of FA catabolism in macrophages to prevent them from lipid overload.

Like in macrophages, the role of PPARδ in keratinocytes is very complex. All three PPAR subtypes are usually undetectable in the adult epidermis, but the PPARδ gene gets upregulated by pro-inflammatory cytokines such as tumor necrosis factor- (TNF)-α. The epidermis in which keratinocytes are the predominant cell-type is characterized by a lifelong polarized pattern of epithelial growth and differentiation. Injury or other pathological conditions lead to activation of keratinocytes; they become migratory, produce and respond to cytokines [22]. This activation is attended by activation of the PPARδ gene itself and the production of endogenous ligands for the receptor [21]. This take-off of PPARδ, in turn, further enhances the differentiation of the keratinocytes and boosts their response to apoptotic signals. These results conform to the observation that the lack of one PPARδ allele results in impeded wound healing [86]. Tan et al. [87] demonstrated that the anti-inflammatory cytokine TGFβ1, which is also produced at wound sites, is able to inhibit inflammation induced PPARδ expression. This indicates (at least in part) a PPARδ-mediated crosstalk between pro- and anti-inflammatory signaling pathways in keratinocytes.

3.6. *Conclusions and outlook. The ugly duckling PPARδ: a potent secret agent in metabolic active tissue?*

The past 10 years have seen considerable progress in unravelling the mechanisms of PPARδ. Agonists for PPARγ and PPARα are already established as insulin sensitizers and hypolipidemic drugs, respectively, and are used in the treatment of metabolic diseases, such as hyperinsulinemia, insulin resistance and type-II diabetes, dyslipidemia, obesity, and inflammation. The recent development of synthetic and specific agonists for PPARδ provides a novel therapeutic concept to pursue these medical conditions. PPARδ is expressed in a variety of tissues, often at a higher level than PPARα or PPARγ, where it activates genes that increase lipid absorption, preferential lipid utilization, lipid catabolism and β-oxidation, and energy expenditure (Fig. 1). This review summarizes striking evidence that specific agonists for PPARδ ameliorate cholesterol homeostasis, have great potential in treating hyperlipidemia, cardiovascular disease, hypertension, and other metabolic diseases associated with obesity and the metabolic syndrome.

Activation of PPARδ in skeletal muscle results in remodeling of this major peripheral mass tissue, increasing its oxidative fibers and thereby contributing to the reduction of overall body-fat content. Recently, it has been reported that PPARδ is also a potential therapeutic target in treating lipotoxic cardiomyopathy and other heart diseases, excluding side effects observed with agents that activate PPARα [88]. Furthermore, positive effects on biological processes like inflammation and wound healing have also been demonstrated.

Unfortunately, there is also evidence that activation of this receptor also may lead to tumor development, especially in colorectal cancers. This involvement of PPARδ in cancer promotion is still controversial, as a number of conflicting reports exist [24,25,73]. The Food and Drug Administration (FDA) of the USA is particularly concerned about safety of PPAR-related compounds and has published specific standards for preclinical and clinical safety assessments for PPAR agonists that recommend two-year carcinogenity studies [89]. GW501516 is currently undergoing clinical trials and the outcome of these is of great interest, especially in Westernized societies like the USA, where 55% of the population was considered overweight or obese in 1998 [90] and where the costs for treatment of diseases associated with dyslipidemia certainly exceed the cost of therapeutic intervention with drugs like PPARδ agonists.

Dyslipidemia, hyperinsulinemia, blood glucose levels (and glucose tolerance), diabetes, inflammation, and obesity are all serious risk factors for cardiovascular and metabolic disease. PPARδ has been reported to ameliorate many of these metabolic perturbations. However, the promise and potential of PPARδ agonists in the therapeutic setting remains to be determined.

Acknowledgements

We thank Sue Conrad and Michael Pearen for carefully reading the manuscript. Uwe Dressel was a University of Queensland Postdoctoral Research Fellow. George E.O. Muscat is a Professorial Research Fellow at the University of Queensland, and a Principal Research Fellow of the National Health and Medical Research Council (NHMRC).

References

[1] AH Association, Heart disease and stroke statistics – 2004 update. American Heart Association, 2004. URL: www.americanheart.org/downloadable/heart/1079736729696HDSStats2004UpdateREV3-19-04.pdf.

[2] AO Association, AOA fact sheets: "obesity in the US," 2004. http://www.obesity.org/subs/fastfacts/obesity_US.shtml, accessed February 2004.

[3] T. Prentice, World Health Organization: world health report. Overview, World Health Organization, Geneva, 2002, p. 8.

[4] K.M. Narayan, J.P. Boyle, T.J. Thompson, S.W. Sorensen, D.F. Williamson, Lifetime risk for diabetes mellitus in the United States, JAMA 290 (2003) 1884–1890.

[5] Federation WHOID, Diabetes action now, 2004. World URL: www.who.int/entity/diabetes/actionnow/en/DANbooklet.pdf.

[6] A. Chawla, J.J. Repa, R.M. Evans, D.J. Mangelsdorf, Nuclear receptors and lipid physiology: opening the X-files, Science 294 (2001) 1866–1870.

[7] T.T. Lu, J.J. Repa, D.J. Mangelsdorf, Orphan nuclear receptors as eLiXiRs and FiXeRs of sterol metabolism, J. Biol. Chem. 276 (2001) 37735–37738.

[8] A.K. Hihi, L. Michalik, W. Wahli, PPARs: transcriptional effectors of fatty acids and their derivatives, Cell Mol. Life Sci. 59 (2002) 790–798.

 [9] C. Dreyer, G. Krey, H. Keller, F. Givel, G. Helftenbein, W. Wahli, Control of the peroxisomal
     beta-oxidation pathway by a novel family of nuclear hormone receptors, Cell 68 (1992) 879–887.
[10] S.A. Kliewer, B.M. Forman, B. Blumberg, E.S. Ong, U. Borgmeyer, D.J. Mangelsdorf, K. Umesono,
     R.M. Evans, Differential expression and activation of a family of murine peroxisome proliferator-
     activated receptors, Proc. Natl. Acad. Sci. USA 91 (1994) 7355–7359.
[11] A. Schmidt, E. Endo, S.J. Rutledge, R. Vogel, D. Shinar, G.A. Rodan, Identification of a new
     member of the steroid hormone receptor superfamily that is activated by a peroxisome proliferator
     and fatty acids, Mol. Endocrinol. 6 (1992) 1634–1641.
[12] E.Z. Amri, F. Bonino, G. Ailhaud, N.A. Abumrad, P.A. Grimaldi, Cloning of a protein that mediates
     transcriptional effects of fatty acids in preadipocytes. Homology to peroxisome proliferator-activated
     receptors, J. Biol. Chem. 270 (1995) 2367–2371.
[13] W.R. Oliver Jr., J.L. Shenk, M.R. Snaith, C.S. Russell, K.D. Plunket, N.L. Bodkin, M.C. Lewis,
     D.A. Winegar, M.L. Sznaidman, M.H. Lambert, H.E. Xu, D.D. Sternbach, S.A. Kliewer, B.C.
     Hansen, T.M. Willson, A selective peroxisome proliferator-activated receptor delta agonist promotes
     reverse cholesterol transport, Proc. Natl. Acad. Sci. USA 98 (2001) 5306–5311.
[14] O. Braissant, F. Foufelle, C. Scotto, M. Dauca, W. Wahli, Differential expression of peroxisome
     proliferator-activated receptors (PPARs): tissue distribution of PPAR-alpha,-beta, and -gamma in the
     adult rat, Endocrinology 137 (1996) 354–366.
[15] P.R. Devchand, H. Keller, J.M. Peters, M. Vazquez, F.J. Gonzalez, W. Wahli, The PPARalpha-
     leukotriene B4 pathway to inflammation control, Nature 384 (1994) 39–43.
[16] E.D. Rosen, P. Sarraf, A.E. Troy, G. Bradwin, K. Moore, D.S. Milstone, B.M. Spiegelman, R.M.
     Mortensen, PPAR gamma is required for the differentiation of adipose tissue *in vivo* and *in vitro*, Mol.
     Cell 4 (1999) 611–617.
[17] H.E. Xu, M.H. Lambert, V.G. Montana, D.J. Parks, S.G. Blanchard, P.J. Brown, D.D. Sternbach,
     J.M. Lehmann, G.B. Wisely, T.M. Willson, S.A. Kliewer, M.V. Milburn, Molecular recognition of
     fatty acids by peroxisome proliferator-activated receptors, Mol. Cell 3 (1999) 397–403.
[18] H. Lim, R.A. Gupta, W.G. Ma, B.C. Paria, D.E. Moller, J.D. Morrow, R.N. DuBois, J.M. Trzaskos,
     S.K. Dey, Cyclo-oxygenase-2-derived prostacyclin mediates embryo implantation in the mouse via
     PPARdelta, Genes Dev. 13 (1999) 1561–1574.
[19] Y.X. Wang, C.H. Lee, S. Tiep, R.T. Yu, J. Ham, H. Kang, R.M. Evans, Peroxisome-proliferator-
     activated receptor delta activates fat metabolism to prevent obesity, Cell 113 (2003) 159–170.
[20] U. Dressel, T.L. Allen, J.B. Pippal, P.R. Rohde, P. Lau, G.E. Muscat, The peroxisome proliferator-
     activated receptor beta/delta agonist, GW501516, regulates the expression of genes involved in
     lipid catabolism and energy uncoupling in skeletal muscle cells, Mol. Endocrinol. 17 (2003) 2477–2493.
[21] N.S. Tan, L. Michalik, N. Noy, R. Yasmin, C. Pacot, M. Heim, B. Fluhmann, B. Desvergne,
     W. Wahli, Critical roles of PPAR beta/delta in keratinocyte response to inflammation, Genes Dev. 15
     (2001) 3263–3277.
[22] N.S. Tan, L. Michalik, N. Di-Poi, B. Desvergne, W. Wahli, Critical roles of the nuclear receptor
     PPARbeta (peroxisome-proliferator-activated receptor beta) in skin wound healing, Biochem. Soc.
     Trans. 32 (2004) 97–102.
[23] C.H. Lee, A. Chawla, N. Urbiztondo, D. Liao, W.A. Boisvert, R.M. Evans, L.K. Curtiss, Transcrip-
     tional repression of atherogenic inflammation: modulation by PPARdelta, Science 302 (2003) 453–457.
[24] B.H. Park, B. Vogelstein, K.W. Kinzler, Genetic disruption of PPARdelta decreases the tumori-
     genicity of human colon cancer cells, Proc. Natl. Acad. Sci. USA 98 (2001) 2598–2603.
[25] R.A. Gupta, D. Wang, S. Katkuri, H. Wang, S.K. Dey, R.N. DuBois, Activation of nuclear hormone
     receptor peroxisome proliferator-activated receptor-delta accelerates intestinal adenoma growth, Nat.
     Med. 10 (2004) 245–247.
[26] R.M. Evans, G.D. Barish, Y.X. Wang, PPARs and the complex journey to obesity, Nat. Med. 10
     (2004) 355–361.
[27] L. Jow, R. Mukherjee, The human peroxisome proliferator-activated receptor (PPAR) subtype
     NUC1 represses the activation of hPPAR alpha and thyroid hormone receptors, J. Biol. Chem. 270
     (1995) 3836–3840.

[28] Y. Shi, M. Hon, R.M. Evans, The peroxisome proliferator-activated receptor delta, an integrator of transcriptional repression and nuclear receptor signaling, Proc. Natl. Acad. Sci. USA 99 (2002) 2613–2618.

[29] J. Aubert, O. Champigny, P. Saint-Marc, R. Negrel, S. Collins, D. Ricquier, G. Ailhaud, Up-regulation of UCP-2 gene expression by PPAR agonists in preadipose and adipose cells, Biochem. Biophys. Res. Commun. 238 (1997) 606–611.

[30] I. Nagase, S. Yoshida, X. Canas, Y. Irie, K. Kimura, T. Yoshida, M. Saito, Up-regulation of uncoupling protein 3 by thyroid hormone, peroxisome proliferator-activated receptor ligands and 9-cis retinoic acid in L6 myotubes, FEBS Lett. 461 (1999) 319–322.

[31] R.P. Brun, P. Tontonoz, B.M. Forman, R. Ellis, J. Chen, R.M. Evans, B.M. Spiegelman, Differential activation of adipogenesis by multiple PPAR isoforms, Genes Dev. 10 (1996) 974–984.

[32] C. Bastie, D. Holst, D. Gaillard, C. Jehl-Pietri, P.A. Grimaldi, Expression of peroxisome proliferator-activated receptor PPARdelta promotes induction of PPARgamma and adipocyte differentiation in 3T3C2 fibroblasts, J. Biol. Chem. 274 (1999) 21920–21925.

[33] H.M. Guardiola-Diaz, S. Rehnmark, N. Usuda, T. Albrektsen, D. Feltkamp, J.A. Gustafsson, S.E. Alexson, Rat peroxisome proliferator-activated receptors and brown adipose tissue function during cold acclimatization, J. Biol. Chem. 274 (1999) 23368–23377.

[34] K. Matsusue, J.M. Peters, F.J. Gonzalez, PPARbeta/delta potentiates PPARgamma-stimulated adipocyte differentiation, FASEB J. 18 (2004) 1477–1479.

[35] A. Schmidt, R.L. Vogel, K.M. Witherup, S.J. Rutledge, S.M. Pitzenberger, M. Adam, G.A. Rodan, Identification of fatty acid methyl ester as naturally occurring transcriptional regulators of the members of the peroxisome proliferator-activated receptor family, Lipids 31 (1996) 1115–1124.

[36] B.M. Forman, J. Chen, R.M. Evans, Hypolipidemic drugs, polyunsaturated fatty acids, and eicosanoids are ligands for peroxisome proliferator-activated receptors alpha and delta, Proc. Natl. Acad. Sci. USA 94 (1997) 4312–4317.

[37] G. Krey, O. Braissant, F. L'Horset, E. Kalkhoven, M. Perroud, M.G. Parker, W. Wahli, Fatty acids, eicosanoids, and hypolipidemic agents identified as ligands of peroxisome proliferator-activated receptors by coactivator-dependent receptor ligand assay, Mol. Endocrinol. 11 (1997) 779–791.

[38] K. Schoonjans, G. Martin, B. Staels, J. Auwerx, Peroxisome proliferator-activated receptors, orphans with ligands and functions, Curr. Opin. Lipidol. 8 (1997) 159–166.

[39] T.E. Johnson, M.K. Holloway, R. Vogel, S.J. Rutledge, J.J. Perkins, G.A. Rodan, A. Schmidt, Structural requirements and cell-type specificity for ligand activation of peroxisome proliferator-activated receptors, J. Steroid. Biochem. Mol. Biol. 63 (1997) 1–8.

[40] A. Schmidt, R. Vogel, M.K. Holloway, S.J. Rutledge, O. Friedman, Z. Yang, G.A. Rodan, E. Friedman, Transcription control and neuronal differentiation by agents that activate the LXR nuclear receptor family, Mol. Cell. Endocrinol. 155 (1999) 51–60.

[41] P.J. Brown, T.A. Smith-Oliver, P.S. Charifson, N.C. Tomkinson, A.M. Fivush, D.D. Sternbach, L.E. Wade, L. Orband-Miller, D.J. Parks, S.G. Blanchard, S.A. Kliewer, J.M. Lehmann, T.M. Willson, Identification of peroxisome proliferator-activated receptor ligands from a biased chemical library, Chem. Biol. 4 (1997) 909–918.

[42] R.L. Rosenfield, A. Kentsis, D. Deplewski, N. Ciletti, Rat preputial sebocyte differentiation involves peroxisome proliferator-activated receptors, J. Invest. Dermatol. 112 (1999) 226–232.

[43] R.L. Rosenfield, D. Deplewski, A. Kentsis, N. Ciletti, Mechanisms of androgen induction of sebocyte differentiation, Dermatology 196 (1998) 43–46.

[44] J.M. Peters, T. Aoyama, A.M. Burns, F.J. Gonzalez, Bezafibrate is a dual ligand for PPARalpha and PPARbeta: studies using null mice, Biochim. Biophys. Acta 1632 (2003) 80–89.

[45] J. Berger, M.D. Leibowitz, T.W. Doebber, A. Elbrecht, B. Zhang, G. Zhou, C. Biswas, C.A. Cullinan, N.S. Hayes, Y. Li, M. Tanen, J. Ventre, M.S. Wu, G.D. Berger, R. Mosley, R. Marquis, C. Santini, S.P. Sahoo, R.L. Tolman, R.G. Smith, D.E. Moller, Novel peroxisome proliferator-activated receptor (PPAR) gamma and PPARdelta ligands produce distinct biological effects, J. Biol. Chem. 274 (1999) 6718–6725.

[46] S. Basu-Modak, O. Braissant, P. Escher, B. Desvergne, P. Honegger, W. Wahli, Peroxisome pro-liferator-activated receptor beta regulates acyl-CoA synthetase 2 in reaggregated rat brain cell cul-tures, J. Biol. Chem. 274 (1999) 35881–35888.

[47] M.D. Leibowitz, C. Fievet, N. Hennuyer, J. Peinado-Onsurbe, H. Duez, J. Bergera, C.A. Cullinan, C.P. Sparrow, J. Baffic, G.D. Berger, C. Santini, R.W. Marquis, R.L. Tolman, R.G. Smith, D.E. Moller, J. Auwerx, Activation of PPARdelta alters lipid metabolism in db/db mice, FEBS Lett. 473 (2000) 333–336.

[48] R.L. Stephen, M.C. Gustafsson, M. Jarvis, R. Tatoud, B.R. Marshall, D. Knight, E. Ehrenborg, A.L. Harris, C.R. Wolf, C.N. Palmer, Activation of peroxisome proliferator-activated receptor delta stimulates the proliferation of human breast and prostate cancer cell lines, Cancer Res. 64 (2004) 3162–3170.

[49] M. Schmuth, C.M. Haqq, W.J. Cairns, J.C. Holder, S. Dorsam, S. Chang, P. Lau, A.J. Fowler, G. Chuang, A.H. Moser, B.E. Brown, M. Mao-Qiang, Y. Uchida, K. Schoonjans, J. Auwerx, P. Chambon, T.M. Willson, P.M. Elias, K.R. Feingold, Peroxisome proliferator-activated receptor (PPAR)-beta/delta stimulates differentiation and lipid accumulation in keratinocytes, J. Invest. Dermatol. 122 (2004) 971–983.

[50] T. Tanaka, J. Yamamoto, S. Iwasaki, H. Asaba, H. Hamura, Y. Ikeda, M. Watanabe, K. Magoori, R.X. Ioka, K. Tachibana, Y. Watanabe, Y. Uchiyama, K. Sumi, H. Iguchi, S. Ito, T. Doi, T. Hamakubo, M. Naito, J. Auwerx, M. Yanagisawa, T. Kodama, J. Sakai, Activation of peroxisome proliferator-activated receptor delta induces fatty acid beta-oxidation in skeletal muscle and atten-uates metabolic syndrome, Proc. Natl. Acad. Sci. USA 100 (2003) 15924–15929.

[51] Z.L. Wei, A.P. Kozikowski, A short and efficient synthesis of the pharmacological research tool GW501516 for the peroxisome proliferator-activated receptor delta, J. Org. Chem. 68 (2003) 9116–9118.

[52] B. Glinghammar, J. Skogsberg, A. Hamsten, E. Ehrenborg, PPARdelta activation induces COX-2 gene expression and cell proliferation in human hepatocellular carcinoma cells, Biochem. Biophys. Res. Commun. 308 (2003) 361–368.

[53] A.J. Gilde, K.A. van der Lee, P.H. Willemsen, G. Chinetti, F.R. van der Leij, G.J. van der Vusse, B. Staels, M. van Bilsen, Peroxisome proliferator-activated receptor (PPAR) alpha and PPARbeta/delta, but not PPARgamma, modulate the expression of genes involved in cardiac lipid metabolism, Circ. Res. 92 (2003) 518–524.

[54] M.L. Sznaidman, C.D. Haffner, P.R. Maloney, A. Fivush, E. Chao, D. Goreham, M.L. Sierra, C. LeGrumelec, H.E. Xu, V.G. Montana, M.H. Lambert, T.M. Willson, W.R. Oliver Jr., D.D. Sternbach, Novel selective small molecule agonists for peroxisome proliferator-activated receptor delta (PPARdelta) – synthesis and biological activity, Bioorg. Med. Chem. Lett. 13 (2003) 1517–1521.

[55] S.A. Smith, G.R. Monteith, J.A. Robinson, N.G. Venkata, F.J. May, S.J. Roberts-Thomson, Effect of the peroxisome proliferator-activated receptor beta activator GW0742 in rat cultured cerebellar granule neurons, J. Neurosci. Res. 77 (2004) 240–249.

[56] L. Cheng, G. Ding, Q. Qin, Y. Xiao, D. Woods, Y.E. Chen, Q. Yang, Peroxisome proliferator-activated receptor delta activates fatty acid oxidation in cultured neonatal and adult cardiomyocytes, Biochem. Biophys. Res. Commun. 313 (2004) 277–286.

[57] Y. Lin, X. Zhu, F.L. McLntee, H. Xiao, J. Zhang, M. Fu, Y.E. Chen, Interferon regulatory factor-1 mediates PPARgamma-induced apoptosis in vascular smooth muscle cells, Arterioscler. Thromb. Vasc. Biol. 24 (2004) 257–263.

[58] D.M. Muoio, P.S. MacLean, D.B. Lang, S. Li, J.A. Houmard, J.M. Way, D.A. Winegar, J.C. Corton, G.L. Dohm, W.E. Kraus, Fatty acid homeostasis and induction of lipid regulatory genes in skeletal muscles of peroxisome proliferator-activated receptor (PPAR) alpha knock-out mice. Evidence for compensatory regulation by PPAR delta,, J. Biol. Chem. 277 (2002) 26089–26097.

[59] M.D. Leibowitz, J.P. Berger, D.E. Moller, J. Auwerx, G.D. Berger, Compound F. International patent publication no. WO 97/28149, 1997.

[60] H. Vosper, G.A. Khoudoli, C.N. Palmer, The peroxisome proliferator activated receptor delta is required for the differentiation of THP-1 monocytic cells by phorbol ester, Nucl. Recept. 1 (2003) 9.

[61] H. Vosper, L. Patel, T.L. Graham, G.A. Khoudoli, A. Hill, C.H. Macphee, I. Pinto, S.A. Smith, K.E. Suckling, C.R. Wolf, C.N. Palmer, The peroxisome proliferator-activated receptor delta promotes lipid accumulation in human macrophages, J. Biol. Chem. 276 (2001) 44258–44265.

[62] R. Epple, M. Azimioara, R. Russo, B. Bursulaya, S.S. Tian, A. Gerken, M. Iskandar, 1,3,5-Trisubstituted aryls as highly selective PPARdelta agonists, Bioorg. Med. Chem. Lett. March 17.

[63] A. Chawla, C.H. Lee, Y. Barak, W. He, J. Rosenfeld, D. Liao, J. Han, H. Kang, R.M. Evans, PPARdelta is a very low-density lipoprotein sensor in macrophages, Proc. Natl. Acad. Sci. USA 100 (2003) 1268–1273.

[64] T.E. Akiyama, G. Lambert, C.J. Nicol, K. Matsusue, J.M. Peters, H.B. Brewer Jr., F.J. Gonzalez, Peroxisome proliferator-activated receptor beta/delta regulates very low density lipoprotein production and catabolism in mice on a Western diet, J. Biol. Chem. 279 (2004) 20874–20881.

[65] C. Bastie, S. Luquet, D. Holst, C. Jehl-Pietri, P.A. Grimaldi, Alterations of peroxisome proliferator-activated receptor delta activity affect fatty acid-controlled adipose differentiation, J. Biol. Chem. 275 (2000) 38768–38773.

[66] J. Eriksson, A. Franssila-Kallunki, A. Ekstrand, C. Saloranta, E. Widen, C. Schalin, L. Groop, Early metabolic defects in persons at increased risk for non-insulin-dependent diabetes mellitus, N. Engl. J. Med. 321 (1989) 337–343.

[67] E. Chevillotte, J. Rieusset, M. Roques, M. Desage, H. Vidal, The regulation of uncoupling protein-2 gene expression by omega-6 polyunsaturated fatty acids in human skeletal muscle cells involves multiple pathways, including the nuclear receptor peroxisome proliferator-activated receptor beta, J. Biol. Chem. 276 (2001) 10853–10860.

[68] D. Holst, S. Luquet, V. Nogueira, K. Kristiansen, X. Leverve, P.A. Grimaldi, Nutritional regulation and role of peroxisome proliferator-activated receptor delta in fatty acid catabolism in skeletal muscle, Biochim. Biophys. Acta 1633 (2003) 43–50.

[69] D. Holst, S. Luquet, K. Kristiansen, P.A. Grimaldi, Roles of peroxisome proliferator-activated receptors delta and gamma in myoblast transdifferentiation, Exp. Cell. Res. 288 (2003) 168–176.

[70] S. Luquet, J. Lopez-Soriano, D. Holst, A. Fredenrich, J. Melki, M. Rassoulzadegan, P.A. Grimaldi, Peroxisome proliferator-activated receptor delta controls muscle development and oxidative capability, FASEB J. 17 (2003) 2299–2301.

[71] M. Loviscach, N. Rehman, L. Carter, S. Mudaliar, P. Mohadeen, T.P. Ciaraldi, J.H. Veerkamp, R.R. Henry, Distribution of peroxisome proliferator-activated receptors (PPARs) in human skeletal muscle and adipose tissue: relation to insulin action, Diabetologia 43 (2000) 304–311.

[72] J.M. Peters, S.S. Lee, W. Li, J.M. Ward, O. Gavrilova, C. Everett, M.L. Reitman, L.D. Hudson, F.J. Gonzalez, Growth, adipose, brain, and skin alterations resulting from targeted disruption of the mouse peroxisome proliferator-activated receptor beta(delta), Mol. Cell. Biol. 20 (2000) 5119–5128.

[73] Y. Barak, D. Liao, W. He, E.S. Ong, M.C. Nelson, J.M. Olefsky, R. Boland, R.M. Evans, Effects of peroxisome proliferator-activated receptor delta on placentation, adiposity, and colorectal cancer, Proc. Natl. Acad. Sci. USA 99 (2002) 303–308.

[74] H. Chen, O. Charlat, L.A. Tartaglia, E.A. Woolf, X. Weng, S.J. Ellis, N.D. Lakey, J. Culpepper, K.J. Moore, R.E. Breitbart, G.M. Duyk, R.I. Tepper, J.P. Morgenstern, Evidence that the diabetes gene encodes the leptin receptor: identification of a mutation in the leptin receptor gene in db/db mice, Cell 84 (1996) 491–495.

[75] G.H. Lee, R. Proenca, J.M. Montez, K.M. Carroll, J.G. Darvishzadeh, J.I. Lee, J.M. Friedman, Abnormal splicing of the leptin receptor in diabetic mice, Nature 379 (1996) 632–635.

[76] Y.X. Wang, C.L. Zhang, R.T. Yu, H.K. Cho, M.C. Nelson, C.R. Bayuga-Ocampo, J. Ham, H. Kang, R.M. Evans, Regulation of muscle fiber type and Running Endurance by PPARdelta, PLoS Biol. 2 (2004) E294.

[77] J.C. Clapham, J.R. Arch, H. Chapman, A. Haynes, C. Lister, G.B. Moore, V. Piercy, S.A. Carter, I. Lehner, S.A. Smith, L.J. Beeley, R.J. Godden, N. Herrity, M. Skehel, K.K. Changani, P.D. Hockings, D.G. Reid, S.M. Squires, J. Hatcher, B. Trail, J. Latcham, S. Rastan, A.J. Harper, S. Cadenas, J.A. Buckingham, M.D. Brand, A. Abuin, Mice overexpressing human uncoupling protein-3 in skeletal muscle are hyperphagic and lean, Nature 406 (2000) 415–418.

[78] G.I. Shulman, Cellular mechanisms of insulin resistance, J. Clin. Invest. 106 (2000) 171–176.

[79] C.H. Lee, P. Olson, A. Hevener, I. Mehl, L.W. Chong, J.M. Olefsky, F.J. Gonzalez, J. Ham, H. Kang, J.M. Peters, R.M. Evans, PPARdelta regulates glucose metabolism and insulin sensitivity, Proc. Natl. Acad. Sci. USA 103 (2006) 3444–3449 Epub 2006 Feb 21.

[80] A. Dresner, D. Laurent, M. Marcucci, M.E. Griffin, S. Dufour, G.W. Cline, L.A. Slezak, D.K. Andersen, R.S. Hundal, D.L. Rothman, K.F. Petersen, G.I. Shulman, Effects of free fatty acids on glucose transport and IRS-1-associated phosphatidylinositol 3-kinase activity, J. Clin. Invest. 103 (1999) 253–259.

[81] G. Perseghin, P. Scifo, F. De Cobelli, E. Pagliato, A. Battezzati, C. Arcelloni, A. Vanzulli, G. Testolin, G. Pozza, A. Del Maschio, L. Luzi, Intramyocellular triglyceride content is a determinant of *in vivo* insulin resistance in humans: a 1H-13C nuclear magnetic resonance spectroscopy assessment in offspring of type 2 diabetic parents, Diabetes 48 (1999) 1600–1606.

[82] M. Manco, M. Calvani, G. Mingrone, Effects of dietary fatty acids on insulin sensitivity and secretion, Diabetes Obes Metab 6 (2004) 402–413.

[83] H.D. Shin, B.L. Park, L.H. Kim, H.S. Jung, Y.M. Cho, M.K. Moon, Y.J. Park, H.K. Lee, K.S. Park, Genetic polymorphisms in peroxisome proliferator-activated receptor delta associated with obesity, Diabetes 53 (2004) 847–851.

[84] N. Marx, H. Duez, J.C. Fruchart, B. Staels, Peroxisome proliferator-activated receptors and atherogenesis: regulators of gene expression in vascular cells, Circ. Res. 94 (2004) 1168–1178.

[85] C.H. Lee, K. Kang, I.R. Mehl, R. Nofsinger, W.A. Alaynick, L.W. Chong, J.M. Rosenfeld, R.M. Evans, Peroxisome proliferator-activated receptor delta promotes very low-density lipoprotein-derived fatty acid catabolism in the macrophage, Proc Natl Acad Sci. USA 103 (2006) 2434–2439.

[86] L. Michalik, B. Desvergne, N.S. Tan, S. Basu-Modak, P. Escher, J. Rieusset, J.M. Peters, G. Kaya, F.J. Gonzalez, J. Zakany, D. Metzger, P. Chambon, D. Duboule, W. Wahli, Impaired skin wound healing in peroxisome proliferator-activated receptor (PPAR)alpha and PPARbeta mutant mice, J. Cell Biol. 154 (2001) 799–814.

[87] N.S. Tan, L. Michalik, N. Di-Poi, C.Y. Ng, N. Mermod, A.B. Roberts, B. Desvergne, W. Wahli, Essential role of Smad3 in the inhibition of inflammation-induced PPARbeta/delta expression, EMBO J. 23 (2004) 4211–4221.

[88] L. Cheng, G. Ding, Q. Qin Y. Huang, W. Lewis, N. He, R.M. Evans, M.D. Schneider, F.A. Brako, Y. Xiao, Y.E. Chen, Q. Yang, Cardiomyocyte-restricted peroxisome proliferator-activated receptor-delta deletion perturbs myocardial fatty acid oxidation and leads to cardiomyopathy, Nat. Med. (2004).

[89] J. El-Hage, Preclinical and Clinical Safety Assessments for PPAR Agonists. URL: www.fda.gov/cder/present/DIA2004/elhage_files/frame.htm.

[90] P. Abelson, D. Kennedy, The obesity epidemic, Science 304 (2004) 1413.

Chapter 4

Liver X receptors as potential drug targets for diabetes and its disorders

Knut R. Steffensen

Receptor Biology Unit, Department of Biosciences at NOVUM, Karolinska Institute, S–14157 Huddinge, Sweden

Summary

The liver X receptors (LXR) are a subclass of nuclear receptors (NRs), which are activated by specific oxysterols. These receptors have recently gained much attention as a potential drug target for diseases affecting metabolic processes, such as diabetes and its associated disorders. When oxysterols were identified as activators of the LXRs these NRs were suggested to play an important role as sensors of cholesterol metabolism. Huge research efforts were put into investigating the LXRs and their involvement in various metabolic processes revealing that the LXRs also play important roles in fatty acid biosynthesis, triglyceride biosynthesis, carbohydrate metabolism, atherosclerosis and inflammation. Dysregulation or dysfunction of one or more of these biological processes is often the cause or a consequence of developing diabetes. Several studies also reported cross-talk between LXR signaling and other NRs including the peroxisome proliferator-activated receptor (PPAR) and the glucocorticoid receptor (GR) which are also important regulators of metabolic processes. Hence, developing drugs that target LXR might provide new therapeutic interventions against several metabolic disorders. This chapter focuses on the physiological roles of the LXRs, particularly in carbohydrate-, lipid- and cholesterol metabolism, atherosclerosis and subsequent development of cardiovascular disease and their underlying molecular mechanisms. Particular attention will be paid to why these NRs are such highly attractive drug targets for the treatment of diabetes and its associated metabolic disorders.

1. Introduction to LXR

1.1. *General mechanisms of LXR signaling*

The LXRs are members of the nuclear receptor (NR) superfamily consisting of 48 family members in humans, 21 members in *Drosophila melanogaster* and 250

ADVANCES IN MOLECULAR AND CELLULAR ENDOCRINOLOGY
VOLUME 5 ISSN 1569-2566/DOI 10.1016/S1569-2566(06)05004-6

members in *Caenorhabditis elegans* [1]. The NR superfamily is the most abundant family of transcription factors that, in general, are ligand activated transcription factors. Their natural ligands are lipophilic endocrine hormones and small signaling molecules like fatty acids, cholesterol derivatives, retinoic acid, prostaglandins and leukotrienes [1,2]. These signaling molecules easily penetrate the cellular membrane and bind their cognate NR. NR target genes are involved in diverse biological functions, such as aging, reproduction, development and metabolism pointing to paramount biological roles of the NRs. Most NRs share a common structural organization [1] (Fig. 1). The N-terminal domain is the least conserved domain and contains a ligand-independent transactivation function (AF-1). The DNA-binding domain (DBD) responsible for sequence specific binding by the NRs to DNA and dimerization with other NRs. The DBD is highly conserved among the NRs. The moderately conserved C-terminal domain contains a strong dimerization interface for other NRs, a ligand-binding domain (LBD) and a ligand-dependent transactivation domain. The hinge domain between DBD and LBD allows a flexible three-dimensional structure of the NR. Two nuclear localization signal (NLS) sequences are found in the hinge and C-terminal domain. Some NRs have an additional domain at the extreme C-terminal (F-domain). The function of this domain is poorly

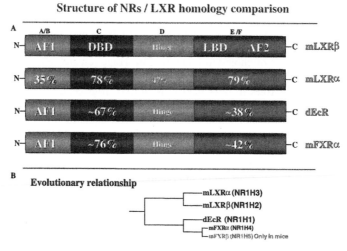

Fig. 1. A. The primary structure of NRs is divided into several domains (A-F). The A and B domains contain the activator function 1 (AF1; a ligand-independent transcription activator function), the C domain contains the DNA binding domain (DBD; a zink-finger domains which contacts the major groove of the DNA helix), the D domain that bridges the rigid N-terminal part from the more flexible C-terminal part and the E and F domain containing the ligand binding domain (LBD) as well as the activator function 2 (AF2; a ligand-dependent transcription activator function). The amino acid sequence homology between mouse LXRβ and the mouse LXRα, *Drosophila* EcR and mouse FXR is also indicated for different domains. B. The evolutionary relationship between these receptors (the official nomenclature of the respective receptors in brackets) is presented in a hierarchical tree. The existence of a second FXR paralog is still debated but is so far only identified in mouse.

elucidated and is still not fully understood. Most NRs bind to their cognate response element as homo- or heterodimers [3].

The LXR subfamily consists of two members, LXRα and LXRβ. LXRα (RLD-1) was cloned in 1994 from a rat liver cDNA library [4] and from a human liver cDNA library in 1995 [5]. LXRβ was cloned in 1994 from a human bone cDNA library (NER) [6] and from a rat vagina cDNA library in 1994 (UR) [7]. Two additional LXRβ cDNAs were also reported in 1995 from a rat liver cDNA library (OR-1) [8] and from a mouse liver library using yeast two hybrid screening (RIP15) [9]. The existence of a truncated pseudogene of LXRβ has also been proposed in the mouse genome [10]. At the present time, their common names are LXRα and LXRβ although they were given the official names, NR1H3 (LXRα) and NR1H2 (LXRβ), in 1999 by *The Nuclear Receptor Nomenclature Committee*. The LXR paralogs are highly conserved between rodents and humans. Human LXRα and rat LXRα show close to 100% homology in amino acid composition in the DNA and LBDs and human LXRα and LXRβ show almost 80% homology in the same domains [5]. This indicates that both LXR paralogs belong to the same family of NRs and that they might serve the same biological functions. There is a close evolutionary relationship between the LXRs and both ecdysone receptor (EcR; the Drosophila paralog of LXR) and the farnesoid X receptor (FXR) (Fig. 1). The LXRs and FXR work in concert as sensors of cholesterol homeostasis as they both regulate transcription of genes involved in cholesterol-, bile acid-, lipoprotein- and lipid metabolism [11] but other NRs including the GR, PPAR, liver receptor homologue 1 (LRH1) and short heterodimer partner (SHP) also have important roles in nutrient metabolism [12].

High expression of LXRα is restricted to tissues with high metabolic activity including liver, kidney, adipose tissue, small intestine and macrophages whereas LXRβ is ubiquitously expressed [5,13]. The increasing number of identified LXR target genes demonstrates that the LXRs regulate expression of genes with multiple biological functions (Table 1). However, the fact that most of the identified target genes are involved in metabolic processes indicates that proper LXR signaling is pivotal to metabolic homeostasis in the body.

1.2. *Molecular mechanisms underlying LXR signaling*

The LXRs bind to their cognate liver X response element (LXRE), consisting of two direct hexanucleotide repeats separated by 4 nucleotides (DR4), in the promoter of the target gene where they preferentially heterodimerize with the RXR. The LXR/RXR heterodimer is activated upon binding of either 9-cis-retinoic acid (RXR agonist), LXR agonist or synergistically by binding of both ligands [14]. A dimerization-induced transactivation of RXR/LXR in the absence of ligand, that is mainly dependent on the LBD of LXR, has also been proposed [15]. Subtle alterations of the hexamer repeat, spacer sequence or flanking regions, led to changes in the transactivation potential indicating highly sequence specific interaction of the RXR/LXR heterodimer [16]. The RXRα/LXRβ heterodimer, but not the RXRα/LXRα heterodimer, was shown to bind a DR1 element in a DNA-binding site selection assay suggesting different binding properties between the LXR-paralogs [17]. A unique

Table 1
Reported LXR target genes with an LXRE (LXR response element) found in the promoter or regulated by exposure to an LXR agonist is listed. ↑ upregulated and ↓ downregulated. SR-B1 (scavenger receptor B1), FPPS (farnesyl pyrophosphate synthase), AKR-B7 (aldo–keto reductase 1-B7), Cyp7α (cholesterol 7-alpha hydroxylase), I-BABP (ileal-bile acid binding protein), CETP (cholesterol ester transfer protein), PLTP (phospholipid transfer protein), apo (apolipoprotein) AIV-V/E/CI-II-IV/D/E, ABC (ATP binding cassette transporter), A1/G1-4-5-8, SREBP1c (sterol regulatory element binding protein 1c), FAS (fatty acid synthase), ACC (acetyl CoA carboxylase), SCD (stearoyl coA desaturase) 1/2, Angptl3 (angiopoietin-like protein 3), Spot14 (thyroid hormone responsive spot 14), LPL (lipoprotein lipase), LXR (liver X receptor) α, PPARγ (peroxisome proliferator-activated receptor γ), FTF (alpha1-fetoprotein transcription factor), SHP (short heterodimer partner), PEPCK (phosphoenylpyruvate carboxykinase), Fbp1 (fructose-1, 6-biphosphatase), G6P (glucose-6-phosphatase), PGC1 (PPARγ coactivator 1), Pfkfb3 (6-phosphofructo-2-kinase 3), PDK4 (pyruvate dehydrogenase kinase 4), GK (glucokinase), GLUT1/4 (glucose transporter 1/4), TNFα (tumor necrosis factor alpha), IL-6 (interleukin-6), iNOS (inducible nitric oxide synthase), Cox-2 (cycloxygenase-2), sPLA$_2$ (group IIA secretory phospholipase A2), UCP (uncoupling protein) 1/3, AdipoR1/R2 (adiponectin receptor 1/2), 11β-HSD1 (11-beta-hydroxysteroid dehydrogenase 1), VEGF-A (vascular endothelial growth factor A)

Gene	Function	Direction	Ref
	Lipid biosynthesis and cholesterol metabolism		
SR-B1	HDL-receptor involved in reverse cholesterol transport	↑ LXRE	[85]
FPPS	Cholesterol synthesis	↑ LXRE	[138]
AKR1-B7	side-chain cleavage of cholesterol; the first step of steroidogenesis	↑ LXRE	[139]
Cyp7α[a]	Rate-limiting enzyme in the conversion of cholesterol to bile acids.	↑ LXRE	[36]
I-BABP	Cholesterol metabolism; binds bile acid	↑ LXRE[b]	[20]
CETP	Mediates transfer of cholesterol esters from HDL to triglyceride rich lipoproteins	↑ LXRE	[97]
PLTP	Transfer phospholipids from triglyceride-rich lipoproteins to HDL	↑	[96]
ApoAIV	Facilitates lipid and cholesterol transport particularly in intestines	↑ LXRE	[93]
ApoAV	Involved in plasma triglyceride metabolism	↓	[94]
ApoC-I/IV/II	Cofactor for LPL in hydrolysis of triglyceride	↑ LXRE	[91]
ApoD	Facilitates lipid and cholesterol transport	↑ LXRE	[75]
ApoE	Facilitates cholesterol efflux outside the enterohepatic axis	↑ LXRE	[91,92]
ABCA1	Mediates the active efflux of cholesterol and phospholipids from cells to apolipoproteins	↑ LXRE	[43,87–89]
ABCG1	Mediates the active efflux of cholesterol and phospholipids from cells to apolipoproteins	↑	[90]
ABCG4	Cellular transmembrane transport of endogenous lipid substrates	↑	[140]
ABCG5/8	Important role in entero-hepatic sterol transport	↑	[86]
SREBP1c	Transcription factor that regulates expression of lipogenic enzymes	↑ LXRE	[68–70]
FAS	Catalyzes the formation of long-chain fatty acids from acetyl-CoA	↑ LXRE	[72]
ACC	Carboxylation of acetyl-CoA to malonyl-CoA for the synthesis of long-chain fatty acids	↑ T3RE[c]	[71]
SCD-1/2	Rate-limiting enzyme in the cellular synthesis of monounsaturated fatty acids from saturated fatty acids that is an important step in producing triglycerides	↑	[67,77,78]

Table 1 (*continued*)

Gene	Function	Direction	Ref
Angptl3	A family member of the secreted growth factor angiopoietins involved in synthesis of triglycerides	↑ LXRE	[80]
Spot14	Fatty acid biosynthesis	↑	[75]
LPL	Hydrolyzes triglycerides in circulating large lipoproteins	↑ LXRE	[76]
LXRα	Autoregulation	↑ LXRE	[33,34,141]
PPARγ	Nuclear receptor particularly involved in adipocytes	↑ LXRE	[106]
FTF	Nuclear receptor with multiple functions – also involved in cholesterol metabolism	↑ LXRE	[142]
SHP	Atypical nuclear receptor that antagonize signaling of several other nuclear receptors	↑ LXRE	[84]
	Carbohydrate metabolism		
PEPCK	Gluconeogenic enzyme	↓	[59,61,62]
Fbp1	Gluconeogenic enzyme	↓	[59]
G6P	Gluconeogenic enzyme	↓	[59,61,62]
PGC1	Coactivator involved in gluconeogenesis	↓	[62]
Pfkfb3	Glycolytic enzyme	↓	[59]
PDK4	Glycolysis inhibitor	↑	[59]
GK	Stimulates glycolysis and glycogen synthesis	↑	[62]
GLUT1	Glucose transporter	↑	[65]
GLUT4	Glucose transporter	↑ LXRE	[59,62,64]
	Inflammatory response		
TNFα	Pro-inflammatory cytokine	↑/↓ LXRE	[111,143]
IL-6	Pro-inflammatory cytokine	↓	[113]
INOS	Inflammatory mediator	↓	[113]
Cox-2	Inflammatory mediator	↓	[113]
sPLA$_2$	Inflammatory mediator	↑ LXRE	[115]
SPα	Anti-apoptotic factor involved in immune responses	↑ LXRE	[32]
	Energy homeostasis		
UCP-1/3	Proton carrier in the mitochondrial membrane	↓	[59,78]
	Others		
AdipoR1/R2	Receptor for adiponectin a hormone secreted by adipocytes with multiple biological functions	↑	[137]
Renin	Generate angiotensin from angiotensinogen, initiating a cascade of reactions that produces an elevation of blood pressure and increased sodium retention by the kidney.	↑ CNRE[d]	[19]
c-myc	Transcription factor that seems to activate the transcription of growth-related genes.	↑ CNRE[d]	[19]
11β-HSD1	Catalyzes the conversion of inactive cortisone to active cortisol	↓	[60]
VEGF-A	Growth factor particularly involved in angiogenesis	↑ LXRE	[144]
Fra1, JunD, cFos	Transcription factors of the Fos and Jun family making up the AP1 complexes binding AP1 elements	↑	[145]

[a]Not directly LXR regulated in humans (84).
[b]LXR binds via a FXR response element.
[c]LXR is involved in a complex that binds a thyroid hormone (triiodothyronine, T3) response element.
[d]Response to LXR mediated through a cis-acting DNA element (CNRE).

LXR response element where LXRα binds as a monomer has also been reported [18,19]. The human intestinal bile acid binding protein (I-BABP) was induced by LXR via an IR1 (inverted repeat) FXRE, introducing a novel response element for the LXRs [20].

Principally, ligand-activated NRs bind to their cognate response element, which then interact with several coactivator complexes to activate transcription. In contrast unliganded NRs interact with corepressors complexes to repress transcription, however, other mechanisms also exist [21]. Numerous cofactor proteins have been identified as participants of transcriptional complexes that mediate the transcriptional activity of NRs on target genes but few findings have reported LXR-cofactor interactions. LXRα interacts with the atypical NR SHP that lacks a DBD and works as one of the few repressors of ligand-activated NRs [22]. Furthermore, LXRα was shown to interact with the PPARγ coactivator 1α (PGC-1α) leading to increased LXRα-mediated transactivation [23]. The coactivator activating signal cointegrator 2 (ASC-2) (also called nuclear receptor-activating protein 250 (RAP250)) [24] contains an NR box (nuclear receptor box; interaction surface present in cofactors), which selectively binds the LXRs, but not any other of the NRs [25]. Transgenic mice that express a fragment of RAP250 encompassing this selective NR box in the liver showed accumulation of cholesterol, the same phenotype as observed in LXRα$^{-/-}$ mice. This indicates an important physiological role of the LXRα–RAP250 interaction in cholesterol metabolism. Both steroid receptor coactivator -1 (SRC-1) and receptor interacting protein 140 (RIP140) were shown to interact with LXRβ in a ligand dependent manner [26]. However, ligand dependency was more pronounced for SRC-1 than RIP140. They could not bind simultaneously and the interaction was competitive i.e. excess of one factor replaced the other and vice versa. The SRC-1, SRC-2 (GRIP1), p300 and CREB-binding protein (CBP) coactivators interacts with LXRα on the identified LXRE in the human ABCA1 promoter and induce transcriptional activity of LXRα [27]. Vitamin D receptor-interacting protein (DRIP), a member of the mediator complex, is also recruited by LXRα [28]. Whereas LXRα showed a strong interaction with both nuclear corepressor (NCoR) and silencing mediator for retinoid and thyroid hormone receptor (SMRT), a weak interaction was observed between LXRβ and NCoR or SMRT in mammalian two-hybrid assays and chromatin immunoprecipitating assays [29,30]. Both the NRs showed a preference for NCoR over SMRT. Furthermore, the recruitment of the corepressors only led to repressed mRNA expression of ABCA1, but not SREBP1c, indicating promoter specific activities of the LXRs. Another study has indicated different transactivation potentials on common target genes as well as the existence of different target genes of the two LXR paralogs [31]. A plausible explanation for this might be found in the different affinity toward transcriptional comodulators and/or different affinity of the two paralogs to LXREs [32–34]. Although still poorly investigated these observations open a multitude of possibilities to modulate LXR signaling with specific drugs targeting LXR-cofactor interactions.

1.3. *LXR agonists and antagonists*

Only a few natural and potent LXR agonists have been identified. Both LXR paralogs are activated upon binding of certain mono-oxygenated cholesterol derivatives (oxysterols). These are suggested to be natural ligands for the LXRs with 22(R)-hydroxycholesterol, 24(S)-hydroxycholesterol and 24(S),25-epoxycholesterol and 20(S)-hydroxycholesterol being the most potent natural activators of the LXRs [35–37]. Binding assays showed that these oxysterols bind directly to either of the LXR paralogs at physiological concentrations that occure *in vivo* [38]. 24(S),25-epoxycholesterol and 20(S)-hydroxycholesterol are highly abundant in the liver where both cholesterol metabolism and LXR expression is high, 22(R)-hydroxycholesterol is an intermediate of steroid hormone production and 24(S)-hydroxycholesterol is the main oxysterol present in brain. The oxysterol 27-hydroxycholesterol, produced in macrophages in response to cholesterol loading, has also been identified as an endogenous LXR ligand [39].

In addition to the natural oxysterols described above the 24(S),25-epoxycholesterol, highly abundant in liver, is also a potent activator of the LXRs [36]. While none of these oxysterols show any bias toward any of the LXR paralogs, three LXRα selective compounds were identified; 5,6-24(S),25-diepoxycholesterol, 6α-hydroxy bile acid and cholestenoic acid [38,40,41], but the physiological significance of these observations have not been elucidated. Acetyl podocarpic dimer (APD) [42], T0901317 [43] and GW3965 [44] are synthetic ligands which activate both LXR paralogs where the two latter ones have been widely used in studies to characterize biological functions of the LXRs. GW3965 activate LXRα has a lower transcription potential in liver than T0901317 activated LXRα, probably because of their difference in recruiting coactivators [28] while in other tissues activation by either two compounds were similar. The GW3965 agonist was shown to raise HDL-bound cholesterol without increasing hepatic triglyceride levels while the T0901317 agonist induced both. However, the T0901317 agonist has been shown to activate FXR as well [45]. Another synthetic oxysterol compound, N,N-dimethyl-3β-hydroxycholenamide (DMHCA), was proposed as a gene selective LXR agonist [46]. The agonist selectively induced transcriptional activation of the ABCA1 but not SREBP-1c, thus, inducing reverse cholesterol transport from macrophages and reduced cholesterol absorption from intestines but avoiding increased plasma triglyceride levels. Paxilline, a natural non-oxysterol fungal metabolite that inhibits calcium-activated potassium channels, was identified as an agonist for both LXRs [47]. 1-pyridyl hydantoin (1-PH), a small synthetic compound, was proposed as a LXRα selective agonist that does not alter the transactivation potential of LXRβ [48]. In a cell-based reporter gene assay the plant sterol sigmasterol but not sitosterol, induced transcriptional activation of LXRα [49].

Several compounds with antagonistic effect have been reported. Polyunsaturated fatty acids are competitive inhibitors to LXR ligands, antagonizing LXR activity [50,51] by inhibiting binding of the RXR/LXR heterodimer to the LXRE, while geranylgeranyl pyrophosphate disrupts interaction between coactivators and the

LXRs leading to the inhibition of LXR transcriptional activity [37,52]. Oxidized cholesterol sulfates found in human plasma can act as antagonists of the LXRs by disrupting coactivator recruitment [53]. It was shown that fibrate esters bound the LXRs and antagonize the receptors while fibrate acids did not [54]. However, the fibrate acids bound PPARα. Fenofibrate, a PPARα agonist used clinically to treat hypertriglyceridemia, antagonized LXR-induced mRNA expression of hepatic lipogenic genes, but not ABCA1 mRNA. Thus, addition of a acid/ester moiety to fibrates acts as a chemical switch regulating specificity for PPARα versus the LXRs.

Crystal structures of the human LBD of LXRβ binding the naturally occurring 24(S),25-epoxycholesterol, the T0901317 compound or the GW3965 compound revealed a large and flexible ligand-binding pocket [55,56]. These findings indicated that a variety of structurally different compounds can act as ligands for the LXRs. Similar observations were made when the crystal structure of the LXRα-RXRβ heterodimer was resolved [57]. The ligand-binding pockets of the LXRα and LXRβ suggested a common anchoring of the oxysterols to essential amino acids in the pockets. Moreover, comparisons of LXRα and LXRβ showed very similar ligand-binding features indicating that the development of a selection of selective LXR agonists can be challenging. More detailed information will be available when the three-dimensional crystal structures of the full-length receptors have been analysed. However, structure analysis of the *Drosophila* EcR (the closest NR to LXR in sequence homology) showed that the ligand-binding pocket adopted different structural conformations to different ligands that could not be predicted by molecular modeling and docking studies [58]. This implies that large scale screening of putative LXR ligands is the only way to pick up all possible agonists and antagonists for the LXRs. Amino acid 267 in the ligand-binding pocket of LXRα was shown to be important for mediating the antagonistic effect of polyunsaturated fatty acids [57] providing vital information for the process of developing LXR antagonists.

2. LXR signaling in carbohydrate metabolism

The first reports suggesting an important role of the LXRs in carbohydrate metabolism came from genome wide expression profiling studies, a very powerful method to discover genes responsive to a particular treatment or genes differently expressed in two or more samples. This method was used to identify putative LXR target genes in mice and resulted in the identification of several novel LXR target genes [59,60]. Feeding mice an LXR agonist significantly inhibited mRNA expression of gluconeogenic enzymes in liver including phosphoenolpyruvate carboxykinase (PEPCK) (the rate-limiting enzyme in gluconeogenesis), fructose 1,6-biphosphatase 1 (FBP1) and glucose-6-phosphatase (G6P), indicating that the LXRs might suppress hepatic gluconeogenesis. These studies also indicated the involvement of the LXRs in various aspects of glucose metabolism in white and brown adipose tissue as mRNA expression of several glycolytic genes was suppressed and the mRNA expression of the glucose transporter gene, GLUT4, was induced in these tissues.

Several excellent reports were soon published emphasizing the physiological consequences on carbohydrate metabolism of administrating LXR agonists to rodents. Diabetic mice (db/db mice), insulin resistant Zucker diabetic fatty (ZDF) rats (fa/fa rats) as well as wild type C57BL/6 mice were used to investigate *in vivo* effects of an LXR agonist [61]. Activating the LXRs significantly decreased glucose levels in db/db mice and improved insulin sensitivity in insulin-resistant rats but did not cause hypoglycemia in normal mice. Glucose output was dramatically reduced from liver samples isolated from ZDF rats treated with an LXR agonist consistent with a significant decrease in mRNA expression of gluconeogenetic enzymes including PEPCK, G6P, pyruvate carboxylase and fructose 1,6-biphosphatase 1. Another study showed that treatment of murine models of diet-induced obesity and insulin resistance with an LXR agonist improved glucose tolerance significantly compared to untreated controls [62]. Convincingly, mRNA expression of gluconeogenetic enzymes including PEPCK, G6P and PGC1α was suppressed while mRNA expression of glucokinase, which promotes glucose utilization, was induced in livers of these mice. Improved glucose tolerance in LXR agonist-treated db/db mice has later been confirmed [63]. The insulin sensitivity was not changed in these mice as was observed in insulin resistant ZDF rats mentioned above, likely due to the lipogenic promoting aspects for the drug. LXRβ$^{-/-}$ mice, but not LXRα$^{-/-}$ mice are glucose intolerant due to impaired insulin secretion of pancreatic β-cells of LXRβ$^{-/-}$ mice [64]. This is in agreement with a study showing that activated LXRs increase glucose-induced insulin secretion by pancreatic β-cells [65] Intriguingly, LXRα$^{-/-}$LXRβ$^{-/-}$ mice are not glucose intolerant indicating that absence of LXRα rescues this phenotype observed in LXRβ$^{-/-}$ mice [64,66]. These observations strongly indicate that the LXRs are involved in many processes of carbohydrate metabolism.

The insulin sensitive glucose transporter GLUT4 is also under transcriptional control of LXR in white adipose tissue [62,67]. An LXR agonist induced mRNA expression of GLUT4 via an LXRE identified in the promoter of the *glut4* gene. Basal mRNA expression of GLUT4 was decreased in LXRα$^{-/-}$ mice but not LXRβ$^{-/-}$ and LXRα$^{-/-}$LXRβ$^{-/-}$ mice and insulin-induced expression of GLUT4 was dependent on LXRα. There was also less LXRα mRNA expressed in the liver of obese ZDF rats than in lean ZDF rats. This is also seen for GLUT4 mRNA suggesting that low expression level of LXRα might lead to suppressed expression of GLUT4. Furthermore, the LXR agonist also improved glucose uptake in NIH-3T3 adipocytes [62] and activation of ectopically expressed LXRα in NIH-3T3 adipocytes resulted in increased synthesis of glycogen [68]. Overexpression and activation of LXRα increased basal uptake of glucose in the NIH-3T3 adipocytes cell line [68] probably mediated mainly through the GLUT1 glucose transporter as GLUT1 mRNA expression as well as protein levels was induced by treatment with an LXR agonist. This was not seen in a cell line without overexpression of LXRα or in white adipose tissue from mice fed an LXR agonist [62].

Skeletal muscle constitutes 40% of the human body weight and is the major site for glucose utilization and lipid oxidation. Both LXRα and a subset of LXR target genes are induced during myogenesis and activation of the LXRs led to induction of genes involved in cholesterol metabolism as well as efflux of intracellular cholesterol

[69]. Furthermore, activated LXRs increase glucose uptake, glucose oxidation and GLUT4 expression as well as lipid metabolism in muscle cells [70] suggesting an important role(s) of LXRs in muscle cells.

The above effects seen using an LXR agonist are also seen in response to insulin and in line with this it was observed that mRNA expression of LXRα was induced in livers of rats injected with insulin as well as in insulin-treated primary heptocytes [71]. mRNA expression of several insulin target genes involved in lipogenesis in livers from LXRα$^{-/-}$LXRβ$^{-/-}$ mice were non-responsive to insulin treatment. This observation indicates that LXRα is a mediator of insulin action on lipogenic enzymes. The physiological importance of LXR in carbohydrate metabolism is clearly demonstrated in these studies. They show that the LXRs suppress gluconeogenesis, increase glucose uptake and is possibly involved in intra-cellular utilization of glucose and glycogen production; all of which speaks in favor of an important anti-diabetic effect of LXR.

3. LXR signaling in lipid and cholesterol metabolism

3.1. *Lipid and triglyceride biosynthesis*

There is a large body of evidence that activation of the LXRs leads to increased lipid and triglyceride production rendering the LXRs as important lipogenic factors. Administration of an LXR agonist to both mice and hamsters increased plasma and hepatic triglyceride levels as well as plasma phospholipid levels. This was accompanied with increased mRNA expression of sterol regulatory element-binding protein-1 (SREBP-1), acetyl CoA carboxylase (ACC), fatty acid synthase (FAS) and stearoyl CoA desaturase (SCD-1) [72]. SREBP-1c (a splice variant of the srebp1 gene) is a lipogenic transcription factor, which under conditions of lipid demand, induces expression of several enzymes in the lipogenic program including ACC, FAS and SCD-1. All of these enzymes are also induced by LXR in keeping with the identification of LXREs in the gene-promoter regions of ACC and FAS [59,72–77]. Increased plasma and hepatic triglyceride levels have also been reported in both the diabetic mice (db/db mice) and in the insulin-resistant ZDF rats after administration of an LXR agonist [61]. Basal serum and hepatic triglyceride levels were dramatically reduced in LXRα$^{-/-}$LXRβ$^{-/-}$ mice and LXR-induced triglyceride levels are completely abolished in these mice as was the induction of lipogenic enzymes by administration of an LXR agonist [72]. LXRα$^{-/-}$ mice fed a high cholesterol diet had significantly lower hepatic triglyceride levels compared to wild type mice but serum triglyceride levels were unchanged between the mice strains [78]. Reduced serum triglycerides, triglycerides in lipoproteins and triglycerides in tissues were observed in LXRα$^{-/-}$LXRβ$^{-/-}$ but not LXRα$^{-/-}$ or LXRβ$^{-/-}$ mice compared to wild type mice when these mice were fed a normal diet [79]. Moreover, increased levels of non-esterified fatty acids (NEFA) and glycerol were observed in serum and cell growth medium after treatment of wild type mice or the NIH-3T3 adipocyte cell line with an

LXR agonist, respectively. Thus in-cellulo and *in vivo* data suggest lipolysis in adipocytes is mediated via LXR activation [68].

Other LXR target genes involved in lipid and triglyceride biosynthesis and metabolism have been identified (Table 1). These genes include *spot14* in adipocytes, implicated in lipogenesis [80], and lipoprotein lipase (*lpl*) in liver and macrophages but not in adipose tissue and muscle [81]. LPL is a key enzyme for lipoprotein metabolism and is responsible for the hydrolysis of triglycerides in circulating lipoproteins leading to the release of free fatty acids to peripheral tissues. In liver, LPL is also believed to promote uptake of high-density lipoprotein (HDL)-cholesterol.

The LXR-induced mRNA expression of SCD-1 and SCD-2 [82,83] and proper control of these enzymes might be highly important for triglyceride production. The SCDs are the rate-limiting enzymes in the conversion of saturated fatty acids to monounsaturated fatty acids, an important step in the generation of triglycerides. Increased SCD activity leads to high levels of plasma triglycerides, which has been linked to the development of cardiovascular disease and obesity. Obese hyperglycemic mice (ob/ob mice) have an elevated activity of SCD and higher depositions of body fats compared to their lean counterparts. In type 2 diabetes SCD activity is increased, probably in response to increased levels of insulin [84]. SCD might therefore significantly contribute to hyperlipidemia often seen in diabetes. The LXRs also induced mRNA expression of the angiopoietin-like protein 3 (Angptl3) [85]. Angptl3 facilitates synthesis of triglycerides and in the KK/San mouse strain, which has low levels of plasma triglycerides, total cholesterol and NEFAs due to a mutation in the *angptl3* gene, overexpression of Angptl3 resulted in increased circulating levels of plasma cholesterol, triglycerides and NEFAs [86]. It is clear that triglyceride production and both serum and tissue triglyceride levels are elevated by activation of LXR via induced expression of key lipogenic enzymes. However, it was reported that elevated plasma triglyceride levels and induced hepatic mRNA expression of the lipogenic enzymes are transient in response to an LXR agonist [77]. Administration of an LXR agonist to C57BL/6 mice for 3 days significantly increased plasma triglyceride levels and hepatic mRNA expression of FAS and SREBP-1c, which, surprisingly, was almost diminished after 7 days. While plasma triglyceride levels normalized after 7 days and stayed normal for up to 4 weeks, another study reported increased hepatic triglyceride accumulation in response to an LXR agonist persistent for 4 weeks in C57BLKS/J mice [63]. Moreover, administration of an LXR agonist led to a much higher increase in plasma cholesterol, phospholipids, and triacylglycerol in db/db mice than normal C57BLKS/J mice. These observations point toward exacerbated lipogenic effects of the LXRs when the physiological conditions of the mice are changed. This is an important observation and if this holds true for humans with metabolic disturbances, the LXRs are attractive drug targets for the treatment of these conditions.

3.2. *Cholesterol metabolism*

Gene targeted deletion of the *lxra* and *lxrb* genes have severe implications on hepatic cholesterol metabolism and transport of cholesterol in the body. Impaired mRNA expression of hepatic genes involved in cholesterol and fatty acid metabolism like cholesterol 7α-hydroxylase (Cyp7α), hydroxymethyl glutaryl–coenzyme A (HMG–CoA) synthase/reductase, farnesyl pyrophosphate synthase (FPPS), squalene synthase, SREBPs, SCD1 and FAS was seen in LXRα$^{-/-}$ mice [78]. When fed a high cholesterol diet LXRα$^{-/-}$ mice fail to induce transcription of Cyp7α, the rate-limiting enzyme in bile acid synthesis from cholesterol leading to accumulation of large amounts of cholesterol in the liver, with impaired hepatic function as a consequence. This phenotype was not observed in LXRβ$^{-/-}$ mice [87]. However, several lines of evidence suggest that there are differences between how species regulate conversion and clearance of hepatic cholesterol. In mice, the LXRs induce mRNA expression of CYP7α via an LXRE in the promoter [36] promoting conversion of cholesterol to bile acids while FXR suppresses bile acid synthesis by inhibiting expression of the same enzyme. FXR induces expression of SHP leading to inhibition of LRH-1, where the latter is necessary for expression of Cyp7α [12]. No functional LXRE has been identified in the gene promoter of human Cyp7α but, surprisingly, LXRα suppresses the mRNA expression of human Cyp7α, opposite to what was observed in mouse [88,89]. Furthermore, LXRα induced the mRNA expression of SHP in humans, but not in rodents suggesting completely different pathways of LXR signaling on the conversion of hepatic cholesterol to bile acids in rodents and humans. Hence, observations and conclusions made in rodent models do not necessarily reflect the metabolic processes occurring in humans.

How the circulating blood cholesterol are distributed in the various apolipoprotein particles is also affected by LXR signaling. An increase in LDL cholesterol content and a decrease in HDL cholesterol content was observed in LXRα$^{-/-}$ and LXR-α$^{-/-}$β$^{-/-}$ but not LXRβ$^{-/-}$ mice [79] while administration of an LXR agonist to wild type C57BL/6 mice led to increased total plasma cholesterol, mainly in HDL particles [72]. Uptake of cholesterol in the liver is facilitated by the LXRs as expression of the HDL-receptor, scavenger receptor-B1 (SR-B1), in humans is induced by the LXRs via an LXRE in its promoter [90]. Taken together these observations indicate that the LXRs control circulating cholesterol levels in the blood and hepatic conversion of cholesterol to bile acid; a process also involving LXR-induced expression of transmembrane transporters, lipid exchange proteins and apolipoproteins.

3.3. *Lipid and cholesterol transport*

Dietary lipid and cholesterol are transported via chylomicrons, produced in the intestines, to other peripheral tissues including muscle and adipose tissue. The remnant chylomicron particle is then taken up by the liver. In addition, the liver supplies peripheral tissue with lipids and cholesterol via VLDL and LDL particles (Fig. 2). The transport of cholesterol from peripheral tissues to the liver via pre-HDL and HDL particles are called reverse cholesterol transport. Transport and exchange of lipids and cholesterol between lipoprotein particles as well as between lipoprotein particles and tissues involves many different genes and some of these have been identified as LXR target genes.

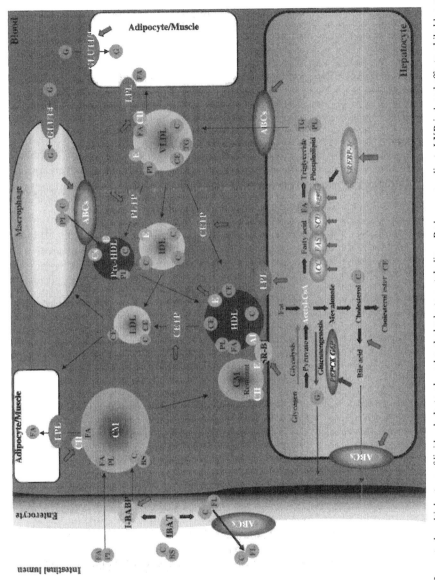

Fig. 2. The LXRs control multiple steps of lipid-, cholesterol- and carbohydrate metabolism. Red arrows indicate LXR induced effects while blue arrows indicate LXR repressed effects. C: cholesterol, CE: cholesterol ester, FA: fatty acid, PL: phospholipid, TG: triglyceride, BS: bile salt, G: glucose, AI: apolipoprotein AI, Cs: apolipoprotein C-I/C-IV/ C-II, C-II: apolipoprotein C-II, E: apolipoprotein E. See text for further details. See Plate 1 in Colour Plate Section.

Numerous observations show that the LXRs induce mRNA expression of many family members of the ATP-binding cassette (ABC) transmembrane transporters that facilitate unidirectional substrate translocation across the lipid bilayer membrane. Administration of an LXR agonist induced mRNA expression of ABCA1- and ABCG5/8 in the intestines leading to decreased cholesterol absorption from the intestinal lumen while LXR agonist induced ABCA5/8 in the liver led to increased biliary cholesterol levels [43,91]. Treatment with an LXR agonist also induced mRNA expression of ABCA1 and ABCG1 in many tissues facilitating efflux of cholesterol and phospholipids [43,83,92–95]. Transport of lipid and cholesterol between tissues depends on various apolipoproteins, which are associated with different lipoprotein particles. Both apoE mRNA levels which aids cholesterol efflux from cells outside the enterohepatic axis [96,97] and the ApoC-I/C-IV/C-II mRNA levels which are involved in hydrolysis of triglycerides [96] are induced by an LXR agonist. Moreover, apoD mRNA levels whose potential physiological ligands are cholesterol and certain fatty acids is an LXR target gene in adipose tissue [80] and apoAIV mRNA levels which is highly expressed in intestines and believed to be involved in lipid absorption to chylomicrons [98] are induced by activation of the LXRs. Hepatic mRNA expression and plasma levels of apoAV was reduced in response to treatment with an LXR agonist mediated via the SREBP-1c signaling pathway [99]. Reduced apoAV levels have been associated with increased plasma triglyceride levels [100] providing yet another mechanism for the elevated triglyceride levels seen when challenging LXR signaling. Expression of the HDL associated phospholipid transfer protein (PLTP) and cholesterol ester transport protein (CETP) is induced by activation of the LXRs [101,102]. PLTP primarily transports phospholipids and apolipoproteins from triglyceride rich lipoproteins to HDL particles while CETP facilitates transfer of lipids, cholesterol esters and triglycerides between lipoproteins [103]. Hence, the LXRs are important players in reverse cholesterol transport mechanisms.

4. The LXRs control energy homeostasis

Most animal species have the ability to convert excess dietary nutrients into high-energy stores such as fat and then utilize the fat as an energy source in times of need. This important feature for survival is also a major cause of obesity and increased risk of developing diabetes and its disorders. Recent observations suggest that LXRβ is an important player in the control of energy metabolism. Adipose tissues of LXR$\beta^{-/-}$ mice have reduced weight and mice lacking LXRβ do not increase adipocyte fat storage when fed a high fat diet [64]. Expression of UCP-1 is highly induced in adipose tissue of LXR$\beta^{-/-}$ mice leading to increased energy expenditure by UCP-1 mediated uncoupling of mitochondria which is in concordance with reports that activation of the LXRs lead to suppressed expression of UCP-1 [59,104]. These observations indicate that increased UCP-1 expression and, hence, increased energy expenditure in LXR$\beta^{-/-}$ mice may protect against diet-induced obesity. However, increased fat depots in non-adipose tissue were observed in LXR$\beta^{-/-}$ mice and total body fat was not reduced in these mice. Interestingly, it seems that cholesterol is a prerequisite constituent in the diet for the resistance to diet-induced obesity as a high lipid diet without high cholesterol does not protect LXR deficient mice against obesity [66]. An increase in UCP-1 expression was also seen in skeletal muscle of LXR$\alpha^{-/-}$LXR$\beta^{-/-}$ mice and uncoupled respiration was increased in skeletal muscle fibers. LXR$\alpha^{-/-}$LXR$\beta^{-/-}$ mice also have increased oxygen consumption, however, there was no increase in plasma levels of ketone bodies. This confirms that increased energy consumption take place in peripheral tissues, not in liver [66]. Surprisingly, expression of UCP-1 was not observed in brown adipose tissue. Taken together, these observations suggest that the LXRs are involved in controlling energy homeostasis, probably via transcriptional control of UCP-1 expression in adipose tissue and muscle [66].

5. The LXRs are anti-atherosclerotic and anti-inflammatory factors

An increased risk of developing atherosclerosis and subsequent cardiovascular disease as well as development of type 2 diabetes is often observed over time in obese individuals. Although incompletely assessed, both lowering lipid and carbohydrate intake in severely obese individuals seem beneficiary to reduce atherosclerosis [105,106]. These are processes in which the LXRs are highly involved and several observations speak in favor of the LXRs as anti-atherogenic factors. As described above, the LXRs induce reverse cholesterol transport from peripheral tissue by stimulating the production of apolipoproteins and ABC-transporters. Pre-HDL particles are loaded with cholesterol to form HDL particles. Cholesterol is then transported to the liver via HDL-cholesterol-mediated uptake, converted to bile acids and finally excess cholesterol and/or bile acids are transferred to the intestinal lumen for excretion out of the body. The LXR-induced removal of cholesterol via reverse cholesterol transport from macrophages has been proposed to be of principal importance in reducing the development of atherosclerosis.

One of the first indications that the LXRs might be involved in atherosclerosis came from a study in which an activator of RXR was shown to reduce development of atherosclerosis and that an LXR agonist induced mRNA expression of ABCA1 in macrophages from wild type mice but not from LXR$\alpha^{-/-}$LXR$\beta^{-/-}$ mice [107]. Furthermore, transplantation of macrophages from LXR$\alpha^{-/-}$LXR$\beta^{-/-}$ mice into two different murine models of atherosclerosis (LDLR$^{-/-}$ and apoE$^{-/-}$ mice) led to a significant increase of atherosclerosis in both mice strains [108]. Other studies corroborated these observations in which significant decreases in atherosclerotic lesions were seen in the aorta of both LDLR$^{-/-}$ and apoE$^{-/-}$ murine atherosclerotic models treated with an LXR agonist and mRNA expression of both ABCA1 and ABCG1 was induced in the lesions and macrophages [109,110]. It was shown that oxidized LDL was taken up by the CD36 receptor in macrophages, which subsequently presented lipid components in the cells that activated PPARγ. PPARγ then induced expression of CD36 pointing toward a feed forward mechanism of PPARγ, accelerating macrophage foam cell formation. Surprisingly, PPARγ also activated

LXRα signaling that led to reverse cholesterol transport [111]. A response element for PPAR (PPRE) was identified in both the mouse and human lxra genes [33,111] and an LXRE was identified in the promoter of the *pparg* gene [112] indicating a reciprocal action of LXRα and PPARγ. Another indirect mechanism of cross-talk also exists. Activated PPARγ in macrophages upregulated Cyp27 activity leading to production of 27-hydroxycholesterol from cholesterol [113]. 27-hydroxycholesterol is an activator of LXR, which in turn activated downstream effects of LXR signaling (Fig. 3). Together with the anti-inflammatory effects of the LXRs (see below) these observations provide a teasing model for drug discovery to develop drugs that selectively activate LXR signaling in machrophages.

Atherosclerotic processes are often associated with inflammatory processes mediated partly by macrophages located in the lesions [114]. Several elegant studies have reported anti-inflammatory effects of the LXRs proposed to be beneficial for reducing development of atherosclerosis. The anti-inflammatory effect of the LXRs might prove to be important to prevent or at least attenuate the progress of type 1 Diabetes, an autoimmune disease in which pro-inflammatory cytokines including interferon γ (INFγ), tumor necrosis factor α (TNFα) and interleukin-4 (IL-4) play important roles. Inflammatory responses, particularly by TNFα, have been linked to increased insulin resistance and several studies in rodent models have revealed that manipulation of the cytokine network can delay or prevent diabetes. There are also indications that chronic inflammation leads to a condition of insulin insensitivity with TNFα having a central role [115,116]. Mechanistically, it has been suggested that TNFα may downregulate genes required for insulin action but the molecular mechanisms behind this are far from fully understood. The LXRs have anti-inflammatory effects in models of contact dermatitis in rodents. Addition of an LXR agonist on foci of the skin showed inhibited production of TNFα and interleukin-1α (IL-1α). It was also reported that an LXR agonist induced TNFα in macrophages and primary monocytes [117] so the effect of the LXRs on TNFα remains equivocal. The LXRs inhibit mRNA expression of the matrix metalloproteinase 9 (MMP9) in macrophages [118]. MMP9 is a endopeptidase induced by pro-inflammatory signals which is necessary for adequate immune response and cell migration. Transcriptional profiling of lipopolysaccharide-induced macrophages showed an LXR dependent downregulation of the expression of inflammatory mediators such as cyclooxygenase-2 (COX-2), inducible nitric oxide synthase (iNOS) and IL-6 [119]. The inhibitory effect of the LXRs were due to interference and crosstalk with the transcription factor NF-kB on target promoters. Furthermore, toll-like receptor (TLR) signaling, via TLR3 and TLR4, inhibited induction of LXR induced target genes [120]. The molecular mechanism underlying this cross-talk seems to be competition for cofactors between LXR and IRF3 on the common target promoters where IRF3 is the transcription factor mediating TLR3 and TLR4 signaling on the target genes. Moreover, it was proposed that LXRα has a more pronounced impact on anti-microbal responses in macrophages than LXRβ where LXRα regulates the innate immune response of macrophages in response to bacterial infection by *Listeria monocytogenes* (LM), a bacteria implicated in several food-borne human illnesses [32]. Infection by LM induced expression of LXRα, but not LXRβ. LXRα$^{-/-}$ and

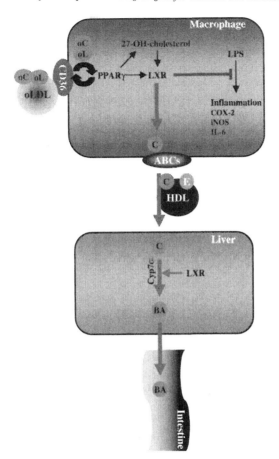

Fig. 3. The LXRs promote reverse cholesterol transport from peripheral tissues, including machrophages, to the liver. On machrophages oxidized LDL (oLDL) docks at the CD36 receptor off loading oxidized cholesterol (oC) and oxidized lipids (oL). OoL activates PPARγ which induces expression of CD36 further enhancing uptake of oC and oL. This indicates a pro-atherosclerotic effect of PPARγ also activates. However, PPARγ induces LXRα expression directly via a PPAR response element in the promoter of LXRα. It also activates the LXR by inducing expression of Cyp27 thereby producing the 27-hydroxy-cholesterol (27-OH-cholesterol) LXR agonist. Activated LXRs then induce expression of apoE and ABCA1 promoting efflux of intracellular cholesterol (C) to the HDL particle which transport cholesterol to the liver. In liver, the LXRs induce expression of Cyp7α which is the rate-limiting enzyme in the conversion of cholesterol to bile acid (BA) and subsequently BA is excreted out of the body via the intestines. Lipopolysaccaride (LPS), a highly potent inducer of inflammatory responses, induce expression of inflammatory responsive genes in macrophages including Cox-2, iNOS and IL-6. Activation of the LXRs suppresses the LPS-induced expression of these inflammatory mediators pointing towards an anti-inflammatory role of the LXR. Hence, the LXRs are both anti-atherosclerotic and anti-inflammatory mediators which suggest a positive effect of these receptors in terms of cardiovascular diseases. See Plate 2 in Colour Plate Section.

LXRα$^{-/-}$LXRβ$^{-/-}$ mice were more susceptible to infection than LXRβ$^{-/-}$ mice. An LXRE in the promoter of the anti-apoptotic factor SPα was preferably responsive to LXRα compared to LXRβ and the presence of LXRα and induction of SPα inhibited macrophage apoptosis, thereby promoting both macrophage survival and destruction of bacteria. This study adds to the growing line of evidence that the LXR paralogs have different biological activity, emphasizing the importance of developing LXR paralog-specific drugs. Surprisingly, the group IIA secretory phospholipase A2 (sPLA2), which is induced in inflammatory reactions seen in rheumatoid arthritis and atherosclerosis, is induced by the LXRs [121]. sPLA2 generates proinflammatory lipid mediators from phospholipids implying that LXR could mediate pro-inflammatory actions which is in sharp contrast to the other observations. These reports establishing the LXRs as, preferably, anti-inflammatory mediators open new and exciting prospects for therapeutic intervention of the highly complex inflammatory signaling network.

6. Cross-talk between the LXRs and other NRs regulates overall body homeostasis

There is a large and growing body of evidence that the LXRs work in concert with several other members of the NR family to control homeostatic processes in the body. The cross-talk between LXR- and PPAR signaling largely affect lipid and cholesterol metabolism in macrophages, adipocytes and liver as they reciprocally induce each others expression levels (described above). However, many studies support additional mechanisms of cross-talk between the LXRs and the PPARs. Coadministration of an LXR agonist and a PPARα agonist in mice led to synergistic elevation of HDL cholesterol [122]. Coadministration of a PPARα agonist did not normalize the increase in liver triglyceride levels caused by the LXR agonist. However, the PPARα agonist normalized plasma triglyceride levels increased by the LXR agonist. Interestingly, PPARα and the LXRs showed overlapping transcriptional programs in the liver where they regulate several common target genes involved in lipid and cholesterol metabolism [123]. Caloric restriction has been suggested to have beneficial effects on metabolic syndromes including obesity, diabetes and cardiovascular disease. Activation of both PPARα- and LXR signaling in mouse liver showed altered mRNA expression of several common genes. mRNA expression of these common genes were also altered in mice undergoing caloric restriction [124]. Thus, activation of PPARα and the LXRs in liver might mimic the effects of caloric restriction, at least at the gene expression level. While these observations suggest that LXRs and PPARα may have a common action on a set of liver genes, observations have also been made to suggest opposing effects of PPARα and LXR cross-talk. Coadministration of an LXR agonist in liver cells treated with a PPARα agonist reduced mRNA expression of PPARα target genes [125] and coadministration of a PPARα agonist in liver cells treated with an LXR agonist reduced mRNA expression of LXR targets genes such as SREBP-1c [126]. The inhibitory effects were most probably due to competition for their common heterodimeric partner retinoic X receptor (RXR) as overexpression of RXR attenuated the inhibitory effect. A direct interaction of PPARα–LXR generating an antagonizing heterodimer has also been proposed by several studies [125–129].

Glucocorticoids regulate a variety of metabolic processes in the body such as energy-, carbohydrate-, lipid- and cholesterol metabolism as well as inflammatory responses via activation of the GR [130]. Overactivity of the adrenal cortex generates high levels of glucocorticoids, as seen in Cushing's syndrome, and can lead to visceral obesity (central obesity or abdominal obesity) and metabolic disorders including hypertension, insulin resistance and diabetes [131]. Both $LXR\alpha^{-/-}LXR\beta^{-/-}$ mice and administration of an LXR agonist to wild type mice resulted in a dramatic increase in plasma corticosterone levels suggesting that these mice have a glucocorticoid profile resembling Cushing's syndrome [83]. However, contrary to developing visceral obesity which is often associated with elevated levels of glucocorticoids, LXR $\alpha^{-/-}LXR\beta^{-/-}$ mice did not develop visceral obesity but showed less peritoneal adipose tissue [132]. Although overall plasma levels of glucocorticoids are altered, the local action of glucocorticoids seems to be repressed by the LXRs. Conversion of inactive forms of glucocorticoids (cortisone in humans and 11-dehydrocorticosterone in rodents) to active forms (cortisol in humans and corticosterone in rodents) is enzymatically carried out by 11β-hydroxysteroid dehydrogenase type-1 (11β-HSD-1) while conversion of active forms to inactive forms of glucocorticoids are carried out by 11βHSD-2. Both mRNA levels and activity of 11β-HSD-1 is significantly suppressed by activated LXRs [60]. Higher basal mRNA levels and activity of 11β-HSD-1 is observed in visceral adipose tissue than in subcutaneous adipose tissue and [133] and overexpressing 11β-HSD-1 in adipocytes of mice yielded increased corticosterone levels in these adipocytes and subsequently development of visceral obesity, insulin resistance and diabetes in these mice [134]. Moreover, inhibition of 11β-HSD-1 activity in livers of humans increased insulin sensitivity [135]. The ability of the LXRs to repress 11β-HSD-1 suggests that the LXRs might prevent such a progression. These observations indicate a dual effect of the LXRs on glucocorticoid signaling. The anticipated increase in glucocorticoid signaling by the increased plasma glucocorticoid levels is antagonized in tissues expressing 11β-HSD-1 where glucocorticoid signaling is repressed by activated LXRs. In mice with targeted deletion of the *11bhsd1* gene local glucocorticoid effects in the liver of these mice were attenuated despite increased plasma glucocorticoid levels [136] indicating the importance of tissue specific control of glucocorticoid signaling. 11β-HSD-1 is expressed in several tissues but high expression is observed in adipose tissue and liver [137]. The LXRs are also highly expressed in adipose tissue and liver suggesting that the LXRs can suppress glucocorticoid signaling in these tissues.

Cross-talk with other NRs has also been described. For instance, estrogen signaling has been linked to reduced activity of LXR signaling which might have important effects in adipocytes tissue, liver and macrophages [138,139]. Cross-talk between LXR signaling and FXR signaling influences enterohepatic cholesterol and bile acid metabolism. Surprisingly, the LXRs bound to a previously identified FXR response element (a DR1 element) in the promoter of I-BABP leading to increased mRNA expression of I-BABP [20]. It was shown that the unliganded thyroid hormone receptor (TR) β1 isoform could bind to the LXRE in SERBP-1c and thereby inhibit

SREBP-1c induction by LXR signaling [140]. TRβ1 is ubiquitously expressed and the above observation indicates that cross-talk between thyroid hormone signaling and LXR signaling regulate lipid metabolism in tissues where both receptors are expressed. A comprehensive understanding of NR cross-talk would greatly enhance our ability to develop specific drugs for the various metabolic processes where NRs are involved.

7. Perspectives

The many roles of the LXRs including suppression of gluconeogenesis, reduced absorption of cholesterol from the intestines, induced reverse cholesterol transport, anti-atherosclerotic effect and anti-inflammatory effect make the LXRs highly interesting drug targets for therapeutic intervention and treatment of metabolic disorders. However, the increased fatty acid biosynthesis and triglyceride levels observed through activated LXR signaling are unwanted effects. Due to the partial different biological functions of the LXRs, future challenges in drug development would be to identify LXR-paralog specific drugs, tissue specific drugs or gene selective drugs. The pharmaceutical industry is very much engaged in screenings for putative drugs working through the LXRs. Few candidates have been reported and all without any accompanying clinical observations. As the ligand-binding pocket is very flexible and quite similar between LXRα and LXRβ, predicting putatitive drug candidates may be difficult and large high-throughput screenings may be the easiest way to identify such candidates.

The causality between development of type 2 diabetes and obesity, insulin resistance, hyperlipidemia, hyperglycemia as well as atherosclerosis is far from solved and we still do not know for certain what is the cause and what is the consequence in disease progression, but these are processes where modification of LXR signaling could be highly beneficial. The less common form, type 1 diabetes, is a multifactorial autoimmune disease characterized by serious damage of the insulin producing β-cells in the islet of Langerhans of the pancreas [141]. Hence, drugs targeting LXR signaling might prove beneficial in type 1 diabetes since there is a increasing amount of evidence that the LXRs mediate anti-inflammatory effects.

The observed beneficial effects of LXR are sometimes marginal and might not be enough to completely reverse the development of metabolic disorders. However, since these processes are probably both synergized and antagonized by additional NRs working in concert with the LXRs to regulate metabolic processes, modifying LXR signaling might be one important target in a mix of drugs for treatment of metabolic disorders including diabetes.

The interest in the LXRs has drastically increased during the last decade and as more research efforts are made, new and interesting biological functions of the LXR will surely emerge. For instance, reduced levels of the hormone adiponectin secreted from adipocytes has been linked to insulin resistance and obesity [142] and the LXRs were shown to induce receptors for adiponectin providing yet another mechanism for the LXRs to affect metabolic processes [143]. Moreover, association studies of single nucleotide polymorphisms (SNPs) in the LXR genes of patient with diabetes and its disorders versus case control groups will yield further insight into the pathophysiology of the LXRs. These and other future studies will add to the already existing evidence that the LXRs are highly valid drug targets for combating the epidemic development of metabolic disorders, particularly in the Western world.

References

[1] M. Robinson-Rechavi, H.E. Garcia, V. Laudet, The nuclear receptor superfamily, J. Cell Sci. 116 (2003) 585–586.

[2] H. Escriva, F. Delaunay, V. Laudet, Ligand binding and nuclear receptor evolution, Bioessays 22 (2000) 717–727.

[3] J.M. Olefsky, Nuclear receptor minireview series, J. Biol. Chem. 276 (2001) 36863–36864.

[4] R. Apfel, D. Benbrook, E. Lernhardt, M.A. Ortiz, G. Salbert, M. Pfahl, A novel orphan receptor specific for a subset of thyroid hormone-responsive elements and its interaction with the retinoid/thyroid hormone receptor subfamily, Mol. Cell. Biol. 14 (1994) 7025–7035.

[5] P.J. Willy, K. Umesono, E.S. Ong, R.M. Evans, R.A. Heyman, D.J. Mangelsdorf, LXR, a nuclear receptor that defines a distinct retinoid response pathway, Genes Dev. 9 (1995) 1033–1045.

[6] D.M. Shinar, N. Endo, S.J. Rutledge, R. Vogel, G.A. Rodan, A. Schmidt, NER, a new member of the gene family encoding the human steroid hormone nuclear receptor, Gene 147 (1994) 273–276.

[7] C. Song, R.A. Hiipakka, J.M. Kokontis, S. Liao, Ubiquitous receptor: structures, immunocytochemical localization, and modulation of gene activation by receptors for retinoic acids and thyroid hormones, Ann. NY Acad. Sci. 761 (1995) 38–49.

[8] M. Teboul, E. Enmark, Q. Li, A.C. Wikstrom, M. Pelto-Huikko, J.A. Gustafsson, OR-1, a member of the nuclear receptor superfamily that interacts with the 9-cis-retinoic acid receptor, Proc. Natl. Acad. Sci. USA 92 (1995) 2096–2100.

[9] W. Seol, H.S. Choi, D.D. Moore, Isolation of proteins that interact specifically with the retinoid X receptor: two novel orphan receptors, Mol. Endocrinol. 9 (1995) 72–85.

[10] S. Alberti, K.R. Steffensen, J.A. Gustafsson, Structural characterisation of the mouse nuclear oxysterol receptor genes LXRalpha and LXRbeta, Gene 243 (2000) 93–103.

[11] P.A. Edwards, H.R. Kast, A.M. Anisfeld, BAREing it all: the adoption of LXR and FXR and their roles in lipid homeostasis, J. Lipid Res. 43 (2002) 2–12.

[12] G.A. Francis, E. Fayard, F. Picard, J. Auwerx, Nuclear receptors and the control of metabolism, Annu. Rev. Physiol. 65 (2003) 261–311.

[13] D. Auboeuf, J. Rieusset, L. Fajas, et al., Tissue distribution and quantification of the expression of mRNAs of peroxisome proliferator-activated receptors and liver X receptor-alpha in humans: no alteration in adipose tissue of obese and NIDDM patients, Diabetes 46 (1997) 1319–1327.

[14] D.J. Peet, B.A. Janowski, D.J. Mangelsdorf, The LXRs: a new class of oxysterol receptors, Curr. Opin. Genet. Dev. 8 (1998) 571–575.

[15] F.F. Wiebel, J.A. Gustafsson, Heterodimeric interaction between retinoid X receptor alpha and orphan nuclear receptor OR1 reveals dimerization-induced activation as a novel mechanism of nuclear receptor activation, Mol. Cell. Biol. 17 (1997) 3977–3986.

[16] P.J. Willy, D.J. Mangelsdorf, Unique requirements for retinoid-dependent transcriptional activation by the orphan receptor LXR, Genes Dev. 11 (1997) 289–298.

[17] D. Feltkamp, F.F. Wiebel, S. Alberti, J.A. Gustafsson, Identification of a novel DNA binding site for nuclear orphan receptor OR1, J. Biol. Chem. 274 (1999) 10421–10429.

[18] L.M. Anderson, S.E. Choe, R.Y. Yukhananov, et al., Identification of a novel set of genes regulated by a unique liver X receptor-alpha -mediated transcription mechanism, J. Biol. Chem. 278 (2003) 15252–15260.

[19] K. Tamura, Y.E. Chen, M. Horiuchi, et al., LXRalpha functions as a cAMP-responsive transcriptional regulator of gene expression, Proc. Natl. Acad. Sci. USA 97 (2000) 8513–8518.

[20] J.F. Landrier, J. Grober, J. Demydchuk, P. Besnard, FXRE can function as an LXRE in the promoter of human ileal bile acid-binding protein (I-BABP) gene, FEBS Lett. 553 (2003) 299–303.

[21] C.K. Glass, M.G. Rosenfeld, The coregulator exchange in transcriptional functions of nuclear receptors, Genes Dev. 14 (2000) 121–141.

[22] C. Brendel, K. Schoonjans, O.A. Botrugno, E. Treuter, J. Auwerx, The small heterodimer partner interacts with the liver X receptor alpha and represses its transcriptional activity, Mol. Endocrinol. 16 (2002) 2065–2076.

[23] H. Oberkofler, E. Schraml, F. Krempler, W. Patsch, Potentiation of liver X receptor transcriptional activity by peroxisome-proliferator-activated receptor gamma co-activator 1 alpha, Biochem. J. 371 (2003) 89–96.

[24] F. Caira, P. Antonson, M. Pelto-Huikko, E. Treuter, J.A. Gustafsson, Cloning and characterization of RAP250, a novel nuclear receptor coactivator, J. Biol. Chem. 275 (2000) 5308–5317.

[25] S.W. Kim, K. Park, E. Kwak, et al., Activating signal cointegrator 2 required for liver lipid metabolism mediated by liver X receptors in mice, Mol. Cell Biol. 23 (2003) 3583–3592.

[26] F.F. Wiebel, K.R. Steffensen, E. Treuter, D. Feltkamp, J.A. Gustafsson, Ligand-independent coregulator recruitment by the triply activatable OR1/retinoid X receptor-alpha nuclear receptor heterodimer, Mol. Endocrinol. 13 (1999) 1105–1118.

[27] J. Huuskonen, P.E. Fielding, C.J. Fielding, Role of p160 coactivator complex in the activation of liver X receptor, Arterioscler. Thromb. Vasc. Biol. 24 (2004) 703–708.

[28] B. Miao, S. Zondlo, S. Gibbs, et al., Raising HDL cholesterol without inducing hepatic steatosis and hypertriglyceridemia by a selective LXR modulator, J. Lipid Res. 45 (2004) 1410–1417.

[29] X. Hu, S. Li, J. Wu, C. Xia, D.S. Lala, Liver x receptors interact with corepressors to regulate gene expression, Mol. Endocrinol. 17 (2003) 1019–1026.

[30] B.L. Wagner, A.F. Valledor, G. Shao, et al., Promoter-specific roles for liver X receptor/corepressor complexes in the regulation of ABCA1 and SREBP1 gene expression, Mol. Cell Biol. 23 (2003) 5780–5789.

[31] K.R. Steffensen, M. Nilsson, G.U. Schuster, T.M. Stulnig, K. Dahlman-Wright, J.A. Gustafsson, Gene expression profiling in adipose tissue indicates different transcriptional mechanisms of liver X receptors alpha and beta, respectively, Biochem. Biophys. Res. Commun. 310 (2003) 589–593.

[32] S.B. Joseph, M.N. Bradley, A. Castrillo, et al., LXR-dependent gene expression is important for macrophage survival and the innate immune response, Cell 119 (2004) 299–309.

[33] B.A. Laffitte, S.B. Joseph, R. Walczak, et al., Autoregulation of the human liver X receptor alpha promoter, Mol. Cell Biol. 21 (2001) 7558–7568.

[34] Y. Li, C. Bolten, B.G. Bhat, et al., Induction of human liver X receptor alpha gene expression via an autoregulatory loop mechanism, Mol. Endocrinol. 16 (2002) 506–514.

[35] B.A. Janowski, P.J. Willy, T.R. Devi, J.R. Falck, D.J. Mangelsdorf, An oxysterol signalling pathway mediated by the nuclear receptor LXR alpha, Nature 383 (1996) 728–731.

[36] J.M. Lehmann, S.A. Kliewer, L.B. Moore, et al., Activation of the nuclear receptor LXR by oxysterols defines a new hormone response pathway, J. Biol. Chem. 272 (1997) 3137–3140.

[37] B.M. Forman, B. Ruan, J. Chen, G.J. Schroepfer Jr., R.M. Evans, The orphan nuclear receptor LXRalpha is positively and negatively regulated by distinct products of mevalonate metabolism, Proc. Natl. Acad. Sci. USA 94 (1997) 10588–10593.

[38] B.A. Janowski, M.J. Grogan, S.A. Jones, et al., Structural requirements of ligands for the oxysterol liver X receptors LXRalpha and LXRbeta, Proc. Natl. Acad. Sci. USA 96 (1999) 266–271.

[39] X. Fu, J.G. Menke, Y. Chen, et al., 27-hydroxycholesterol is an endogenous ligand for liver X receptor in cholesterol-loaded cells, J. Biol. Chem. 276 (2001) 38378–38387.

[40] C. Song, R.A. Hiipakka, S. Liao, Selective activation of liver X receptor alpha by 6alpha-hydroxy bile acids and analogs, Steroids 65 (2000) 423–427.

[41] C. Song, S. Liao, Cholestenoic acid is a naturally occurring ligand for liver X receptor alpha, Endocrinology 141 (2000) 4180–4184.

[42] C.P. Sparrow, J. Baffic, M.H. Lam, et al., A potent synthetic LXR agonist is more effective than cholesterol loading at inducing ABCA1 mRNA and stimulating cholesterol efflux, J. Biol. Chem. 277 (2002) 10021–10027.

[43] J.J. Repa, S.D. Turley, J.A. Lobaccaro, et al., Regulation of absorption and ABC1-mediated efflux of cholesterol by RXR heterodimers, Science 289 (2000) 1524–1529.

[44] J.L. Collins, A.M. Fivush, M.A. Watson, et al., Identification of a nonsteroidal liver X receptor agonist through parallel array synthesis of tertiary amines, J. Med. Chem. 45 (2002) 1963–1966.

[45] K.A. Houck, K.M. Borchert, C.D. Hepler, et al., T0901317 is a dual LXR/FXR agonist, Mol. Genet. Metab. 83 (2004) 184–187.

[46] E.M. Quinet, D.A. Savio, A.R. Halpern, L. Chen, C.P. Miller, P. Nambi, Gene-selective modulation by a synthetic oxysterol ligand of the liver X receptor, J. Lipid Res. 45 (2004) 1929–1942.

[47] K.S. Bramlett, K.A. Houck, K.M. Borchert, et al., A natural product ligand of the oxysterol receptor, liver X receptor, J. Pharmacol. Exp. Ther. 307 (2003) 291–296.

[48] J. Chin, A.D. Adams, A. Bouffard, et al., Miniaturization of cell-based beta-lactamase-dependent FRET assays to ultra-high throughput formats to identify agonists of human liver X receptors, Assay Drug Dev. Technol. 1 (2003) 777–787.

[49] C. Yang, L. Yu, W. Li, F. Xu, J.C. Cohen, H.H. Hobbs, Disruption of cholesterol homeostasis by plant sterols, J. Clin. Invest. 114 (2004) 813–822.

[50] T. Yoshikawa, H. Shimano, N. Yahagi, et al., Polyunsaturated fatty acids suppress sterol regulatory element-binding protein 1c promoter activity by inhibition of liver X receptor (LXR) binding to LXR response elements, J. Biol. Chem. 277 (2002) 1705–1711.

[51] J. Ou, H. Tu, B. Shan, et al., Unsaturated fatty acids inhibit transcription of the sterol regulatory element-binding protein-1c (SREBP-1c) gene by antagonizing ligand-dependent activation of the LXR, Proc. Natl. Acad. Sci. USA 98 (2001) 6027–6032.

[52] X. Gan, R. Kaplan, J.G. Menke, et al., Dual mechanisms of ABCA1 regulation by geranylgeranyl pyrophosphate, J. Biol. Chem. 276 (2001) 48702–48708.

[53] C. Song, R.A. Hiipakka, S. Liao, Auto-oxidized cholesterol sulfates are antagonistic ligands of liver X receptors: implications for the development and treatment of atherosclerosis, Steroids 66 (2001) 473–479.

[54] J. Thomas, K.S. Bramlett, C. Montrose, et al., A chemical switch regulates fibrate specificity for peroxisome proliferator-activated receptor alpha (PPARalpha) versus liver X receptor, J. Biol. Chem. 278 (2003) 2403–2410.

[55] M. Farnegardh, T. Bonn, S. Sun, et al., The three-dimensional structure of the liver X receptor beta reveals a flexible ligand-binding pocket that can accommodate fundamentally different ligands, J. Biol. Chem. 278 (2003) 38821–38828.

[56] S. Williams, R.K. Bledsoe, J.L. Collins, et al., X-ray crystal structure of the liver X receptor beta ligand binding domain: regulation by a histidine-tryptophan switch, J. Biol. Chem. 278 (2003) 27138–27143.

[57] S. Svensson, T. Ostberg, M. Jacobsson, et al., Crystal structure of the heterodimeric complex of LXRalpha and RXRbeta ligand-binding domains in a fully agonistic conformation, Embo. J. 22 (2003) 4625–4633.

[58] I.M. Billas, T. Iwema, J.M. Garnier, A. Mitschler, N. Rochel, D. Moras, Structural adaptability in the ligand-binding pocket of the ecdysone hormone receptor, Nature 426 (2003) 91–96.

[59] T.M. Stulnig, K.R. Steffensen, H. Gao, et al., Novel roles of liver X receptors exposed by gene expression profiling in liver and adipose tissue, Mol. Pharmacol. 62 (2002) 1299–1305.

[60] T.M. Stulnig, U. Oppermann, K.R. Steffensen, G.U. Schuster, J.A. Gustafsson, Liver X receptors downregulate 11beta-hydroxysteroid dehydrogenase type 1 expression and activity, Diabetes 51 (2002) 2426–2433.

[61] G. Cao, Y. Liang, C.L. Broderick, et al., Antidiabetic action of a liver x receptor agonist mediated by inhibition of hepatic gluconeogenesis, J. Biol. Chem. 278 (2003) 1131–1136.

[62] B.A. Laffitte, L.C. Chao, J. Li, et al., Activation of liver X receptor improves glucose tolerance through coordinate regulation of glucose metabolism in liver and adipose tissue, Proc. Natl. Acad. Sci. USA 100 (2003) 5419–5424.

[63] J.W. Chisholm, J. Hong, S.A. Mills, R.M. Lawn, The LXR ligand T0901317 induces severe lipogenesis in the db/db diabetic mouse, J. Lipid Res. 44 (2003) 2039–2048.

[64] I. Gerin, V.W. Dolinsky, J.G. Shackman, et al., LXRbeta is required for adipocyte growth, glucose homeostasis and beta cell function, J. Biol. Chem. 280 (2005) 23024–23031.

[65] A.M. Efanov, S. Sewing, K. Bokvist, J. Gromada, Liver X receptor activation stimulates insulin secretion via modulation of glucose and lipid metabolism in pancreatic beta-cells, Diabetes 53 (Suppl. 3) (2004) S75–S78.

[66] N.Y. Kalaany, K.C. Gauthier, A.M. Zavacki, et al., LXRs regulate the balance between fat storage and oxidation, Cell Metabolism 1 (2005) 231–244.

[67] K.T. Dalen, S.M. Ulven, K. Bamberg, J.A. Gustafsson, H.I. Nebb, Expression of the insulin-responsive glucose transporter GLUT4 in adipocytes is dependent on liver X receptor alpha, J. Biol. Chem. 278 (2003) 48283–48291.

[68] S.E. Ross, R.L. Erickson, I. Gerin, et al., Microarray analyses during adipogenesis: understanding the effects of Wnt signaling on adipogenesis and the roles of liver X receptor alpha in adipocyte metabolism, Mol. Cell. Biol. 22 (2002) 5989–5999.

[69] G.E. Muscat, B.L. Wagner, J. Hou, et al., Regulation of cholesterol homeostasis and lipid metabolism in skeletal muscle by liver X receptors, J. Biol. Chem. 277 (2002) 40722–40728.

[70] E.T. Kase, A.J. Wensaas, V. Aas, et al., Skeletal muscle lipid accumulation in type 2 diabetes may involve the liver x receptor pathway, Diabetes 54 (2005) 1108–1115.

[71] K.A. Tobin, S.M. Ulven, G.U. Schuster, et al., Liver X receptors as insulin-mediating factors in fatty acid and cholesterol biosynthesis, J. Biol. Chem. 277 (2002) 10691–10697.

[72] J.R. Schultz, H. Tu, A. Luk, et al., Role of LXRs in control of lipogenesis, Genes Dev. 14 (2000) 831–838.

[73] R.A. DeBose-Boyd, J. Ou, J.L. Goldstein, M.S. Brown, Expression of sterol regulatory element-binding protein 1c (SREBP-1c) mRNA in rat hepatoma cells requires endogenous LXR ligands, Proc. Natl. Acad. Sci. USA 98 (2001) 1477–1482.

[74] J.J. Repa, G. Liang, J. Ou, et al., Regulation of mouse sterol regulatory element-binding protein-1c gene (SREBP-1c) by oxysterol receptors, LXRalpha and LXRbeta, Genes Dev. 14 (2000) 2819–2830.

[75] T. Yoshikawa, H. Shimano, M. Amemiya-Kudo, et al., Identification of liver X receptor-retinoid X receptor as an activator of the sterol regulatory element-binding protein 1c gene promoter, Mol. Cell. Biol. 21 (2001) 2991–3000.

[76] Y. Zhang, L. Yin, F.B. Hillgartner, Thyroid hormone stimulates acetyl-coA carboxylase-alpha transcription in hepatocytes by modulating the composition of nuclear receptor complexes bound to a thyroid hormone response element, J. Biol. Chem. 276 (2001) 974–983.

[77] S.B. Joseph, B.A. Laffitte, P.H. Patel, et al., Direct and indirect mechanisms for regulation of fatty acid synthase gene expression by liver X receptors, J Biol. Chem. 277 (2002) 11019–11025.

[78] D.J. Peet, S.D. Turley, W. Ma, et al., Cholesterol and bile acid metabolism are impaired in mice lacking the nuclear oxysterol receptor LXR alpha, Cell 93 (1998) 693–704.

[79] G.U. Schuster, P. Parini, L. Wang, et al., Accumulation of foam cells in liver X receptor-deficient mice, Circulation 106 (2002) 1147–1153.

[80] S. Hummasti, B.A. Laffitte, M.A. Watson, et al., Liver X receptors are regulators of adipocyte gene expression but not differentiation: identification of apoD as a direct target, J. Lipid Res. 45 (2004) 616–625.

[81] Y. Zhang, J.J. Repa, K. Gauthier, D.J. Mangelsdorf, Regulation of lipoprotein lipase by the oxysterol receptors, LXRalpha and LXRbeta, J. Biol. Chem. 276 (2001) 43018–43024.

[82] Y. Wang, B. Kurdi-Haidar, J.F. Oram. LXR-mediated activation of macrophage stearoyl-CoA desaturase generates unsaturated fatty acids that destabilize ABCA1, J. Lipid Res. 45 (2004) 972–980.

[83] K.R. Steffensen, E. Holter, K.A. Tobin, et al., Members of the nuclear factor 1 family reduce the transcriptional potential of the nuclear receptor LXRalpha promoter, Biochem. Biophys. Res. Commun. 289 (2001) 1262–1267.

[84] J.M. Ntambi, Regulation of stearoyl-CoA desaturase by polyunsaturated fatty acids and cholesterol, J. Lipid Res. 40 (1999) 1549–1558.

[85] R. Kaplan, T. Zhang, M. Hernandez, et al., Regulation of the angiopoietin-like protein 3 gene by LXR, J. Lipid Res. 44 (2003) 136–143.

[86] R. Koishi, Y. Ando, M. Ono, et al., Angptl3 regulates lipid metabolism in mice, Nat. Genet. 30 (2002) 151–157.

[87] S. Alberti, G. Schuster, P. Parini, et al., Hepatic cholesterol metabolism and resistance to dietary cholesterol in LXRbeta-deficient mice, J. Clin. Invest. 107 (2001) 565–573.

[88] J.Y. Chiang, R. Kimmel, D. Stroup, Regulation of cholesterol 7alpha-hydroxylase gene (CYP7A1) transcription by the liver orphan receptor (LXRalpha), Gene 262 (2001) 257–265.

[89] B. Goodwin, M.A. Watson, H. Kim, J. Miao, J.K. Kemper, S.A. Kliewer, Differential Regulation of Rat and Human CYP7A1 by the Nuclear Oxysterol Receptor Liver X Receptor-{alpha}, Mol. Endocrinol. 17 (2003) 386–394.

[90] L. Malerod, L.K. Juvet, A. Hanssen-Bauer, W. Eskild, T. Berg, Oxysterol-activated LXRalpha/ RXR induces hSR-BI-promoter activity in hepatoma cells and preadipocytes, Biochem. Biophys. Res. Commun. 299 (2002) 916–923.

[91] L. Yu, J. York, K. von Bergmann, D. Lutjohann, J.C. Cohen, H.H. Hobbs, Stimulation of cholesterol excretion by the liver X receptor agonist requires ATP-binding cassette transporters G5 and G8, J. Biol. Chem. 278 (2003) 15565–15570.

[92] P. Costet, Y. Luo, N. Wang, A.R. Tall, Sterol-dependent transactivation of the ABC1 promoter by the liver X receptor/retinoid X receptor, J. Biol. Chem. 275 (2000) 28240–28245.

[93] A. Venkateswaran, B.A. Laffitte, S.B. Joseph, et al., Control of cellular cholesterol efflux by the nuclear oxysterol receptor LXR alpha, Proc. Natl. Acad. Sci. USA 97 (2000) 12097–12102.

[94] K. Schwartz, R.M. Lawn, D.P. Wade, ABC1 gene expression and ApoA-I-mediated cholesterol efflux are regulated by LXR, Biochem. Biophys. Res. Commun. 274 (2000) 794–802.

[95] M.A. Kennedy, A. Venkateswaran, P.T. Tarr, et al., Characterization of the human ABCG1 gene: liver X receptor activates an internal promoter that produces a novel transcript encoding an alternative form of the protein, J. Biol. Chem. 276 (2001) 39438–39447.

[96] P.A. Mak, B.A. Laffitte, C. Desrumaux, et al., Regulated expression of the apolipoprotein E/C-I/ C-IV/C-II gene cluster in murine and human macrophages. A critical role for nuclear liver X receptors alpha and beta, J. Biol. Chem. 277 (2002) 31900–31908.

[97] B.A. Laffitte, J.J. Repa, S.B. Joseph, et al., LXRs control lipid-inducible expression of the apolipoprotein E gene in macrophages and adipocytes, Proc. Natl. Acad. Sci. USA 98 (2001) 507–512.

[98] Y. Liang, X.C. Jiang, R. Liu, et al., Liver X receptors (LXRs) regulate apolipoprotein AIV-implications of the antiatherosclerotic effect of LXR agonists, Mol. Endocrinol. 18 (2004) 2000–2010.

[99] H. Jakel, M. Nowak, E. Moitrot, et al., The LXR ligand T0901317 down-regulates APOA5 gene expression through activation of SREBP-1c, J. Biol. Chem. 279 (2004) 45462–45469.

[100] L.A. Pennacchio, M. Olivier, J.A. Hubacek, et al., An apolipoprotein influencing triglycerides in humans and mice revealed by comparative sequencing, Science 294 (2001) 169–173.

[101] G. Cao, T.P. Beyer, X.P. Yang, et al., Phospholipid transfer protein is regulated by liver X receptors *in vivo*, J. Biol. Chem. 277 (2002) 39561–39565.

[102] Y. Luo, A.R. Tall, Sterol upregulation of human CETP expression in vitro and in transgenic mice by an LXR element, J. Clin. Invest. 105 (2000) 513–520.

[103] D.S. Ory, Nuclear receptor signaling in the control of cholesterol homeostasis: have the orphans found a home? Circ. Res. 95 (2004) 660–670.

[104] K.R. Steffensen, S.Y. Neo, T.M. Stulnig, et al., Genome-wide expression profiling; a panel of mouse tissues discloses novel biological functions of liver X receptors in adrenals, J. Mol. Endocrinol. 33 (2004) 609–622.

[105] F.F. Samaha, N. Iqbal, P. Seshadri, et al., A low-carbohydrate as compared with a low-fat diet in severe obesity, N. Engl. J. Med. 348 (2003) 2074–2081.

[106] L. Stern, N. Iqbal, P. Seshadri, et al., The effects of low-carbohydrate versus conventional weight loss diets in severely obese adults: one-year follow-up of a randomized trial, Ann. Intern. Med. 140 (2004) 778–785.

[107] T. Claudel, M.D. Leibowitz, C. Fievet, et al., Reduction of atherosclerosis in apolipoprotein E knockout mice by activation of the retinoid X receptor, Proc. Natl. Acad. Sci. USA 98 (2001) 2610–2615.

[108] R.K. Tangirala, E.D. Bischoff, S.B. Joseph, et al., Identification of macrophage liver X receptors as inhibitors of atherosclerosis, Proc. Natl. Acad. Sci. USA 99 (2002) 11896–11901.

[109] S.B. Joseph, E. McKilligin, L. Pei, et al., Synthetic LXR ligand inhibits the development of atherosclerosis in mice, Proc. Natl. Acad. Sci. USA 99 (2002) 7604–7609.

[110] N. Terasaka, A. Hiroshima, T. Koieyama, et al., T-0901317, a synthetic liver X receptor ligand, inhibits development of atherosclerosis in LDL receptor-deficient mice, FEBS Lett 536 (2003) 6–11.

[111] A. Chawla, W.A. Boisvert, C.H. Lee, et al., A PPAR gamma-LXR-ABCA1 pathway in macrophages is involved in cholesterol efflux and atherogenesis, Mol. Cell. 7 (2001) 161–171.

[112] J.B. Seo, H.M. Moon, W.S. Kim, et al., Activated liver X receptors stimulate adipocyte differentiation through induction of peroxisome proliferator-activated receptor gamma expression, Mol. Cell. Biol. 24 (2004) 3430–3444.

[113] A. Szanto, S. Benko, I. Szatmari, et al., Transcriptional regulation of human CYP27 integrates retinoid, peroxisome proliferator-activated receptor, and liver X receptor signaling in macrophages, Mol. Cell. Biol. 24 (2004) 8154–8166.

[114] C.K. Glass, J.L. Witztum, Atherosclerosis. the road ahead. Cell 104 (2001) 503–516.

[115] R. Tisch, H. McDevitt, Insulin-dependent diabetes mellitus, Cell 85 (1996) 291–297.

[116] R.F. Grimble, Inflammatory status and insulin resistance, Curr. Opin. Clin. Nutr. Metab. Care 5 (2002) 551–559.

[117] M.S. Landis, H.V. Patel, J.P. Capone, Oxysterol activators of liver X receptor and 9-cis-retinoic acid promote sequential steps in the synthesis and secretion of tumor necrosis factor-alpha from human monocytes, J. Biol. Chem. 277 (2002) 4713–4721.

[118] A. Castrillo, S.B. Joseph, C. Marathe, D.J. Mangelsdorf, P. Tontonoz, Liver X receptor-dependent repression of matrix metalloproteinase-9 expression in macrophages, J. Biol. Chem. 278 (2003) 10443–10449.

[119] S.B. Joseph, A. Castrillo, B.A. Laffitte, D.J. Mangelsdorf, P. Tontonoz, Reciprocal regulation of inflammation and lipid metabolism by liver X receptors, Nat. Med. 9 (2003) 213–219.

[120] A. Castrillo, S.B. Joseph, S.A. Vaidya, et al., Crosstalk between LXR and toll-like receptor signaling mediates bacterial and viral antagonism of cholesterol metabolism, Mol. Cell 12 (2003) 805–816.

[121] V. Antonio, B. Janvier, A. Brouillet, M. Andreani, M. Raymondjean, Oxysterol and 9-cis-retinoic acid stimulate the group IIA secretory phospholipase A2 gene in rat smooth muscle cells, Biochem. J. 376 (2003) 351–360.

[122] T.P. Beyer, R.J. Schmidt, P. Foxworthy, et al., Coadministration of a liver X receptor agonist and a peroxisome proliferator activator receptor-alpha agonist in Mice: effects of nuclear receptor interplay on high-density lipoprotein and triglyceride metabolism in vivo, J. Pharmacol. Exp. Ther. 309 (2004) 861–868.

[123] S.P. Anderson, C. Dunn, A. Laughter, et al., Overlapping Transcriptional Programs Regulated by the Nuclear Receptors Peroxisome Proliferator-Activated Receptor {alpha}, Retinoid X Receptor and Liver X Receptor in Mouse Liver, Mol. Pharmacol. 66 (2004) 1440–1452.

[124] J.C. Corton, U. Apte, S.P. Anderson, et al., Mimetics of caloric restriction include agonists of lipid-activated nuclear receptors, J. Biol. Chem. 279 (2004) 46204–46212.

[125] T. Ide, H. Shimano, T. Yoshikawa, et al., Cross-Talk between Peroxisome Proliferator-Activated Receptor (PPAR) {alpha} and Liver X Receptor (LXR) in Nutritional Regulation of Fatty Acid Metabolism. II. LXRs Suppress Lipid Degradation Gene Promoters through Inhibition of PPAR Signaling, Mol. Endocrinol. 17 (2003) 1255–1267.

[126] T. Yoshikawa, T. Ide, H. Shimano, et al., Cross-Talk between Peroxisome Proliferator-Activated Receptor (PPAR) {alpha} and Liver X Receptor (LXR) in Nutritional Regulation of Fatty Acid Metabolism. I. PPARs Suppress Sterol Regulatory Element Binding Protein-1c Promoter through Inhibition of LXR Signaling, Mol. Endocrinol. 17 (2003) 1240–1254.

[127] G.F. Gbaguidi, L.B. Agellon, The inhibition of the human cholesterol 7alpha-hydroxylase gene (CYP7A1) promoter by fibrates in cultured cells is mediated via the liver x receptor alpha and peroxisome proliferator-activated receptor alpha heterodimer, Nucleic Acids Res. 32 (2004) 1113–1121.

[128] G.F. Gbaguidi, L.B. Agellon, The atypical interaction of peroxisome proliferator-activated receptor alpha with liver X receptor alpha antagonizes the stimulatory effect of their respective ligands on the murine cholesterol 7alpha-hydroxylase gene promoter, Biochim. Biophys. Acta 1583 (2002) 229–236.

[129] K.S. Miyata, S.E. McCaw, H.V. Patel, R.A. Rachubinski, J.P. Capone, The orphan nuclear hormone receptor LXR alpha interacts with the peroxisome proliferator-activated receptor and inhibits peroxisome proliferator signaling, J. Biol. Chem. 271 (1996) 9189–9192.

[130] M.U. De Martino, S. Alesci, G.P. Chrousos, T. Kino, Interaction of the glucocorticoid receptor and the chicken ovalbumin upstream promoter-transcription factor II (COUP-TFII): implications for the actions of glucocorticoids on glucose, lipoprotein, and xenobiotic metabolism, Ann. NY Acad. Sci. 1024 (2004) 72–85.

[131] H. Raff, J.W. Findling, A physiologic approach to diagnosis of the Cushing syndrome, Ann. Intern. Med. 138 (2003) 980–991.

[132] L.K. Juvet, S.M. Andresen, G.U. Schuster, et al., On the role of liver x receptors in lipid accumulation in adipocytes, Mol. Endocrinol. 17 (2003) 172–182.

[133] I.J. Bujalska, S. Kumar, P.M. Stewart, Does central obesity reflect Cushing's disease of the omentum? Lancet 349 (1997) 1210–1213.

[134] H. Masuzaki, J. Paterson, H. Shinyama, et al., A transgenic model of visceral obesity and the metabolic syndrome, Science 294 (2001) 2166–2170.

[135] B.R. Walker, A.A. Connacher, R.M. Lindsay, D.J. Webb, C.R. Edwards, Carbenoxolone increases hepatic insulin sensitivity in man: a novel role for 11-oxosteroid reductase in enhancing glucocorticoid receptor activation, J. Clin. Endocrinol. Metab. 80 (1995) 3155–3159.

[136] Y. Kotelevtsev, M.C. Holmes, A. Burchell, et al., 11beta-hydroxysteroid dehydrogenase type 1 knockout mice show attenuated glucocorticoid-inducible responses and resist hyperglycemia on obesity or stress, Proc. Natl. Acad. Sci. USA 94 (1997) 14924–14929.

[137] J.W. Tomlinson, E.A. Walker, I.J. Bujalska, et al., 11beta-hydroxysteroid dehydrogenase type 1: a tissue-specific regulator of glucocorticoid response, Endocr. Rev. 25 (2004) 831–866.

[138] L. Lundholm, S. Moverare, K.R. Steffensen, et al., Gene expression profiling identifies liver X receptor alpha as an estrogen-regulated gene in mouse adipose tissue, J. Mol. Endocrinol. 32 (2004) 879–892.

[139] P.R. Kramer, S. Wray, 17-Beta-estradiol regulates expression of genes that function in macrophage activation and cholesterol homeostasis, J. Steroid Biochem. Mol. Biol. 81 (2002) 203–216.

[140] K. Kawai, S. Sasaki, H. Morita, et al., Unliganded thyroid hormone receptor {beta}1 represses liver X receptor {alpha}/oxysterol-dependent transactivation. Endocrinology, 145 (2004) 5515–5524.

[141] D. Mathis, L. Vence, C. Benoist, Beta-cell death during progression to diabetes, Nature 414 (2001) 792–798.

[142] M. Gil-Campos, R.R. Canete, A. Gil, Adiponectin, the missing link in insulin resistance and obesity, Clin. Nutr. 23 (2004) 963–974.

[143] G. Chinetti, C. Zawadski, J.C. Fruchart, B. Staels, Expression of adiponectin receptors in human macrophages and regulation by agonists of the nuclear receptors PPARalpha, PPARgamma, and LXR, Biochem. Biophys. Res. Commun. 314 (2004) 151–158.

Chapter 5

SREBP-1c regulation of nutrient homeostasis and lipid accumulation

Pascal Ferré, Delphine Eberlé, Bronwyn Hegarty, Fabienne Foufelle

INSERM U671, Université Pierre et Marie Curie, 15 rue de l'Ecole de médecine, 75270 Paris Cedex 06, France

Summary

The regulation of metabolism involves short-term regulation of enzymes and transporters as well as changes in the transcription rate of their genes. In the last decade, the transcription factor Sterol Regulatory Element Binding Protein (SREBP)-1c has emerged as a major protein involved not only in the regulation of genes involved in carbohydrate and lipid metabolism in the liver, but also in adipose tissue, muscle and pancreatic β-cells. SREBP-1c is synthetized as a precursor bound to the membranes of the endoplasmic reticulum. Its mature, transcriptionally active nuclear form is released from this precursor by a proteolytic cleavage process, regulated in part by insulin and cholesterol. SREBP isoforms, SREBP-2 and -1a, are involved in the regulation of genes in the pathway of cholesterol metabolism. In contrast, SREBP-1c transduces the effects of insulin on gene expression and thus favors glucose utilization and glycogen synthesis, as well as lipid synthesis from glucose and triglyceride storage into adipocytes (SREBP-1c is also a transcription factor favoring adipocyte differentiation). Insulin not only stimulates the expression of the SREBP-1c gene, but activates also its cleavage into its nuclear mature form. Changes in SREBP-1c expression as well as polymorphisms in the gene have been associated with a number of pathologies linked to lipotoxicity, such as hyper-triglyceridemia, insulin resistance, and type 2 diabetes. Due to its anabolic effect on genes involved in glucose and lipid storage, SREBP-1c can be considered as a thrifty gene.

1. Introduction

Energy storage during caloric excess is critical for survival in periods of increased energy expenditure or decreased nutrient availability. Quantitatively, the major form

ADVANCES IN MOLECULAR AND CELLULAR ENDOCRINOLOGY
VOLUME 5 ISSN 1569-2566/DOI 10.1016/S1569-2566(06)05005-8

of energy storage is lipids in adipose tissue. However, glucose metabolism also has a crucial role in these adaptations since glucose is an obligatory substrate for a number of tissues including the brain. When a meal containing carbohydrate is absorbed, it induces several metabolic events aimed at decreasing endogenous glucose production by the liver (glycogenolysis and gluconeogenesis), and increasing glucose uptake and storage in the form of glycogen in the liver and muscle. If glucose is delivered into the portal vein in large quantities and hepatic glycogen stores are full, then it can be converted in the liver into lipids (*de-novo* lipogenesis), which are subsequently exported as VLDL and ultimately stored as triglycerides in adipose tissue. Glucose is the main insulin secretagogue, and as such it has an important role in lipid anabolism, which is absolutely dependent upon the presence of this hormone. Thus, glucose and lipid metabolism are tightly linked, especially in the liver, which has the property of storing or producing glucose, synthetizing lipids (fatty acids, cholesterol) from glucose or oxidizing fatty acids. Glucose and lipid metabolism are controlled at least in part by a common family of transcription factors designated SREBPs. SREBPs transcriptionally activate a cascade of genes that code for critical enzymes required for glucose utilization and cholesterol, fatty acids, triglycerides (TG) and phospholipid synthesis. Although the specificities of the different SREBP isoforms will be addressed, we will emphasize the regulation of SREBP-1c, its role in the control of glucose and lipid homeostasis and its relationship with metabolic diseases such as obesity and type 2 diabetes.

2. Structure, genes and tissue distribution of SREBP isoforms

SREBP-1c belongs to a family of transcription factors originally described as regulating genes via changes in the cellular availability in cholesterol [1]. Three members of the SREBP family have been described in several mammalian species (mice, rat, hamster and human). SREBP-1a and -1c are encoded by a single gene through the use of alternative transcription start sites and differ in their first exon [2]. In mice, the first exon of SREBP-1a is composed of 29 amino acids of which 8 are acidic, whereas the first exon of SREBP-1c is composed of 5 amino acids of which only one is acidic. *In vitro* and *in vivo* experiments expressing identical levels of both isoforms have shown that SREBP-1a is a much more potent activator of cholesterol genes than SREBP-1c [3]. Another major difference between the SREBP-1a and -1c isoform is their tissue distribution. SREBP-1c is expressed in most tissues of mice and human with especially high levels in the liver, white adipose tissue, adrenal gland and brain [4]. SREBP-1c is also expressed in various muscles in adult rats and humans at appreciable levels [5,6]. By contrast, SREBP-1a is mainly expressed in cell lines and tissues with a high capacity for cell proliferation such as spleen and intestine [4]. The third member of the family, SREBP-2 is derived from a different gene and has 50% homology with the SREBP-1 amino acid sequence. The three isoforms have a common structure: (1) an amino-terminal fragment of 480 amino acids which contains the basic domain-helix, loop, helix characteristic of the leucine zipper family, (2) a region of 80 amino acids containing two transmembrane domains separated by 31 amino acids, and (3) a regulatory C-terminal domain of 590 amino acids. These transcription factors are synthetized as a precursor form bound to the endoplasmic reticulum (ER) and nuclear membranes. Brown and Goldstein have elegantly revealed the mechanisms by which the transcriptionally active fragment of SREBP-2 and 1a are liberated [7–9]. When the concentration of cholesterol decreases in the membranes, the precursor form of SREBP-2 and -1a is increased through enhanced gene transcription. This precursor form is cleaved by a complex mechanism involving two proteolytic cleavages catalyzed by two distinct proteases Site1 and Site2 protease (S1P and S2P), a protein "sensor" for the cholesterol concentration SREBP Cleavage Activating Protein (SCAP) and an anchoring protein termed Insulin-signaling Induced Gene (INSIG). The mature form migrates inside the nucleus, where it activates the promoter of genes involved in cholesterol uptake such as the low-density lipoprotein receptor, or in cholesterol synthesis, such as the cytoplasmic hydroxymethylglutaryl-CoA synthase or the hydroxymethylglutaryl-CoA reductase. The cleavage mechanism will be discussed in greater detail in Section 3.2.

3. Regulation of SREBP-1c transcriptional activity

In contrast to SREBP-2 and -1a, SREBP-1c expression and nuclear abundance is not increased in case of low cholesterol availibility. A nutritional protocol aimed at increasing the demand for cholesterol induces a clear-cut increase in the expression and nuclear abundance of SREBP-2 in the hamster liver, whereas SREBP-1c expression and nuclear abundance are rather decreased [10].

3.1. *Regulation of SREBP-1c at the transcriptional level*

The first insights into the transcriptional regulation of SREBP-1c came from fasting/ refeeding regimes in rodents which showed that changes in nutritional status regulate the expression of SREBP-1c in the liver [11], white adipose tissue [12] and more recently, skeletal muscle [13–15]. SREBP-1c expression is depressed during fasting but increases markedly when animals are refed a high carbohydrate diet. In contrast, such manipulations induce only minor effects on the expression of the other SREBP isoforms. Subsequent experiments in isolated adipocytes [12] and hepatocytes [16] showed that the transcription of SREBP-1c is induced by insulin. This induction of SREBP-1c transcription leads to a parallel increase in expression of both the ER membrane-bound precursor and the nuclear form of the transcription factor [17]. Insulin also induces the expression of SREBP-1c in adipose tissue and muscles of healthy human patients participating in a 3 h hyperinsulinemic-euglycemic clamp [5,18]. In a typical counterregulatory fashion, the effects of insulin on SREBP-1c transcription are opposed by glucagon via cAMP [16]. Experiments showing that SREBP-1c mRNA expression is decreased in the livers of streptozotocin (STZ) diabetic rats and near normalized by insulin treatment, confirmed the role of insulin on SREBP-1c transcription *in vivo* [19].

SREBP-1c transcription can also be induced by the activation of Liver X Receptor (LXR)α. LXRα is a nuclear hormone receptor with high hepatic expression that is activated by oxysterols (derivatives of cholesterol) [20,21]. This transcription factor induces expression of a range of genes involved in cholesterol efflux and clearance [22]. In addition, *in vivo* studies have identified a role for LXRα to induce SREBP-1c and lipogenic genes. Animals lacking LXRα exhibit reduced basal expression of SREBP-1c, fatty acid synthase (FAS), acetyl-CoA carboxylase (ACC) and Stearoyl-CoA desaturase 1(SCD-1) [23,24], whereas LXRβ knockout has no such effect. In contrast, animals fed with cholesterol-enriched diets or synthetic LXR agonists, demonstrate a selective increase in SREBP-1c mRNA and nuclear protein, induced expression of lipogenic target genes and elevated rates of fatty acid synthesis [24–26]. It is believed that LXRα acts as a sensor of cholesterol availability. Consistent with this role, it has been proposed that LXRα induces SREBP-1c in order to generate fatty acids needed for the formation of cholesterol esters, which buffer the free cholesterol concentration [27]. There is evidence that LXRα can act directly to induce some individual lipogenic genes such as FAS [28]. However, the secondary induction of lipogenic genes by LXR via SREBP-1c is physiologically important since SREBP-1c null mice show a diminished lipogenic response to LXR agonist treatment [29]. LXRα mediates its induction of SREBP-1c via RXR/LXR DNA-binding sites in the SREBP-1c gene promoter [24,30]. Interestingly, these LXR response elements not only mediate the regulation of SREBP-1c by LXRα but are also required for full induction of SREBP-1c by insulin [31,32]. This has prompted the hypothesis that insulin may in fact induce SREBP-1c by increasing the activity of LXRα, possibly through the production of a LXR ligand [31]. It must be pointed out, however, that during the fetal period in mice, a period characterized by a non-detectable LXR transcriptional activity, SREBP-1c mRNA can be induced by insulin [33]. Tobin et al. [34] have reported that insulin increases the mRNA and protein content of LXR itself, although the effect of insulin on the LXR protein was not found in later studies [32].

The role of glucose in the regulation of SREBP-1c is controversial. It has been reported that glucose can induce the transcription of SREBP-1c in H2-35 hepatocyte derived cells [35] and contracting myotubes [36]. In contrast, we and others have found that glucose has no effect on the transcription of SREBP-1c in rat hepatocytes [16,37–39]. Matsuzaka et al. [40] have recently reported an effect of glucose, fructose and sucrose to induce SREBP-1c in the liver of STZ diabetic mice, but the same study showed that this was not the case in rats.

Finally, SREBP-1c transcription is suppressed by AMP-activated protein kinase (AMPK) [41], which could account for the decrease in lipogenic gene expression observed in rat hepatocytes with prolonged AMPK activation [42].

3.2. *SREBPs activation by proteolytic cleavage*

Following SREBPs mRNA translation, SREBP precursors are retained in the ER membranes through a tight association with SREBP Cleavage Activating Protein (SCAP) [43]. Under the appropriate conditions, SCAP escorts the SREBP precursors

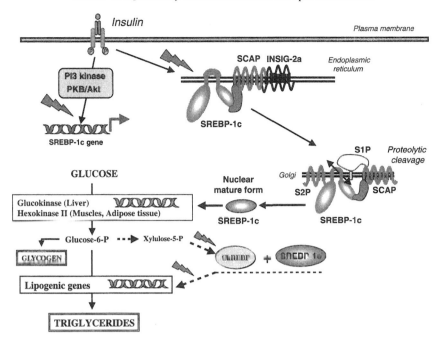

Fig. 1. SREBP-1c synthesis, processing and actions. SREBPs are synthetized as precursors in the ER membranes in tight association with SREBP Cleavage Activating Protein (SCAP). The complex SREBP–SCAP is retained in the ER through an interaction with Insig proteins. When an appropriate stimulus is delivered (decreased cholesterol membrane concentration for SREBP-1a and -2, insulin for SREBP-1c), the SREBP–SCAP complex dissociates from Insig proteins. SCAP then escorts the SREBP precursors from the ER to the Golgi apparatus where two functionally distinct proteases, S1P and S2P, sequentially cleave the precursor protein releasing the mature nuclear SREBPs. SREBP-1c regulates glycolytic and lipogenic gene expression in the liver together with the glucose-dependent ChREBP transcription factor. See Section 5.2 for detailed explanations.

from the ER to Golgi apparatus where two functionally distinct proteases, S1P and S2P, sequentially cleave the precursor protein releasing the mature nuclear SREBPs (nSREBPs) [1,44] (Fig. 1). The group of Brown and Goldstein has demonstrated that SREBP processing can be controlled by the cellular sterol content [8]. In the presence of high-sterol concentrations, the SREBP–SCAP complex is retained in the ER membranes. When sterol content decreases, the SREBP–SCAP complex moves to the Golgi apparatus where the cleavage takes place. It has been shown that this sterol-dependent trafficking requires an intact sterol-sensing domain in the SCAP protein [43]. Cholesterol binds directly the sterol-sensing domain of SCAP [45], and modulates the SCAP conformation [46] suggesting that protein-protein interaction is involved in the ER retention of SREBP–SCAP complex. The recent discovery of Insig proteins as SCAP partners responsible for the ER retention of SREBP–SCAP adds new insights into this mechanism. When sterol levels are high, SCAP interacts strongly with Insig, retaining the SREBP–SCAP complex in the ER [9,47].

However, this sterol-sensitive SREBP process does not apply to the three SREBP isoforms, and other factors such as insulin seem to be involved in the cleavage. All of these studies on SREBP process mechanism and control by sterols were done in cell lines that express SREBP-1a and -2 predominantly [4]. Interestingly, studies done *in vivo* have shown that sterol depletion does not regulate the cleavage of the SREBP-1c isoform [10]. *In vivo*, SREBP-1c is primarily regulated by changes in nutritional status, which has no effects on SREBP-2 expression [11,12]. Recent studies done *in vivo* and *in vitro* have demonstrated that insulin induces the rapid cleavage (minutes) of SREBP-1c, in the absence of variations in sterol concentration [48]. Insulin *per se* is able to rapidly modulate the SREBP-1c concentration in the nucleus, independently of any effect on SREBP-1c transcription [48]. In contrast, activation of SREBP-1c transcription by an LXRα agonist alone increases the precursor form but not the mature nuclear form [48]. This could explain that in suckling rat or mice, a period characterized by a high LXRα transcriptional activity but a low-insulin concentration, the SREBP-1c target genes are not induced despite the presence of a high content of both SREBP-1c mRNA and precursor forms [33,49]. So far, the mechanisms by which insulin acts on SREBP-1c cleavage are not known. But according to recent observations, one could suggest that Insig proteins could be responsible for the differential effects of insulin, LXR agonists and sterols on the cleavage of the SREBP-1c and -2 isoforms. The Insig family is composed of three members: Insig-2a, Insig-2b produced from a single gene by alternative promoters and splicing sites, and Insig-1 from a separate gene [9,47,50]. Insig-2a and 2b differ in their first non-coding exons, thus they produce the same Insig-2 protein. A major difference between Insig-2a and 2b is their tissue distribution; Insig-2a transcripts are mainly expressed in the liver whereas Insig-2b transcripts are ubiquitous.

Interestingly, insulin decreases Insig-2a mRNA expression in the liver while it does not modify Insig-1 mRNA expression [50], suggesting that a decrease in Insig-2a protein leads specifically to the cleavage of SREBP-1c. In contrast, an LXR agonist increases Insig-2a expression [33,48], and this could contribute to the absence of nuclear SREBP-1c in the presence of an LXR agonist and low-insulin concentrations.

3.3. *Post-translational modifications of SREBPs*

Inside the nucleus, the transcriptional activity of mature nuclear SREBP (nSREBP) is regulated by covalent modifications or by interaction with other proteins. The first evidence indicating that SREBPs are modified at a post-translational level came from a study performed by Spiegelman et al. [12], showing that insulin augments the transcriptional activity of nSREBP-1c overexpressed in 3T3-L1 adipocytes.

Further studies (mainly performed in cell lines) have shown that insulin also stimulates the transcriptional activity of nSREBP-2 and -1a through a mitogen-activated protein kinase (MAPK) pathway. The Ser-117 residue has been identified as the major phosphorylation site for MAPK in SREBP-1a [51]. Ser-432 and -455 are described as the MAPK phosphorylation sites [52] *in vitro* and *in vivo* in SREBP-2. These phosphorylations do not modify DNA binding, but enhance SREBP-2 transactivation capacity. A role for MAPK in the modification of SREBP-1c transcriptional activity remains controversial. Although the Ser-117 target of MAPK in

SREBP-1a is also present in the SREBP-1c isoform, the use of inhibitors of the MAPK pathway in cultured hepatocytes do not antagonize the effect of insulin on SREBP-1c target genes [53,54], suggesting that SREBP-1c is not phosphorylated by MAPK in hepatocytes. It was shown recently [55] that glycogen synthase kinase 3 (GSK 3) phosphorylates SREBP-1c and that this phosphorylation decreases nuclear SREBP-1c transcriptional activity. Since insulin inactivates GSK 3, it suggests that insulin could activate nSREBP-1c transcriptional activity through an inhibition of this enzyme [55]. In the nucleus, nSREBPs are modified by ubiquitination and rapidly degraded by the 26 S proteasome [56]. In the presence of the proteasome inhibitors ALLN and lactacystin, nSREBPs are stabilized, and expression of their target genes is enhanced. It has been further demonstrated that SREBP transcription factors are ubiquitinated and degraded through a transcription-dependent pathway involving the proteasome, which thereby terminates the transcriptional signal. These effects require both a functional transactivation and DNA binding domain in SREBPs [57].

In recent years, efforts have been made to identify proteins which interact specifically with SREBP-1c and could modify its transcriptional activity. Kim et al. have shown that SREBP-1c interacts with Twist2, a protein expressed in fat and liver. Overexpression of Twist2 repressed the transcriptional activity of SREBP-1c by inhibiting its binding to target promoters [58].

4. SREBP target genes

While SREBPs display overlapping specificities in trans-activating target genes, several studies demonstrated isoform specific functions. The development of transgenic mice expressing nuclear forms of SREBPs in the liver has been particularly informative in identifying target genes of each individual isoform. Overexpression of the nuclear form of SREBP-1a in mouse liver [59,60] markedly increases the expression of genes involved in cholesterol (for example, 3-hydroxy-3-methylglutaryl-CoA (HMG-CoA) synthase, HMG-CoA reductase, squalene synthase) and fatty acid synthesis (for example, ACC, FAS and SCD-1), and induces a concomitant accumulation of both cholesterol and triglycerides [59,61]. Mice overexpressing hepatic nSREBP-1c demonstrate a selective induction of lipogenic genes, with no effect on genes of cholesterol synthesis [59]. The hepatic overexpression of nSREBP-2 isoform in mice causes a preferential induction of genes involved in cholesterol biosynthesis, although a moderate induction of genes involved in fatty acid synthesis is also observed [60,62]. A comprehensive list of target genes is provided in [63]. Importantly, in addition to genes encoding enzymes of these pathways, SREBPs augment the expression of genes involved in the generation of NADPH, an obligatory co-factor for lipid synthesis [64]. Using luciferase-reporter gene assays in Hep-G2 cells, Amemiya-Kudo et al. [65] showed that the selectivity of the SREBP isoforms for cholesterogenic and/or lipogenic genes is at least partly due to their differing affinities for the various consensus sequences in the target gene DNA.

The selective deletion of the SREBP-1c isoform by homologous recombination leads to a reduction in basal expression of mRNAs encoding enzymes of fatty acids and triglyceride synthesis [29], thus confirming the importance of this isoform in the control of lipogenic genes. Furthermore, the characteristic increase in expression of lipogenic genes in response to a fasting/refeeding regime is severely blunted in SREBP-1c null mice and completely abolished in mice lacking both SREBP-1 isoforms [29,66]. Interestingly, both SREBP-1c -/- and SREBP-1 -/- mice exhibit an increase in hepatic SREBP-2 mRNA. This leads to a corresponding increase in expression of genes encoding cholesterol biosynthetic enzymes and may also partially compensate for the lack of SREBP-1 isoforms in the regulation of lipogenic genes [29,66].

4.1. *SREBP-1c is the mediator of insulin action on hepatic glycolytic and lipogenic genes*

4.1.1. *Long-term regulation of hepatic glycolytic/lipogenic and gluconeogenic enzymes*
The expression of several key glycolytic and lipogenic enzymes is induced by a high-carbohydrate diet in the liver [67]: glucokinase, 6-phosphofructo-1-, 6-phospho-fructo-2-kinase/fructose-2-6-bisphosphatase, aldolase B and L-pyruvate kinase (L-PK) for glycolysis, ATP-citrate lyase, ACC, FAS, SCD-1 for lipogenesis, glucose-6-phosphate dehydrogenase, 6-phosphogluconate dehydrogenase for the pentose-phosphate pathway. High glucose also leads to induction of the S14 gene, which encodes a small acidic polypeptide that is related to lipogenesis although its exact function remains unclear. It is expressed in lipogenic tissues (white and brown adipose tissue, liver, lactating mammary gland) and shares a similar regulation with genes involved in the lipogenic pathway [68–70]. For most of these genes involved in glucose carbon utilisation, the induction of their mRNA expression by a carbohydrate-rich diet is powerful (from 4 to 25 fold), rapid (in the one-two hours range) and involves a transcriptional mechanism. Conversely, the expression of gluconeogenic enzymes such as phosphoenolpyruvate carboxykinase (PEPCK) [71] and glucose-6-phosphatase [72] is strongly repressed after a high carbohydrate meal.

In vitro studies have identified different kinds of gene regulation for genes involved in the lipogenic pathway: purely insulin sensitive genes such as hepatic glucokinase, which can be induced by a high-insulin concentration independently from the presence of glucose [73] and genes that require both increased insulin and glucose concentration in order to be induced, such as L-PK, FAS, ACC, S14 and SCD-1 [74–78]. One potential reason why these genes require both a high-insulin and a high-glucose concentration could be linked to the fact that after a meal the metabolic priority is to replenish glycogen stores, and it is only if glucose is particularly abundant that the glucose carbons are orientated toward lipid synthesis.

4.1.2. *Regulation of Glucokinase transcription by SREBP-1c*
Glucokinase is one of the only hepatic metabolic genes which requires solely insulin as an activator. Glucokinases in hepatic and pancreatic β-cells play a key role in glucose metabolism and β-cell insulin secretion as underlined by the diabetes mellitus

associated with glucokinase mutations or by the consequences of tissue-specific knock-outs [79–82]. In addition to short-term regulation of the enzyme itself by glucose-6-phosphate, glucokinase levels are regulated at a transcriptional level. Two different promoters direct glucokinase transcription in the liver or in pancreatic β-cells [82,83]. The downstream promoter determines the expression of the hepatic GK. In the liver, glucokinase transcription is activated by insulin and is repressed by glucagon via cAMP [73,83,84].

Using dominant positive and negative forms of SREBP-1c cloned in adenoviral vectors [16,85], we have shown in cultured hepatocytes that the transcriptional activity of SREBP-1c was absolutely necessary for insulin action on glucokinase gene expression, and that overexpression of a dominant positive form of SREBP-1c mimicked the effects of insulin on this gene. The importance of SREBP-1c for expression of the glucokinase gene has also been demonstrated *in vivo*. In STZ diabetic mice, adenovirus-mediated overexpression of SREBP-1c in the liver resulted in an increase of glucokinase gene expression and activity as well as an increase in the hepatic glycogen content [86], mimicking the effect of an insulin injection. When mouse livers lack all forms of nuclear SREBP (SCAP or S1P deficient mice) the response of glucokinase to refeeding is abolished [29]. In mice deficient in 3-phosphoinositide-dependent protein kinase (PDK-1), an obligatory step of PI3-kinase mediated insulin action, SREBP-1c expression is not induced by refeeding, and glucokinase expression is severely blunted [87]. The bulk of these studies demonstrated that SREBP-1c is essential for glucokinase expression and that it is a mediator of insulin action on the hepatic gene expression.

4.1.3. SREBP-1c mediates insulin action in liver on lipogenic genes and on a gluconeogenic gene, phosphoenolpyruvate carboxykinase

The involvement of SREBP-1c in insulin action on genes that require for their full expression, both insulin and a high-glucose concentration namely L-PK, FAS, ACC and S14 was also demonstrated [16,85]. It must be pointed out that for lipogenic genes, it acts in concert with another transcription factor, namely Carbohydrate Response Element Binding Protein (ChREBP) (see Section 5).

As described above, the genes encoding gluconeogenic enzymes are negatively controlled by insulin in the liver. Using the dominant positive and negative forms of SREBP-1c, it was confirmed *in vitro* that PEPCK gene transcription is inhibited by SREBP-1c [88].

Further experiments suggested an interaction between SREBP-1c and CBP [88], the transcriptional co-activator critical in coordinating the cAMP stimulation of PEPCK gene transcription [89] and defined a SREBP-1c element in the PEPCK promoter [90]. SREBP-1c was also described as interfering with HNF 4 binding on the PEPCK promoter [91]. However, in cultured primary hepatocytes, we have been unable to show an effect of SREBP-1c on glucose-6-phosphatase gene expression (unpublished results), suggesting that the action of insulin on this gene may be mediated by another factor, probably the factor FOXO1 of the Forkhead family [92].

The importance of SREBP-1c for the expression of lipogenic genes was also demonstrated *in vivo* by showing that their induction by a high-carbohydrate diet was precluded in SREBP-1 knock-out mice [64]. In STZ diabetic mice, adenovirus-mediated overexpression of SREBP-1c in the liver resulted in an increase of lipogenic (FAS, S14) enzyme expression and a dramatic decrease of PEPCK expression [86], mimicking perfectly the effect of an insulin injection. The physiological consequences of SREBP-1c hepatic overexpression include an increase of the glycogen and triglyceride hepatic content and a marked decrease in the hyperglycemia of STZ diabetic mice [86].

4.2. SREBP-1c target genes in non-hepatic tissues

Adipose tissue was the first tissue for which an effect of insulin on SREBP-1c transcriptional activity was described and in which FAS promoter was identified as a SREBP-1c target [12]. The action of insulin on SREBP-1c expression in human adipocytes was also demonstrated [5]. Other genes such as the LDL receptor and SCD-1 have been since characterized as SREBP-1c and insulin target genes, as well as the transcription factor CCAAT/enhancer-binding protein beta [93] and hexokinase II [15], which is the equivalent of liver glucokinase in terms of glucose metabolism. SREBP-1c has been implicated also in adipose tissue differentiation [94]. However, experiments in which SREBP-1c levels have been manipulated in the adipose tissue of mice have been less clear in elucidating a role for this transcription factor in adipogenesis. Overexpression of nSREBP-1c using the adipose-specific aP2 promoter would be expected to promote fat cell development, but instead resulted in the opposite phenotype: lipodystrophy [95]. The mice were also diabetic and had fatty livers, phenotypes also present in humans with lipodystrophy. On the other hand, Horton et al. [61] have shown that overexpression of the nSREBP-1a isoform in adipose tissue of mice resulted in hypertrophy of adipocytes.

In muscles, SREBP-1c expression and nuclear abundance is also stimulated by insulin [5,6,15] and target genes include genes involved in the lipogenic pathway as well as hexokinase II. Hexokinase II has a major role in terms of glucose utilization since it is the first enzyme of glucose metabolism, which feeds both glycogen synthesis as well as glycolysis. It is thus a major component of insulin-induced glucose utilization. Interestingly, insulin-induced down-regulation of UCP3, a protein of the uncoupling protein family, induced by fasting and high-fat feeding, seems too be also mediated by SREBP-1c [6].

In the pancreas or in pancreatic cell lines, overexpression studies have clearly shown that SREBP-1c controls the expression of lipogenic genes [96–99]. Effects on other classes of genes have also been described, for instance an increase in UCP2 [97,99,100]. However, it is difficult to know whether these latter effects are direct or secondary to the large changes in lipid and glucose metabolism observed in the same experimental conditions. At present, whether the control of SREBP-1c by insulin in the pancreas is similar to the liver is not clear.

4.3. *Insulin signaling pathway for SREBP-1c expression*

How does insulin stimulate SREBP-1c expression in the liver? This effect could be mediated through IRS-1 since animal models of insulin resistance presenting a reduced or absent expression of IRS-2 (ob/ob mice, lipodystrophic mice and IRS2-/- mice) are still able to strongly express SREBP-1c and its target genes [101]. In addition, inhibition of insulin-induced IRS-1 phosphorylation abolishes the induction of SREBP-1c gene expression by insulin in cultured rat hepatocytes [102]. Studies using inhibitors of various branches of the insulin signaling pathway have shown that the effect of insulin on SREBP-1c expression and synthesis involves mainly the PI3-kinase pathway [17,103]. The downstream effector(s) remain unclear, with evidence suggesting that both PKB/Akt [103,104] and PKCλ [105] may be involved.

In L-6 skeletal muscle cells, insulin increases skeletal muscle SREBP-1 expression in a dose-dependent fashion via the MAP kinase-dependent signaling pathway whereas in 3T3-L1 adipocytes, insulin action on SREBP-1 expression is mediated via the PI3-kinase signaling pathway [106].

5. Mechanisms involved in glucose action: involvement of the "Carbohydrate Response Element Binding Protein" transcription factor

5.1. *The transcription factor "Carbohydrate response element binding protein"*

As stated above, a subset of glycolytic/lipogenic genes in the liver requires both an increased insulin and glucose concentration to be fully expressed [67]. This regulation involves the stimulation of their transcription rate. In the absence of glucose, insulin by itself is unable to induce their expression. In the absence of insulin, the effect of glucose is greatly reduced in adipose tissue and nearly absent in cultured hepatocytes.

Glucose must be metabolized in order to activate gene expression. Glucose-6-phosphate and xylulose-5-phosphate an intermediate of the non-oxidative branch of the metabolic pathway have both been proposed as the metabolic signal. Glucose or carbohydrate response elements (ChoRE) have been characterized on the promoter of most glucose-responsive genes, L-PK, FAS, S14, ACC [76,107–110]. The group of Uyeda has purified a transcription factor from rat liver, based on its capacity to bind to the ChoRE of the L-PK promoter and named it ChREBP [111]. When transfected in hepatocytes, ChREBP is able to stimulate the L-PK promoter which contains the ChoRE, and this effect is dramatically increased in the presence of glucose. The increase in expression of hepatic glycolytic and lipogenic genes after a high-carbohydrate diet is markedly reduced in mice lacking ChREBP gene expression in comparison to wild type mice [112]. These studies were confirmed in isolated hepatocytes, showing that when the ChREBP transcriptional activity is reduced, glucose is unable to activate genes such as FAS ACC or L-PK [39,113,114].

The mechanism suggested in order to explain the glucose effect on target gene transcription is a translocation of ChREBP between the cytoplasm and the nucleus. ChREBP is located in the cytoplasm when the glucose concentration is low and enters into the nucleus at high glucose [115]. This would be secondary to a dephosphorylation of a specific serine (Ser 196) otherwise phosphorylated by protein kinase A (PKA) in conditions of high-cAMP concentrations such as the fasting state for instance. A second PKA phosphorylation near the DNA-binding domain and which precludes ChREBP binding would also be dephosphorylated in the presence of high glucose [115]. Thus, the main effect of glucose would be to activate a phosphatase counteracting the effect of cAMP, inducing the translocation of ChREBP in the nucleus and stimulating its DNA-binding activity. This would be consistent with the antagonistic effect of glucagon and insulin/glucose on L-PK and lipogenic genes. Recently, phosphatases activated by xylulose-5-phosphates have been identified [116]. They are able to dephosphorylate Ser 196 of ChREBP, thus favoring its translocation into the nucleus.

5.2. *Integration of insulin/glucose regulation of glycolytic and lipogenic genes in the liver*

When a carbohydrate-rich meal is absorbed, plasma glucose concentration is increased and it induces a secretion of insulin by the pancreatic β-cells. High concentrations of both glucose and insulin then reach the liver through the portal vein. Insulin will induce SREBP-1c transcription by a PI3-kinase dependent mechanism and hence the synthesis of the precursor form in the endoplasmic reticulum (Fig. 1). This precursor form will be then cleaved, a process stimulated by insulin and the mature form of SREBP-1c will translocate into the nucleus and activate glucokinase in the liver (and hexokinase II in muscles). Synthesis of glucokinase increases glucose phosphorylation and glycogen repletion. A signal metabolite downstream of the glucokinase step (like xylulose-5-phosphate) activates a transcription factor (ChREBP) by a dephosphorylation-mediated mechanism. ChREBP then translocates into the nucleus where together with SREBP-1c, it activates genes of the glycolytic/lipogenic pathway such as L-PK, ACC, FAS and S14. This will finally lead to the synthesis of fatty acyl-CoA from glucose carbons and ultimately to triglycerides.

6. SREBPs and physiopathology

6.1. *SREBP-1c and insulin sensitivity*

In terms of relationship with metabolic diseases, SREBP-1c can be considered from two opposite perspectives. First, as a transcription factor central for the genomic actions of insulin on both carbohydrate and lipid metabolism, a loss of function should ultimately lead to a phenomenon of insulin resistance. Interestingly enough, in SREBP-1c knock-out mice there is a tendency for a higher basal plasma glucose when compared to wild type mice and a higher glycemia during a carbohydrate refeeding period [29]. On the other hand, SREBP-1c promotes fatty acid synthesis and lipid deposition. Since lipids have been largely implicated in the development of insulin resistance by mechanisms involving substrate competition, antagonism of insulin signaling or lipotoxicity [117], SREBP-1c could also be considered as a factor responsible for insulin resistance. Liver overexpression of SREBP-1c has indeed been described in several models of insulin resistance such as lipodystrophic and ob/ob mice [101], insulin receptor substrate-2 knock-out mice [118] and Zucker obese fa/fa rats [119]. Thus a mutation inducing a gain of function for SREBP-1c could also be responsible for insulin resistance.

Altogether, SREBPs have been incriminated in the development of human metabolic physiopathology such as obesity, type 2 diabetes, dyslipidemia, atherosclerosis, global syndrome X and lipodystrophy. In adipose tissue of obese and type 2 diabetic patients, SREBP-1c mRNA expression was found to be decreased in comparison with lean subjects [5,18,120–123]. These observations are consistent with DNA microarray studies in animal models showing down-regulation of SREBP-1c in adipose tissue of *ob/ob* mice and obese mice progressing to overt diabetes [124,125]. The resistance to insulin observed in obesity and type 2 diabetes has been involved in order to explain the diminished SREBP-1c expression observed. Consistent with this hypothesis, weight loss in obese patients, which is associated with an improved insulin-sensitivity, is also associated with an increase in SREBP-1c expression in adipose tissue [120–122]. In muscle, SREBP-1c mRNA expression is decreased in type 2 diabetic patients but not in obese patients [5,18]. Many individuals with obesity and insulin resistance also have fatty livers. Due to obvious limitations, SREBP-1c mRNA expression in human liver cannot be studied but data in animal models are available. SREBP-1c levels are elevated in the fatty livers of obese, insulin-resistant and hyperinsulinemic *ob/ob* mice [101,126]. Despite the profound insulin resistance of the liver concerning glucose production in these mice, insulin continues to activate the SREBP-1c transcription and protein expression in their liver. This could be explained by the fact that in the insulin-signaling pathway, SREBP-1c transcription is dependent upon the presence of IRS-1, which is not downregulated in these mice, in contrast with IRS-2, which is down-regulated and mediates the insulin inhibitory effects on glucose production. Thus, the elevated nSREBP-1c increases lipogenic gene expression, enhances fatty acid synthesis and accelerates triglyceride accumulation [101,126].

6.2. SREBP-1c and insulin secretion

Several studies demonstrated that overxpression of SREBP-1c in pancreatic cell lines or islets led to a marked reduction in glucose-stimulated insulin secretion, and this was attributed to the concomitant triglyceride accumulation and the subsequent lipotoxicity [97,98,100].

It has been demonstrated in Zucker diabetic fa/fa rats an inappropriately high expression of SREBP-1c and its target lipogenic genes in islets inducing increased triglycerides storage that could account for the associated alterations of pancreatic β-cells that end up in diabetes [119].

6.3. *Genetic association of SREBP-1c with metabolic diseases*

Genetic approaches have highlighted a contribution of SREBPs transcription factors in the development of metabolic pathology or deleterious metabolic traits. Genome scan studies have linked the 17p11 region, comprising the human *SREBF-1* gene locus [2], to plasma leptin concentrations in American obese families [127] and to body mass index in a combined analysis of four ethnic groups [128]. A meta-analysis performed in four European genome-wide screens demonstrated linkage between the 17p11.2-q22 region and type 2 diabetes [129].

Recently, we performed an extensive molecular screening of the whole *SREBF-1* gene for Single Nucleotide Polymorphisms (SNPs) detection [130]. By case-control and association studies performed in large French obese, diabetic, and non-obese non-diabetic cohorts, we have shown that SNPs of the *SREBF-1* gene were associated with obesity and type 2 diabetes. Moreover, SNPs were associated with male-specific hypertriglyceridemia within the obese group. At the same time, Laudes et al. [131] identified a common variant linked to type 2 diabetes risk in men and plasma cholesterol level. Previous genetic studies of *SREBF-1* SNPs have observed modifications in lipid parameters in predominantly male populations [132–134]. Vedie et al. [132] observed that a *SREBF-1* SNP was associated with an atherogenic lipid profile in men at high-cardiovascular risk. In a study evaluating fluvastatin treatment, patients demonstrated differentially modified lipid parameters according to *SREBF-1* genotypes [134]. Another study of highly active antiretroviral therapy (HAART) in HIV-1-infected patients showed that *SREBF-1* SNP carriers had a high risk of developing hyperlipoproteinemia [133]. SREBP-1 related dyslipidemia thus seem to develop in particular pathophysiological contexts, suggesting that gene–gene and/or gene–environment interactions could be necessary for the phenotype expression.

7. Conclusion

Among the various effectors of insulin, the SREBP-1c pathway can be considered as a system that signals to and prepares the tissues to a period of carbohydrate availability. First, by increasing the glucose-phosphorylating activity in the liver (glucokinase activity) and in muscles, it will contribute to replenish the glycogen stores allowing then during the next interprandial interval to provide glucose to organs such as the brain or to have plenty of fuel in case of an exercise. This is an important role since defects of glycogen metabolism are concomitant with dramatic alterations of glucose homeostasis in humans [135].

The capacity of SREBP-1c of maintaining a lipogenic capacity in the liver in conjunction with ChREBP, extends further its role since glucose carbons will be transformed into lipids ultimately stored in adipose tissue, allowing to face even longer periods of energy deprivation. It is probably not a coincidence if SREBP-1c is also an adipocyte differentiation factor [136]. SREBP-1c can be then considered as a real "thrifty" gene, i.e., a gene favoring storage which has allowed the species survival in the context of successive episodes of food availability and restriction.

As such, it can certainly participate to the dramatic increase of obesity and diabetes prevalence given that the nutritional conditions are now extremely favorable.

Acknowledgments

We gratefully thank the following persons for their contribution to the personal work presented in this review: D. Azzout-Marniche, D. Bécard, A. Bobard, P. Bossard, M. Foretz and I. Hainault.

References

[1] X. Wang, R. Sato, M.S. Brown, X. Hua, J.L. Goldstein, SREBP-1,a membrane-bound transcription factor released by sterol-regulated proteolysis, Cell 77 (1994) 53–62.
[2] X. Hua, J. Wu, J.L. Goldstein, M.S. Brown, H.H. Hobbs, Structure of the human gene encoding sterol regulatory element binding protein-1 (SREBF1) and localization of SREBF1 and SREBF2 to chromosomes 17p11.2 and 22q13, Genomics 25 (1995) 667–673.
[3] H. Shimano, J.D. Horton, I. Shimomura, R.E. Hammer, M.S. Brown, J.L. Goldstein, Isoform 1c of sterol regulatory element binding protein is less active than isoform 1a in livers of transgenic mice and in cultured cells, J. Clin. Invest. 99 (1997) 846–854.
[4] I. Shimomura, H. Shimano, J.D. Horton, J.L. Goldstein, M. Brown, Differential expression of exons1a and 1c in mRNAs for sterol regulatory element binding protein-1 in human and mouse organs and cultured cells, J. Clin. Invest. 99 (1997) 838–845.
[5] P.H. Ducluzeau, N. Perretti, M. Laville, F. Andreelli, N. Vega, J.P. Riou, H. Vidal, Regulation by insulin of gene expression in human skeletal muscle and adipose tissue. Evidence for specific defects in type 2 diabetes, Diabetes 50 (2001) 1134–1142.
[6] I. Guillet-Deniau, V. Mieulet, S. Le Lay, Y. Achouri, D. Carre, J. Girard, F. Foufelle, P. Ferré, Sterol regulatory element binding protein-1c expression and action in rat muscles : insulin-like effects on the control of glycolytic and lipogenic enzymes and UCP3 gene expression, Diabetes 51 (2002) 1722–1728.
[7] M.S. Brown, J.L. Goldstein, The SREBP pathway: regulation of cholesterol metabolism by proteolysis of a membrane-bound transcription factor, Cell 89 (1997) 331–340.
[8] M.S. Brown, J.L. Goldstein, A proteolytic pathway that controls the cholesterol content of membranes, cells, and blood, Proc. Natl. Acad. Sci. USA 96 (1999) 11041–11048.
[9] T. Yang, P.J. Espenshade, M.E. Wright, D. Yabe, Y. Gong, R. Aebersold, J.L. Goldstein, M.S. Brown, Crucial step in cholesterol homeostasis: sterols promote binding of SCAP to INSIG-1, a membrane protein that facilitates retention of SREBPs in ER, Cell 110 (2002) 489–500.
[10] Z. Sheng, H. Otani, M.S. Brown, J.L. Goldstein, Independent regulation of sterol regulatory element binding proteins 1 and 2 in hamster liver, Proc. Natl. Acad. Sci. USA 92 (1995) 935–938.
[11] J.D. Horton, Y. Bashmakov, I. Shimomura, H. Shimano, Regulation of sterol regulatory element binding proteins in livers of fasted and refed mice. Proc, Natl. Acad. Sci. 95 (1998) 5987–5992.
[12] J.B. Kim, P. Sarraf, M. Wright, K.M. Yao, E. Mueller, G. Solanes, B.B. Lowell, B. Spiegelman, Nutritional and insulin regulation of fatty acid synthetase and leptin gene expression through ADD1/SREBP1, J. Clin. Invest. 101 (1998) 1–9.
[13] M.E. Bizeau, P.S. MacLean, G.C. Johnson, Y. Wei, Skeletal muscle sterol regulatory element binding protein-1c decreases with food deprivation and increases with feeding in rats, J. Nutr. 133 (2003) 1787–1792.
[14] S.R. Commerford, L. Peng, J.J. Dube, R.M. O'Doherty, *In vivo* regulation of SREBP-1c in skeletal muscle: effects of nutritional status, glucose, insulin, and leptin, Am. J. Physiol. Regul. Integr. Comp. Physiol. 287 (2004) R218–R227.

[15] Y. Gosmain, N. Dif, V. Berbe, E. Loizon, J. Rieusset, H. Vidal, E. Lefai, Regulation of SREBP-1 expression and transcriptional action on HKII and FAS genes during fasting and refeeding in rat tissues, J. Lipid Res. 1 (2005) 1.

[16] M. Foretz, C. Pacot, I. Dugail, P. Lemarchand, C. Guichard, X. Le Liepvre, C. Berthelier-Lubrano, B. Spiegelman, J.B. Kim, P. Ferre, F. Foufelle, ADD1/SREBP-1c is required in the activation of hepatic lipogenic gene expression by glucose, Mol. Cell. Biol. 19 (1999) 3760–3768.

[17] D. Azzout-Marniche, D. Becard, C. Guichard, M. Foretz, P. Ferre, F. Foufelle, Insulin effects on sterol regulatory-element-binding protein-1c (SREBP-1c) transcriptional activity in rat hepatocytes, Biochem. J. 350 (2000) 389–393.

[18] C. Sewter, D. Berger, R.V. Considine, G. Medina, J. Rochford, T. Ciaraldi, R. Henry, L. Dohm, J.S. Flier, S. O'Rahilly, A.J. Vidal-Puig, Human obesity and type 2 diabetes are associated with alterations in SREBP1 isoform expression that are reproduced ex vivo by tumor necrosis factor-alpha, Diabetes 51 (2002) 1035–1041.

[19] I. Shimomura, Y. Bashmakov, S. Ikemoto, J.D. Horton, M.S. Brown, J.L. Goldstein, Insulin selectively increases SREBP-1c mRNA in the livers of rats with streptozotocin-induced diabetes, Proc. Natl. Acad. Sci. USA 96 (1999) 13656–13661.

[20] J.M. Lehmann, S.A. Kliewer, L.B. Moore, T.A. Smith-Oliver, B.B. Oliver, J.L. Su, S.S. Sundseth, D.A. Winegar, D.E. Blanchard, T.A. Spencer, T.M. Willson, Activation of the nuclear receptor LXR by oxysterols defines a new hormone response pathway, J. Biol. Chem. 272 (1997) 3137–3140.

[21] B.A. Janowski, M.J. Grogan, S.A. Jones, G.B. Wisely, S.A. Kliewer, E.J. Corey, D.J. Mangelsdorf, Structural requirements of ligands for the oxysterol liver X receptors LXRalpha and LXRbeta, Proc. Natl. Acad. Sci. USA 96 (1999) 266–271.

[22] K.R. Steffensen, J.A. Gustafsson, Putative metabolic effects of the liver X receptor (LXR), Diabetes 53 (Suppl 1) (2004) S36–S42.

[23] D.J. Peet, S.D. Turley, W. Ma, B.A. Janowski, J.M. Lobaccaro, R.E. Hammer, D.J. Mangelsdorf, Cholesterol and bile acid metabolism are impaired in mice lacking the nuclear oxysterol receptor LXR alpha, Cell 93 (1998) 693–704.

[24] J.J. Repa, G. Liang, J. Ou, Y. Bashmakov, J.M. Lobaccaro, I. Shimomura, B. Shan, M.S. Brown, J.L. Goldstein, D.J. Mangelsdorf, Regulation of mouse sterol regulatory element-binding protein-1c gene (SREBP-1c) by oxysterol receptors, LXRalpha and LXRbeta, Genes Dev 14 (2000) 2819–2830.

[25] J.R. Schultz, H. Tu, A. Luk, J.J. Repa, J.C. Medina, L. Li, S. Schwendner, S. Wang, M. Thoolen, D.J. Mangelsdorf, K.D. Lustig, B. Shan, Role of LXRs in control of lipogenesis, Genes Dev. 14 (2000) 2831–2838.

[26] B.A. Laffitte, L.C. Chao, J. Li, R. Walczak, S. Hummasti, S.B. Joseph, A. Castrillo, D.C. Wilpitz, D.J. Mangelsdorf, J.L. Collins, E. Saez, P. Tontonoz, Activation of liver X receptor improves glucose tolerance through coordinate regulation of glucose metabolism in liver and adipose tissue, Proc. Natl. Acad. Sci. USA 100 (2003) 5419–5424.

[27] P. Tontonoz, D.J. Mangelsdorf, Liver X receptor signaling pathways in cardiovascular disease, Mol. Endocrinol. 17 (2003) 985–993.

[28] S.B. Joseph, B.A. Laffitte, P.H. Patel, M.A. Watson, K.E. Matsukuma, R. Walczak, J.L. Collins, T.F. Osborne, P. Tontonoz, Direct and indirect mechanisms for regulation of fatty acid synthase gene expression by LXRs, J. Biol. Chem. 14 (2002) 14.

[29] G. Liang, J. Yang, J.D. Horton, R.E. Hammer, J.L. Goldstein, M.S. Brown, Diminished hepatic response to fasting/refeeding and liver X receptor agonists in mice with selective deficiency of sterol regulatory element-binding protein-1c, J. Biol. Chem. 277 (2002) 9520–9528.

[30] T. Yoshikawa, H. Shimano, M. Amemiya-Kudo, N. Yahagi, A.H. Hasty, T. Matsuzaka, H. Okazaki, Y. Tamura, Y. Iizuka, K. Ohashi, J. Osuga, K. Harada, T. Gotoda, S. Kimura, S. Ishibashi, N. Yamada, Identification of liver X receptor-retinoid X receptor as an activator of the sterol regulatory element-binding protein 1c gene promoter, Mol. Cell. Biol. 21 (2001) 2991–3000.

[31] G. Chen, G. Liang, J. Ou, J.L. Goldstein, M.S. Brown, Central role for liver X receptor in insulin-mediated activation of Srebp-1c transcription and stimulation of fatty acid synthesis in liver, Proc. Natl. Acad. Sci. USA 101 (2004) 11245–11250.

[32] L.M. Cagen, X. Deng, H.G. Wilcox, E.A. Park, R. Raghow, M.B. Elam, Insulin activates the rat sterol-regulatory-element-binding protein 1c (SREBP-1c) promoter through the combinatorial actions of SREBP, LXR, Sp-1 and NF-Y cis-acting elements, Biochem. J. 385 (2005) 207–216.

[33] A. Bobard, I. Hainault, P. Ferre, F. Foufelle, P. Bossard, Differential regulation of sterol regulatory element-binding protein 1c transcriptional activity by insulin and liver x receptor during liver development, J. Biol. Chem. 280 (2005) 199–206 Epub 2004 Oct 27.

[34] K.A. Tobin, S.M. Ulven, G.U. Schuster, H.H. Steineger, S.M. Andresen, J.A. Gustafsson, H.I. Nebb, LXRs as insulin mediating factors in fatty acid and cholesterol biosynthesis, J. Biol. Chem. 7 (2002) 7.

[35] A.H. Hasty, H. Shimano, N. Yahagi, M. Amemiya-Kudo, S. Perrey, T. Yoshikawa, J. Osuga, H. Okazaki, Y. Tamura, Y. Iizuka, F. Shionoiri, K. Ohashi, K. Harada, T. Gotoda, R. Nagai, S. Ishibashi, N. Yamada, Sterol regulatory element-binding protein-1 is regulated by glucose at the transcriptional level, J. Biol. Chem. 275 (2000) 31069–31077.

[36] I. Guillet-Deniau, A.L. Pichard, A. Kone, C. Esnous, M. Nieruchalski, J. Girard, C. Prip-Buus, Glucose induces de novo lipogenesis in rat muscle satellite cells through a sterol-regulatory-element-binding protein-1c-dependent pathway, J. Cell. Sci. 117 (2004) 1937–1944.

[37] X. Deng, L.M. Cagen, H.G. Wilcox, E.A. Park, R. Raghow, M.B. Elam, Regulation of the rat SREBP-1c promoter in primary rat hepatocytes, Biochem. Biophys. Res. Commun. 290 (2002) 256–262.

[38] D.K. Scott, J.J. Collier, T.T. Doan, A.S. Bunnell, M.C. Daniels, D.T. Eckert, R.M. O'Doherty, A modest glucokinase overexpression in the liver promotes fed expression levels of glycolytic and lipogenic enzyme genes in the fasted state without altering SREBP-1c expression, Mol. Cell. Biochem. 254 (2003) 327–337.

[39] R. Dentin, J.P. Pegorier, F. Benhamed, F. Foufelle, P. Ferre, V. Fauveau, M.A. Magnuson, J. Girard, C. Postic, Hepatic glucokinase is required for the synergistic action of ChREBP and SREBP-1c on glycolytic and lipogenic gene expression, J. Biol. Chem. 279 (2004) 20314–20326 Epub 2004 Feb 25.

[40] T. Matsuzaka, H. Shimano, N. Yahagi, M. Amemiya-Kudo, H. Okazaki, Y. Tamura, Y. Iizuka, K. Ohashi, S. Tomita, M. Sekiya, A. Hasty, Y. Nakagawa, H. Sone, H. Toyoshima, S. Ishibashi, J. Osuga, N. Yamada, Insulin-independent induction of sterol regulatory element-binding protein-1c expression in the livers of streptozotocin-treated mice, Diabetes 53 (2004) 560–569.

[41] G. Zhou, R. Myers, Y. Li, Y. Chen, X. Shen, J. Fenyk-Melody, M. Wu, J. Ventre, T. Doebber, N. Fujii, N. Musi, M.F. Hirshman, L.J. Goodyear, D.E. Moller, Role of AMP-activated protein kinase in mechanism of metformin action, J. Clin. Invest. 108 (2001) 1167–1174.

[42] M. Foretz, D. Carling, G. Guichard, P. Ferré, F. Foufelle, AMP-activated protein kinase inhibits the glucose-activated expression of fatty acid synthase gene in rat hepatocytes, J. Biol. Chem. 273 (1998) 14767–14771.

[43] A. Nohturfft, M.S. Brown, J.L. Goldstein, Topology of SREBP cleavage-activating protein, a polytopic membrane protein with a sterol-sensing domain, J. Biol. Chem. 273 (1998) 17243–17250.

[44] J. Sakai, R.B. Rawson, P.J. Espenshade, D. Cheng, A.C. Seegmiller, J.L. Goldstein, M.S. Brown, Molecular identification of the sterol-regulated luminal protease that cleaves SREBPs and controls lipid composition of animal cells, Mol. Cell. 2 (1998) 505–514.

[45] A. Radhakrishnan, L.P. Sun, H.J. Kwon, M.S. Brown, J.L. Goldstein, Direct binding of cholesterol to the purified membrane region of SCAP: mechanism for a sterol-sensing domain, Mol. Cell. 15 (2004) 259–268.

[46] A.J. Brown, L. Sun, J.D. Feramisco, M.S. Brown, J.L. Goldstein, Cholesterol addition to ER membranes alters conformation of SCAP, the SREBP escort protein that regulates cholesterol metabolism, Mol. Cell. 10 (2002) 237–245.

[47] D. Yabe, M.S. Brown, J.L. Goldstein, Insig-2, a second endoplasmic reticulum protein that binds SCAP and blocks export of sterol regulatory element-binding proteins, Proc. Natl., Acad. Sci. USA 99 (2002) 12753–12758.

[48] B.D. Hegarty, A. Bobard, I. Hainault, P. Ferre, P. Bossard, F. Foufelle, Distinct roles of insulin and liver X receptor in the induction and cleavage of sterol regulatory element-binding protein-1c, Proc. Natl. Acad. Sci. USA 102 (2005) 791–796.

[49] D. Botolin, D.B. Jump, Selective proteolytic processing of rat hepatic sterol regulatory element binding protein-1 (SREBP-1) and SREBP-2 during postnatal development, J. Biol. Chem. 278 (2003) 6959–6962.

[50] D. Yabe, R. Komuro, G. Liang, J.L. Goldstein, M.S. Brown, Liver-specific mRNA for insig-2 down-regulated by insulin: implications for fatty acid synthesis, Proc. Natl. Acad. Sci. USA 100 (2003) 3155–3160.

[51] G. Roth, J. Kotzka, L. Kremer, S. Lehr, C. Lohaus, H.E. Meyer, W. Krone, D. Muller-Wieland, MAP kinases Erk1/2 phosphorylate sterol regulatory element-binding protein (SREBP)-1a at serine 117 *in vitro*, J. Biol. Chem. 275 (2000) 33302–33307.

[52] J. Kotzka, D. Muller-Wieland, G. Roth, L. Kremer, M. Munck, S. Schurmann, B. Knebel, W. Krone, Sterol regulatory element binding proteins (SREBP)-1a and SREBP-2 are linked to the MAP-kinase cascade, J. Lipid. Res. 41 (2000) 99–108.

[53] D. Wang, H.S. Sul, Insulin stimulation of the fatty acid synthase promoter is mediated by the phosphatidylinositol 3-kinase pathway. Involvement of protein kinase B/Akt,, J. Biol. Chem. 273 (1998) 25420–25426.

[54] P.B. Iynedjian, R.A. Roth, M. Fleischmann, A. Gjinovci, Activation of protein kinase B/cAkt in hepatocytes is sufficient for the induction of expression of the gene encoding glucokinase, Biochem. J. 351 (2000) 621–627.

[55] K.H. Kim, M.J. Song, E.J. Yoo, S.S. Choe, S.D. Park, J.B. Kim, Regulatory role of glycogen synthase kinase 3 for transcriptional activity of ADD1/SREBP1c, J. Biol. Chem. 279 (2004) 51999–52006 Epub.

[56] Y. Hirano, M. Yoshid, M. Shimizu, R. Sato, Direct demonstration of rapid degradation of nuclear sterol regulatory element-binding proteins by the ubiquitin-proteasome pathway, J. Biol. Chem. 276 (2001) 36431–36437.

[57] A. Sundqvist, J. Ericsson, Transcription-dependent degradation controls the stability of the SREBP family of transcription factors, Proc. Natl. Acad. Sci. USA 100 (2003) 13833–13838.

[58] Y.S. Lee, H.H. Lee, J. Park, E.J. Yoo, C.A. Glackin, Y.I. Choi, S.H. Jeon, R.H. Seong, S.D. Park, J.B. Kim, Twist2, a novel ADD1/SREBP1c interacting protein, represses the transcriptional activity of ADD1/SREBP1c, Nucleic Acids Res 31 (2003) 7165–7174.

[59] H. Shimano, J.D. Horton, R.E. Hammer, I. Shimomura, M.S. Brown, J.L. Goldstein, Overproduction of cholesterol and fatty acids causes massive liver enlargement in transgenic mice expressing truncated SREBP-1a, J. Clin. Invest. 98 (1996) 1575–1584.

[60] J.D. Horton, N.A. Shah, J.A. Warrington, N.N. Anderson, S.W. Park, M.S. Brown, J.L. Goldstein, Combined analysis of oligonucleotide microarray data from transgenic and knockout mice identifies direct SREBP target genes, Proc. Natl. Acad. Sci. USA 100 (2003) 12027–12032.

[61] J.D. Horton, I. Shimomura, S. Ikemoto, Y. Bashmakov, R.E. Hammer, Overexpression of SREBP-1a in mouse adipose tissue produces adipocyte hypertrophy, increased fatty acid secretion, and fatty liver, J. Biol. Chem. 278 (2003) 36652–36660.

[62] J.D. Horton, I. Shimomura, M. Brown, R. Hammer, J.L. Goldstein, H. Shimano, Activation of cholesterol synthesis in preference to fatty acid synthesis in liver and adipose tissue of transgenic mice overproducing sterol regulatory element binding protein 2, J. Clin. Invest. 101 (1998) 2331–2339.

[63] J.D. Horton, J.L. Goldstein, M.S. Brown, SREBPs: activators of the complete program of cholesterol and fatty acid synthesis in the liver, J. Clin. Invest. 109 (2002) 1125–1131.

[64] H. Shimano, N. Yahagi, M. Amemiya-Kudo, A.H. Hasty, J. Osuga, Y. Tamura, F. Shionoiri, Y. Iizuka, K. Ohashi, K. Harada, T. Gotoda, S. Ishibashi, N. Yamada, Sterol regulatory

element-binding protein-1 as a key transcription factor for nutritional induction of lipogenic enzyme genes, J. Biol. Chem. 274 (1999) 35832–35839.

[65] M. Amemiya-Kudo, H. Shimano, A.H. Hasty, N. Yahagi, T. Yoshikawa, T. Matsuzaka, H. Okazaki, Y. Tamura, Y. Iizuka, K. Ohashi, J. Osuga, K. Harada, T. Gotoda, R. Sato, S. Kimura, S. Ishibashi, N. Yamada, Transcriptional activities of nuclear SREBP-1a, -1c, and -2 to different target promoters of lipogenic and cholesterogenic genes, J. Lipid Res. 43 (2002) 1220–1235.

[66] H. Shimano, I. Shimomura, R.E. Hammer, J. Herz, J.L. Goldstein, M.S. Brown, J.D. Horton, Elevated levels of SREBP-2 and cholesterol synthesis in livers of mice homozygous for a targeted disruption of the SREBP-1 gene, J. Clin. Invest. 100 (1997) 2115–2124.

[67] F. Foufelle, P. Ferre, New perspectives in the regulation of hepatic glycolytic and lipogenic genes by insulin and glucose: a role for the transcription factor sterol regulatory element binding protein-1c, Biochem. J. 366 (2002) 377–391.

[68] C.N. Mariash, S. Seelig, H.L. Schwartz, J.H. Oppenheimer, Rapid synergistic interaction between thyroid hormone and carbohydrate on mRNAS14 induction, J. Biol. Chem. 261 (1986) 9583–9586.

[69] W.B. Kinlaw, A.M. Perez-Castillo, L.H. Fish, C.N. Mariash, H.L. Schwartz, J.H. Oppenheimer, Interaction of dietary carbohydrate and glucagon in regulation of rat hepatic messenger ribonucleic acid S14 expression: role of circadian factors and 3′,5′-cyclic adenosine monophosphate, Mol. Endocrinol. 1 (1987) 609–613.

[70] S.D. Clarke, M.K. Armstrong, D.B. Jump, Nutritional control of rat liver fatty acid synthase and S14 mRNA abundance, J. Nutr. 120 (1990) 218–224.

[71] R.W. Hanson, L. Reshef, Regulation of phosphoenolpyruvate carboxykinase (GTP) gene expression, Annu. Rev. Biochem. 66 (1997) 581–611.

[72] D. Argaud, Q. Zhang, W. Pan, S. Maitra, S.J. Pilkis, A.J. Lange, Regulation of rat liver glucose-6-phosphatase gene expression in different nutritional and hormonal states: gene structure and 5′-flanking sequence, Diabetes 45 (1996) 1563–1571.

[73] P.B. Iynedjian, D. Jotterand, T. Nouspikel, M. Asfari, P.R. Pilot, Transcriptional regulation of glucokinase gene by insulin in cultured liver cells and its repression by the glucagon-cAMP system, J. Biol. Chem. 264 (1989) 21824–21829.

[74] J.F. Decaux, B. Antoine, A. Kahn, Regulation of the expression of the L-type pyruvate kinase gene in adult rat hepatocytes in primary culture, J. Biol. Chem. 264 (1989) 11584–11590.

[75] K. Prip- Buus, D. Perdereau, F. Foufelle, J. Maury, P. Ferré, J. Girard, Induction of fatty acid synthase gene expression by glucose in primary culture of rat hepatocytes, Eur. J. Biochem. 230 (1995) 309–315.

[76] B.L. O'Callaghan, S.H. Koo, Y. Wu, H.C. Freake, H.C. Towle, Glucose regulation of the acetyl-CoA carboxylase promoter PI in rat hepatocytes, J. Biol. Chem. 276 (2001) 16033–16039.

[77] S.H. Koo, A.K. Dutcher, H.C. Towle, Glucose and insulin function through two distinct transcription factors to stimulate expression of lipogenic enzyme genes in liver, J. Biol. Chem. 276 (2001) 9437–9445.

[78] K.M. Waters, J.M. Ntambi, Insulin and dietary fructose induce stearoyl-CoA desaturase 1 gene expression of diabetic mice, J. Biol. Chem. 269 (1994) 27773–27777.

[79] P. Froguel, M. Vaxillaire, F. Sun, G. Velho, H. Zouali, M.O. Butel, S. Lesage, N. Vionnet, K. Clement, F. Fougerousse, et al., Close linkage of glucokinase locus on chromosome 7p to early onset non- insulin-dependent diabetes mellitus [published erratum appears in Nature 1992 Jun 18;357(6379):607], Nature 356 (1992) 162–164.

[80] P. Froguel, H. Zouali, N. Vionnet, G. Velho, M. Vaxillaire, F. Sun, S. Lesage, M. Stoffel, J. Takeda, P. Passa, et al., Familial hyperglycemia due to mutations in glucokinase. Definition of a subtype of diabetes mellitus [see comments], N. Engl. J. Med. 328 (1993) 697–702.

[81] G. Velho, K.F. Petersen, G. Perseghin, J.H. Hwang, D.L. Rothman, M.E. Pueyo, G.W. Cline, P. Froguel, G.I. Shulman, Impaired hepatic glycogen synthesis in glucokinase-deficient (MODY-2) subjects, J. Clin. Invest. 98 (1996) 1755–1761.

[82] C. Postic, M. Shiota, K.D. Niswender, T.L. Jetton, Y. Chen, J.M. Moates, K.D. Shelton, J. Lindner, A.D. Cherrington, M.A. Magnuson, Dual roles for glucokinase in glucose homeostasis

as determined by liver and pancreatic beta cell-specific gene knock-outs using Cre recombinase, J. Biol. Chem. 274 (1999) 305–315.

[83] M.A. Magnuson, T.L. Andreone, R.L. Printz, S. Koch, D.K. Granner, Rat glucokinase gene: structure and regulation by insulin, Proc Natl Acad Sci USA 86 (1989) 4838–4842.

[84] P.B. Iynedjian, A. Gjinovci, A.E. Renold, Stimulation by insulin of glucokinase gene transcription in liver of diabetic rats, J. Biol. Chem. 263 (1988) 740–744.

[85] M. Foretz, C. Guichard, P. Ferre, F. Foufelle, Sterol regulatory element binding protein-1c is a major mediator of insulin action on the hepatic expression of glucokinase and lipogenesis-related genes [see comments], Proc. Natl. Acad. Sci. USA 96 (1999) 12737–12742.

[86] D. Bécard, I. Hainault, D. A-M, L. Bertry-Coussot, P. Ferré, F. Foufelle, Adenovirus-mediated overexpression of sterol regulatory element binding protein-1c mimics insulin effects on hepatic gene expression and glucose homeostasis in diabetic mice, Diabetes 50 (2001) 2425–2430.

[87] A. Mora, C. Lipina, F. Tronche, C. Sutherland, D.R. Alessi, Deficiency of PDK1 in liver results in glucose intolerance, impairment of insulin regulated gene expression and liver failure, Biochem. J. 23 (2004) 23.

[88] K. Chakravarty, P. Leahy, D. Becard, P. Hakimi, M. Foretz, P. Ferre, F. Foufelle, R.W. Hanson, Sterol regulatory element-binding protein-1c mimics the negative effect of insulin on phosphoenolpyruvate carboxykinase (GTP) gene transcription, J. Biol. Chem. 6 (2001) 6.

[89] P. Leahy, D.R. Crawford, G. Grossman, R.M. Gronostajski, R.W. Hanson, CREB binding protein coordinates the function of multiple transcription factors including nuclear factor I to regulate phosphoenolpyruvate carboxykinase (GTP) gene transcription, J. Biol. Chem. 274 (1999) 8813–8822.

[90] K. Chakravarty, S.Y. Wu, C.M. Chiang, D. Samols, R.W. Hanson, SREBP-1c and Sp1 interact to regulate transcription of the gene for phosphoenolpyruvate carboxykinase (GTP) in the liver, J. Biol. Chem. 279 (2004) 15385–15395 Epub 2004 Jan 26.

[91] T. Yamamoto, H. Shimano, Y. Nakagawa, T. Ide, N. Yahagi, T. Matsuzaka, M. Nakakuki, A. Takahashi, H. Suzuki, H. Sone, H. Toyoshima, R. Sato, N. Yamada, SREBP-1 interacts with hepatocyte nuclear factor-4 alpha and interferes with PGC-1 recruitment to suppress hepatic gluconeogenic genes, J. Biol. Chem. 279 (2004) 12027–12035 Epub 2004 Jan 13.

[92] J. Nakae, T. Kitamura, D.L. Silver, D. Accili, The forkhead transcription factor Foxo1 (Fkhr) confers insulin sensitivity onto glucose-6-phosphatase expression, J. Clin. Invest. 108 (2001) 1359–1367.

[93] S. Le Lay, I. Lefrere, C. Trautwein, I. Dugail, S. Krief, Insulin and sterol-regulatory element-binding protein-1c (SREBP-1C) regulation of gene expression in 3T3-L1 adipocytes. Identification of CCAAT/enhancer-binding protein beta as an SREBP-1C target, J. Biol. Chem. 277 (2002) 35625–35634 Epub 2002 Jun 04.

[94] J.B. Kim, B.M. Spiegelman, ADD1/SREBP1 promotes adipocyte differentiation and gene expression linked to fatty acid metabolism, Genes Dev. 10 (1996) 1096–1107.

[95] I. Shimomura, R.E. Hammer, J.A. Richardson, S. Ikemoto, Y. Bashmakov, J.L. Goldstein, M. Brown, Insulin resistance and diabetes mellitus in transgenic mice expressing nuclear SREBP-1c in adipose tissue: model for congenital generalized lipodystrophy, Genes Dev. 12 (1998) 3182–3194.

[96] C. Andreolas, G. da Silva Xavier, F. Diraison, C. Zhao, A. Varadi, F. Lopez-Casillas, P. Ferre, F. Foufelle, G.A. Rutter, Stimulation of acetyl-CoA carboxylase gene expression by glucose requires insulin release and sterol regulatory element binding protein 1c in pancreatic MIN6 beta-cells, Diabetes 51 (2002) 2536–2545.

[97] H. Wang, P. Maechler, P.A. Antinozzi, L. Herrero, K.A. Hagenfeldt-Johansson, A. Bjorklund, C.B. Wollheim, The transcription factor SREBP-1c is instrumental in the development of beta-cell dysfunction, J. Biol. Chem. 278 (2003) 16622–16629 Epub 2003 Feb 24.

[98] T. Yamashita, K. Eto, Y. Okazaki, S. Yamashita, T. Yamauchi, N. Sekine, R. Nagai, M. Noda, T. Kadowaki, Role of uncoupling protein-2 up-regulation and triglyceride accumulation in impaired glucose-stimulated insulin secretion in a beta-cell lipotoxicity model overexpressing sterol regulatory element-binding protein-1c, Endocrinology 145 (2004) 3566–3577 Epub 2004 Apr 01.

[99] F. Diraison, E. Motakis, L.E. Parton, G.P. Nason, I. Leclerc, G.A. Rutter, Impact of adenoviral transduction with SREBP1c or AMPK on pancreatic islet gene expression profile: analysis with oligonucleotide microarrays, Diabetes 53 (2004) S84–S91.

[100] F. Diraison, L. Parton, P. Ferre, F. Foufelle, C.P. Briscoe, I. Leclerc, G.A. Rutter, Over-expression of sterol-regulatory-element-binding protein-1c (SREBP1c) in rat pancreatic islets induces lipogenesis and decreases glucose-stimulated insulin release: modulation by 5-aminoimidazole-4-carboxamide ribonucleoside (AICAR), Biochem. J. 378 (2004) 769–778.

[101] I. Shimomura, M. Matsuda, R.E. Hammer, Y. Bashmakov, M.S. Brown, J.L. Goldstein, Decreased IRS-2 and increased SREBP-1c lead to mixed insulin resistance and sensitivity in livers of lipodystrophic and ob/ob mice, Mol. Cell. 6 (2000) 77–86.

[102] M. Matsumoto, W. Ogawa, K. Teshigawara, H. Inoue, K. Miyake, H. Sakaue, M. Kasuga, Role of the insulin receptor substrate 1 and phosphatidylinositol 3-kinase signaling pathway in insulin-induced expression of sterol regulatory element binding protein 1c and glucokinase genes in rat hepatocytes, Diabetes 51 (2002) 1672–1680.

[103] M. Fleischmann, P.B. Iynedjian, Regulation of sterol regulatory-element binding protein 1 gene expression in liver: role of insulin and protein kinase B/cAkt, Biochem. J. 349 (2000) 13–17.

[104] P.G. Ribaux, P.B. Iynedjian, Analysis of the role of protein kinase B (cAKT) in insulin-dependent induction of glucokinase and sterol regulatory element-binding protein 1 (SREBP1) mRNAs in hepatocytes, Biochem. J. 376 (2003) 697–705.

[105] M. Matsumoto, W. Ogawa, K. Akimoto, H. Inoue, K. Miyake, K. Furukawa, Y. Hayashi, H. Iguchi, Y. Matsuki, R. Hiramatsu, H. Shimano, N. Yamada, S. Ohno, M. Kasuga, T. Noda, PKClambda in liver mediates insulin-induced SREBP-1c expression and determines both hepatic lipid content and overall insulin sensitivity, J. Clin. Invest. 112 (2003) 935–944.

[106] K.J. Nadeau, J.W. Leitner, I. Gurerich, B. Draznin, Insulin regulation of sterol regulatory element-binding protein-1 expression in L-6 muscle cells and 3T3 L1 adipocytes, J. Biol. Chem. 279 (2004) 34380–34387 Epub 2004 Jun 08.

[107] K.S. Thompson, H.C. Towle, Localization of the carbohydrate response element of the rat L-type pyruvate kinase gene, J. Biol. Chem. 266 (1991) 8679–8682.

[108] M.O. Bergot, M.J.H. Diaz-Guerra, N. Puizenat, M. Raymondjean, A. Kahn, Cis-regulation of the L-type pyruvate kinase gene promoter by glucose, insulin and cyclic AMP, Nucleic Acids Res 20 (1992) 1871–1878.

[109] H.M. Shih, H.C. Towle, Definition of the carbohydrate response element of the rat S14 gene, J. Biol. Chem. 267 (1992) 13222–13228.

[110] C. Rufo, M. Teran-Garcia, M.T. Nakamura, S.H. Koo, H.C. Towle, S.D. Clarke, Involvement of a unique carbohydrate-responsive factor in the glucose regulation of rat liver fatty-acid synthase gene transcription, J. Biol. Chem. 276 (2001) 21969–21975.

[111] H. Yamashita, M. Takenoshita, M. Sakurai, R.K. Bruick, W.J. Henzel, W. Shillinglaw, D. Arnot, K. Uyeda, A glucose-responsive transcription factor that regulates carbohydrate metabolism in the liver, Proc. Natl. Acad. Sci. USA 98 (2001) 9116–9121.

[112] K. Iizuka, R.K. Bruick, G. Liang, J.D. Horton, K. Uyeda, Deficiency of carbohydrate response element-binding protein (ChREBP) reduces lipogenesis as well as glycolysis, Proc. Natl. Acad. Sci. USA 101 (2004) 7281–7286 Epub 2004 Apr 26.

[113] S. Ishii, K. Iizuka, B.C. Miller, K. Uyeda, Carbohydrate response element binding protein directly promotes lipogenic enzyme gene transcription, Proc. Natl. Acad. Sci. USA 101 (2004) 15597–15602 Epub 2004 Oct 20.

[114] L. Ma, N.G. Tsatsos, H.C. Towle, Direct role of ChREBP.Mlx in regulating hepatic glucose-responsive genes,, J. Biol. Chem. 280 (2005) 12019–12027 Epub 2005 Jan 20.

[115] T. Kawaguchi, M. Takenoshita, T. Kabashima, K. Uyeda, Glucose and cAMP regulate the L-type pyruvate kinase gene by phosphorylation/dephosphorylation of the carbohydrate response element binding protein, Proc. Natl. Acad. Sci. USA 98 (2001) 13710–13715.

[116] T. Kabashima, T. Kawaguchi, B.E. Wadzinski, K. Uyeda, Xylulose 5-phosphate mediates glucose-induced lipogenesis by xylulose 5-phosphate-activated protein phosphatase in rat liver, Proc. Natl. Acad. Sci. USA 100 (2003) 5107–5112.

[117] C. Schmitz-Peiffer, Signalling aspects of insulin resistance in skeletal muscle: mechanisms induced by lipid oversupply, Cell. Signal 12 (2000) 583–594.

[118] K. Tobe, R. Suzuki, M. Aoyama, T. Yamauchi, J. Kamon, N. Kubota, Y. Terauchi, J. Matsui, Y. Akanuma, S. Kimura, J. Tanaka, M. Abe, J. Ohsumi, R. Nagai, T. Kadowaki, Increased expression of the sterol regulatory element-binding protein-1 gene in insulin receptor substrate-2(-/-) mouse liver, J. Biol. Chem. 276 (2001) 38337–38340.

[119] T. Kakuma, Y. Lee, M. Higa, Z. Wang, W. Pan, I. Shimomura, R.H. Unger, Leptin, troglitazone, and the expression of sterol regulatory element binding proteins in liver and pancreatic islets, Proc. Natl. Acad. Sci. USA 97 (2000) 8536–8541.

[120] M. Kolehmainen, H. Vidal, E. Alhava, M.I. Uusitupa, Sterol regulatory element binding protein 1c (SREBP-1c) expression in human obesity, Obes. Res. 9 (2001) 706–712.

[121] F. Diraison, E. Dusserre, H. Vidal, M. Sothier, M. Beylot, Increased hepatic lipogenesis but decreased expression of lipogenic gene in adipose tissue in human obesity, Am. J. Physiol. Endocrinol. Metab. 282 (2002) E46–E51.

[122] H. Oberkofler, N. Fukushima, H. Esterbauer, F. Krempler, W. Patsch, Sterol regulatory element binding proteins: relationship of adipose tissue gene expression with obesity in humans, Biochim. Biophys. Acta. 1575 (2002) 75–81.

[123] X. Yang, P.A. Jansson, I. Nagaev, M.M. Jack, E. Carvalho, K.S. Sunnerhagen, M.C. Cam, S.W. Cushman, U. Smith, Evidence of impaired adipogenesis in insulin resistance, Biochem. Biophys. Res. Commun. 317 (2004) 1045–1051.

[124] S.T. Nadler, J.P. Stoehr, K.L. Schueler, G. Tanimoto, B.S. Yandell, A.D. Attie, The expression of adipogenic genes is decreased in obesity and diabetes mellitus, Proc. Natl. Acad. Sci. USA 97 (2000) 11371–11376.

[125] A. Soukas, P. Cohen, N.D. Socci, J.M. Friedman, Leptin-specific patterns of gene expression in white adipose tissue, Genes Dev. 14 (2000) 963–980.

[126] I. Shimomura, Y. Bashmakov, J.D. Horton, Increased levels of nuclear SREBP-1c associated with fatty livers in two mouse models of diabetes mellitus, J. Biol. Chem. 274 (1999) 30028–30032.

[127] A.H. Kissebah, G.E. Sonnenberg, J. Myklebust, M. Goldstein, K. Broman, R.G. James, J.A. Marks, G.R. Krakower, H.J. Jacob, J. Weber, L. Martin, J. Blangero, A.G. Comuzzie, Quantitative trait loci on chromosomes 3 and 17 influence phenotypes of the metabolic syndrome, Proc. Natl. Acad. Sci. USA 97 (2000) 14478–14483.

[128] X. Wu, R.S. Cooper, I. Borecki, C. Hanis, M. Bray, C.E. Lewis, X. Zhu, D. Kan, A. Luke, D. Curb, A combined analysis of genomewide linkage scans for body mass index from the National Heart, Lung, and Blood Institute Family Blood Pressure Program, Am. J. Hum. Genet. 70 (2002) 1247–1256 Epub 2002 Mar 28.

[129] F. Demenais, T. Kanninen, C.M. Lindgren, S. Wiltshire, S. Gaget, C. Dandrieux, P. Almgren, M. Sjogren, A. Hattersley, C. Dina, T. Tuomi, M.I. McCarthy, P. Froguel, L.C. Groop, A meta-analysis of four European genome screens (GIFT Consortium) shows evidence for a novel region on chromosome 17p11.2–q22 linked to type 2 diabetes,, Hum. Mol. Genet. 12 (2003) 1865–1873.

[130] D. Eberle, K. Clement, D. Meyre, M. Sahbatou, M. Vaxillaire, A. Le Gall, P. Ferre, A. Basdevant, P. Froguel, F. Foufelle, SREBF-1 gene polymorphisms are associated with obesity and type 2 diabetes in French obese and diabetic cohorts, Diabetes 53 (2004) 2153–2157.

[131] M. Laudes, I. Barroso, J. Luan, M.A. Soos, G. Yeo, A. Meirhaeghe, L. Logie, A. Vidal-Puig, A.J. Schafer, N.J. Wareham, S. O'Rahilly, Genetic variants in human sterol regulatory element binding protein-1c in syndromes of severe insulin resistance and type 2 diabetes, Diabetes 53 (2004) 842–846.

[132] B. Vedie, X. Jeunemaitre, J.L. Megnien, V. Atger, A. Simon, N. Moatti, A new DNA polymorphism in the 5' untranslated region of the human SREBP-1a is related to development of atherosclerosis in high cardiovascular risk population, Atherosclerosis 154 (2001) 589–597.

[133] A.R. Miserez, P.Y. Muller, L. Barella, M. Schwietert, P. Erb, P.L. Vernazza, M. Battegay, A single-nucleotide polymorphism in the sterol-regulatory element-binding protein 1c gene is predictive of HIV-related hyperlipoproteinaemia, Aids 15 (2001) 2045–2049.

[134] L. Salek, S. Lutucuta, C.M. Ballantyne, A.M. Gotto Jr, A.J. Marian, Effects of SREBF-1a and SCAP polymorphisms on plasma levels of lipids, severity, progression and regression of coronary atherosclerosis and response to therapy with fluvastatin, J. Mol. Med. 80 (2002) 737–744.

[135] R. Gitzelmann, M.A. Spycher, G. Feil, J. Muller, B. Seilnacht, M. Stahl, N.U. Bosshard, Liver glycogen synthase deficiency: a rarely diagnosed entity, Eur. J. Pediatr. 155 (1996) 561–567.

[136] P. Tontonoz, J.B. Kim, R.A. Graves, B.M. Spiegelman, ADD1: a novel helix-loop-helix transcription factor associated with adipocyte determination and differenciation, Mol. Cell. Biol. 13 (1993) 4753–4759.

Chapter 6

The adipocyte and adipose tissue as endocrine organs: Impact on the insulin resistance phenotype

Robert R. Henry[1], Susan A. Phillips[2], Sunder R. Mudaliar[3], Theodore P. Ciaraldi[4]

[1]*Professor of Medicine, University of California, San Diego, Chief, Section of Endocrinology & Metabolism, VA San Diego Healthcare System, CA, USA;*
[2]*Assistant Clinical Professor of Pediatrics, University of California, San Diego, CA, USA;*
[3]*Associate Clinical Professor of Medicine, University of California, San Diego Staff Physician, VA San Diego Healthcare System, CA, USA;*
[4]*Project Endocrinologist, University of California, San Diego, CA, USA*

Summary

Adipose tissue (AT) is an essential metabolic tissue, important for both its role in lipid storage and mobilization. While long considered an inert tissue providing a site for passive fat accumulation, insulation against heat loss and mechanical and/or structural support, newly recognized endocrine, paracrine and autocrine activities of AT have forced a re-evaluation of this static view of AT biology. The effects of factors secreted from AT, termed adipokines, increase the impact of AT on multiple processes in other tissues. Importantly, the role of excess adiposity and alterations in adipokine production and secretion in the development of diabetes, cardiovascular and liver disease necessitates a better understanding of AT biology in general and factors influencing its expansion specifically. The formation and metabolism of AT, as well as the production of adipokines are under multiple forms of regulation. At the transcriptional level peroxisome proliferator-activated receptor peroxisome gamma (PPARγ) plays a key role. These factors will be discussed with particular emphasis on human data and the mechanisms for insulin resistance and the metabolic syndrome.

1. Embryonic development of adipose tissue and the role of angiogenesis

A close temporal and spatial relationship has been observed between adipose tissue (AT) development and blood vessel formation. Early observations suggested a causal relationship between the infiltration of connective tissue by capillaries and the future development of fat lobules [1,2]. In the human fetus, arterioles and venules are found in areas that later differentiate into primitive fat organs [3]. Whether blood vessel development precedes or develops concurrently with adipocyte formation likely depends on the species and depot. Primitive fat organs are notable for their mesenchymal cellular component and for their connection to the vascular system. Histologic analysis of developing AT has shown the presence of tightly clustered cords of immature cells of various sizes including endothelial cells of the vascular bed. These structures are reminiscent of the "blood islands" described by Maximow and Bloom [4]. The simultaneous formation of endothelium and blood cells results when proliferating mesenchyme gives rise to clusters of spherical cells (blood islands) that are interconnected by strands of elongated cells. The peripheral cells of the blood islands flatten to form the lumen of blood vessels and the cells within give rise to various blood cells. It has been speculated that the mesenchymal cells of the blood islands are the progenitors of cells destined to become preadipocytes, which then [5] migrate into defined fat cell clusters. This developmental paradigm is supported by studies in human fetal buccal and gluteal subcutaneous fat depots demonstrating a spatial and temporal relationship between capillary formation and AT development [6]. Important confirmatory data are now available that link increased angiogenesis with weight gain [7] and its inhibition with dose-dependent decreases in weight [8].

Angiogenesis appears to be linked not only to fat cluster formation but also to cluster expansion. Once formed the number of AT cell clusters does not appear to change significantly, rather AT expansion with increasing gestational age is achieved via a steady increase of cluster size. The importance of angiogenesis in cluster expansion is highlighted by the observed associations between capillary density and cluster size [9] and location of the larger clusters at large blood vessels entry sites [10]. Neovascularization appears to be critical to the process of cluster expansion, a point underscored by recent findings that suggest adipocytes and their precursors may be an important source of angiogenic factors, including PAI-1, TGF-β and PGE2.

Although PPARγ ligands are best known for their role as regulators of adipogenesis, they also function as potent modulators of angiogenesis [11]. PPARγ activation by natural or synthetic ligands produces potent inhibition of endothelial differentiation and proliferation *in vitro* [12]. *In vivo*, peroxisome proliferator-activated receptor gamma (PPARγ) suppresses VEGF-induced angiogenesis [12]. Activation of PPARγ by thiazolidinediones (TZDs) inhibits proteolysis, a required first step in angiogenesis [12]. On the basis of these observations it is interesting to speculate whether PPARγ inhibitory effects on angiogenesis could constitute feedback inhibition on adipogenesis.

2. Expansion of adiose tissue mass: hypertrophy versus hyperplasia and impact on adipocyte function

Understanding the mechanisms by which AT expands is essential to the development of successful strategies for the treatment and prevention of obesity. The growth of

AT may occur via increases in cell size (hypertrophy), increases in cell number (hyperplasia) or some combination of both processes. The relative importance of these two processes in normal development and in obesity has been limited by the adequacy of available methods. The recent identification of S-100, a protein specifically expressed by adipocytes and their precursors may simplify the process of distinguishing these small fat cells from pericytes, fibroblasts, endothelial and mesenchymal cells [13].

Despite methodologic difficulties, data exist to support the view that in early life AT expansion is primarily hyperplastic while later expansion is principally hypertrophic. The timing of the putative switch from hyperplastic to hypertrophic expansion is not clear and appears to be species specific. In rodents, when caloric intake is altered during the suckling period, changes in epididymal fat pad weight result and are manifest as changes in fat cell number [14]. In newborn baboons nutrient excess during the first 4 months of life, followed by a normal diet until sacrifice at 5 years led to significant increases in fat mass associated with hypertrophy, not hyperplasia of fat cells, suggesting that in primates post-natal hyperplasia may not be a significant mechanism for AT expansion [15]. Interestingly, studies in human fetal and infant tissues obtained after therapeutic abortion or early demise have identified large numbers of small empty fat cells ($<25 \mu m$), suggesting the possibility that early reports [16,17] of postnatal hyperplasia in humans might actually represent lipid-filling of preexisting fat cells [18]. Finally, studies of young men exposed to famine in utero during the last trimester of pregnancy and the first few months of life had significantly lower rates of obesity, consistent with the inference that undernutrition affected a critical period for the development of AT cellularity [19].

The relative contribution of fat cell hyperplasia to the expansion of AT mass later in life is unclear. Early studies in rodents on a hypercaloric diet suggested that threshold adipocyte size might be a trigger for increases in adipocyte number [20]. This finding is supported by others who observed depot-specific hyperplastic expansion of AT depots (and cellular hypertrophy in others) as a response to epididymal and inguinal lipectomy in rats [21]. In human studies, investigators have failed to demonstrate differences in the proliferation and/or differentiation capacity of preadipocytes isolated from obese and nonobese adult subjects [22]. In human mammary AT, obese subjects with body mass index $(BMI) > 30 \, kg/m^2$ showed a larger fat cell size but no increase in fat cell number when compared to lean controls [23]. Recent publications have begun to shed light on possible mechanisms by which hyperplastic expansion of AT may be occurring. A product of activated macrophages, macrophage colony stimulating factor (MCSF) mRNA and protein is expressed by human adipocytes and significantly upregulated in rapidly growing AT [24]. Although macrophage infiltration can occur in AT, over-expression of MCSF in rabbit sc AT was associated with a 16-fold increase in AT growth. Adipose tissue growth occurred in association with increased nuclear staining of MIB-1, a marker of proliferation and without changes in cell size.

The relationship between cell size and adipocyte metabolic function has long been recognized [25]. Early studies in human AT demonstrated a link between insulin responsiveness of adipocytes and cell size – the larger the fat cells the less sensitive the tissue. Conversely, reductions of cell size were shown to be associated with weight loss and improved insulin responsiveness [26]. Impairment of a number of key adipocyte metabolic functions in obese humans and animals including: the storage and mobilization of lipids [27,28], increased secretion of adipokines including leptin, [29], reduced adiponectin [30], and higher IL-6 [31] and TNFα [32] that impairs insulin-signaling cascades [33], have been related to increases in cell size.

2.1. *Impact of PPARγ on adipocyte function*

PPARγ receptor agonists increase whole body fat mass *in vivo*, while *in vitro* they promote adipogenesis [34]. The promoters of a number of molecules involved in fatty acid uptake and storage contain PPAR response elements and are upregulated in response to PPAR activity (see below). The seemingly contradictory effects of PPARγ agonists to promote lipid storage and weight gain while positively affecting the profile of adipokine release, including increased adiponectin [35] and decreased IL-6 and TNF-α is not well understood [36]. One hypothesis, supported by rodent knock-out data is that TZD promotion of adipocyte differentiation and lipid storage results in a hypercellular expansion of AT with an increased number of small insulin sensitive cells [30]. In support of this hypothesis is the recent observation in obese db/db mice that TZD treatment results in reductions in both cell size and expression of mesoderm-specific transcript (Mest)/paternally expressed gene 1 (Peg1), a newly recognized marker of cell size [37]. Other studies in Zucker (fa/fa) rats treated with pioglitazone showed reductions in cell size and an increase in cell number [38]. Biopsy studies in subcutaneous AT of human subjects following 8 weeks of TZD treatment however failed to show significant decreases in cell size but rather a tendency of PPARγ agonists to increase the number of small adipocytes ($<50\,\mu$m) in subcutaneous AT [39]. It is also possible that the observed increase in fat cells is actually the lipid filling of pre-existing very small fat cells whose presence in both rodents [40] and in humans [41] has been noted.

3. Adipose tissue distribution and its relation to metabolism-depot specificity

Regional differences in AT exist at many levels including: vascularization and blood flow; cell size, steroid and growth factor receptor expression; and capacity for replication, adipogenesis and apoptosis. Developmental studies suggest that many of these differences arise early in development. As discussed, vascular development is of paramount importance in the lobule formation and expansion. The more extensively vascularized the site, the more lobules it will contain and the greater the potential metabolic activity of the depot [6]. Studies correlating blood flow and metabolic activity have confirmed the importance of this relationship, noting that a 67% relative reduction of blood flow to the gluteal depot versus the abdominal depot is associated with an 87% reduction in hormone sensitive lipase (HSL) rate of action and a threefold increase in triglyceride clearance [42] in the abdominal depot.

Regional differences in adipocyte cell size are well established and generally assume the order of omental (om) < subcutaneous (sc) [43]. Fat cell size reflects the integrated effect of a number of factors affecting cellular lipid metabolism. Adipocyte volume has been correlated with lipolytic activity in human AT [44]. Lipogenesis is promoted by insulin via activation of lipoprotein lipase (LPL), and by adenosine, the fat cell autocrine regulator of both lipolysis and blood flow. Adipocytes isolated from femoral and gluteal depots have reduced (via decreased β-1 and β-2 receptor expression) lipolytic response to catecholamines when compared to subcutaneous (sc) abdominal adipocytes (increased β-1 and β-2 and decreased α-2 receptor expression) [45]. Visceral abdominal adipocytes are more sensitive than sc fat cells to catecholamine-induced lipolysis, expressing at least as many β- as α-2 receptors and are less sensitive to adenosine and insulin-mediated suppression of lipolysis [46]. Insulin is a potent lipogenic agent, both by promoting lipid synthesis (LPL activity, glucose transport and triglyceride synthesis) and by reducing catecholamine sensitivity (via down regulation of β-adrenergic receptors) [47]. Sensitivity to the anti-lipolytic effects of insulin is depot-dependent. SC abdominal fat cells have a higher affinity for insulin and are more sensitive than femoral or om fat cells [45]. LPL is a key regulator of fat accumulation and variations in LPL activity parallel fat cell size. There are marked depot differences, particularily in women, in LPL expression (sc > om) and in the sensitivity of AT to insulin-stimulated increases in LPL activity [48].

The expression pattern of steroid and growth factor receptors is another important source of adipose depot specialization. Glucocorticoid (GC) receptors are expressed at higher levels in visceral AT [49] as is 11β-hydroxysteroid dehydrogenase-1 (11β-HSD-1) the enzyme that can convert cortisone into biologically active cortisol [50]. GCs have permissive effects on fat cell responsiveness to adrenergic receptor agonists [51]. GCs in the presence of insulin significantly increase LPL activity in om fat cells [52], presenting a possible mechanism by which this depot is expanded in states of GCs excess. Omental fat cells within the viscera, but not sc fat cells manifest an ~50% suppression of both insulin-stimulated glucose uptake and the expression of insulin-signaling molecules following dexamethasone treatment [53].

The expression of both androgen and estrogen receptors (ERs) are also depot specific. Visceral adipocytes exhibit greater numbers of androgen receptors and increase receptor expression to a greater degree in response to testosterone than do sc adipocytes [54]. *In vitro* testosterone treatment of differentiated sc human preadipocytes causes a reduction in catecholamine-stimulated lipolysis, which is likely due to reduced expression of both β-adrenergic receptors and HSL [55]. *In vivo* prolonged androgen treatment (> 9 months) is associated with decreased uptake and increased turnover rate of triglycerides (TG) [56]. Gender-specific differences in AT distribution are well recognized [55]. Increases in total and sc body fat develop peripubertally in women, implicating estrogen-specific effects on fat accumulation and in regional fat distribution. Although both ER-α and ER-β are expressed in AT, depot-specific effects appear to be mediated via ER-α. Investigations in human AT have demonstrated an interaction of estrogen via ER-α to increase sc α-2 (anti-lipolytic) adrenergic receptor expression, thereby favoring fat accumulation in the sc depot.

Interaction between estrogen and α-2 adrenergic receptors does not appear to occur in the intra-abdominal depot [57]. Regional differences also exist in responsiveness to GH-mediated lipolysis [58]. GH deficiency is associated with increased visceral adiposity that is redistributed to sc depots upon replacement. Administration of GH to non-GH deficient children results in decreased abdominal adipocyte size and increased responsiveness of femoral cells to the lipogenic effects of insulin [59].

Important depot-specific differences exist in replication, adipogenesis and apoptosis. Specifically, human abdominal sc and mesenteric adipocytes have a greater capacity for replication than om fat cells [60,61]. Adipose depots also appear to possess differing proportions of preadipocyte populations [41] with differing capacities for replication and apoptosis [62]. Human preadipocytes and adipocytes from the om depot display greater rates of apoptosis than cells from sc depots of the same subject [63]. Human om adipocytes are also more susceptible to apoptosis induced by TNFα [63]. The inhibitors of apoptosis (IAPs) constitute a family of proteins involved in the regulation of apoptosis. Increased expression of cIAP2 has been shown to protect against apoptosis in NIH 3T3-LI cells [64], while cIAP2 is expressed at increased levels in sc versus omental fat cells [65].

Regional fat distribution and function are significantly altered by PPARγ activation by TZDs. The PPARγ receptor has depot-specific effects on cell size. In sc AT, PPARγ agonists have a tendency to increase the number of cells $<50\,\mu m$, selectively expanding this depot [39]. Gene expression profiling studies in 3T3-L1 cells have indicated that rosiglitazone and pioglitazone each regulate a number of gene products that contribute to regional depot differences. For example, PPARγ downregulates 11β-hydroxy sterol dehydrogenase-1, which is differentially expressed in human visceral AT, increasing the local production of cortisol and impairing insulin sensitivity in this tissue [66]. Increases were also observed in the expression of LPL and genes promoting increased fatty acid uptake and storage (see below). The expression and activity of LPL in response to insulin is sc depot specific [48], hence PPARγ-mediated increases in LPL synthesis would predict selective expansion of this depot. A directed expansion of the sc depot by PPARγ agonists is supported by reports on regional fat redistribution in type 2 diabetic subjects on TZD treatment [67,68]. PPARγ depot-specific effects are also seen on preadipocyte differentiation. In studies involving human preadipocytes derived from sc and om depots, PPARγ preferentially directs the differentiation of sc preadipocytes. Preadipocytes derived from om AT were refractory to TZDs despite similar levels of PPARγ expression [69].

3.1. *PPARs as regulators of adipose tissue metabolism and function*

PPARs are members of the nuclear receptor superfamily. PPARs form obligate heterodimers with the Retinoid X Receptor (RXR). It is these heterodimers that bind to specific DNA sequences termed peroxisome proliferator response elements (PPREs). The heterodimer is complexed with a number of proteins, in the unliganded state most often co-repressors of gene transcription. Upon binding of an activating ligand there is a conformational change in the heterodimer, leading to release of co-repressors and recruitment of a large array of co-activators.

The PPAR subfamily consists of three separate gene products, PPARα, PPARβ/δ and PPARγ (reviewed in [70]). The three PPARs differ in structure, tissue distribution, ligand specificity and target genes [70]. The mRNA for PPARα is distributed amongst human tissues with the order of abundance; heart > skeletal muscle = liver > kidney [71,72]. The message was also detected in human vascular endothelial cells [73]. In humans, PPARα protein was detected in the following abundance: skeletal muscle = liver > kidney [74]. PPARα protein is also present in AT, though at approximately 15% of the abundance in skeletal muscle from the same subjects [75].

PPARβ/δ mRNA has been found to be ubiquitously expressed in all tissues and is most abundant in fat and muscle [72]. PPARβ/δ protein content also appears to be roughly equivalent in fat and skeletal muscle from the same individuals [75].

PPARγ is present in a number of tissues, in the general order of abundance: AT ⩾ large intestine > spleen, heart, liver, kidney, small intestine, testes, brain > skeletal muscle [72,76] Alternative splicing of the PPARγ gene generates isoforms of PPARγ designated as γ1 and γ2; a third isoform, γ3, has also been reported [77]. The predominant isoform in all tissues is γ1, with γ2 limited to AT [78]. The γ3 isoform is expressed in large intestine and AT [77]. As had been noted for PPARα, discrepancies are present between measurements of PPARα mRNA and protein.

3.2. *Transcriptional regulation of metabolic function in adipose tissue*

The major direct metabolic role of AT is as the storage depot for lipids, primarily in the form of TG. Loss of this function, as in states of lipodystrophy, or exceeding the storage capacity of AT, leads to lipids being diverted to other tissues ("ectopic fat") resulting in insulin resistance and hyperlipidemia (reviewed in [79]). As de novo lipogenesis from glucose or other precursors is modest in human AT [80] most of the substrate for storage is obtained from circulating lipids, either in the form of lipoprotein particles or complexed with albumin. The adipocyte has developed a system for the control of the storage from and delivery to the circulation of fatty acids (FA). These specific proteins were selected for discussion because they represent potential targets for therapeutic intervention, where regulation of gene expression and activity would be predicted to have major impacts on insulin sensitivity and circulating lipid levels.

3.2.1. *Lipoprotein lipase*

LPL is abundant in many cell types including adipocytes and macrophages as well as skeletal muscle and liver (reviewed in [81]). LPL on the cell surface catalyzes the release of fatty acids from circulating lipoproteins. LPL activity is greater in sc AT compared to visceral tissue from the same subject [48]. Binding sites for a number of transcription factors have been identified on the promoter for human LPL. Important amongst these are (working upstream from the transcription start site): SP-1- and SP-3-binding sites in the proximal promoter, an octomer which binds TFIIB, a CCAAT box which binds NF-Y, a sterol response element (SRE) which can bind SREBP-1, a PPRE and two sites designated as LP-α and LP-β, which resemble sequences which bind HNF-3/forkhead. The LP-α and LP-β sites appear to be important for the induction of LPL expression that occurs during adipocyte differentiation [82]. The effects of PPARγ agonists display tissue specificity, as pioglitazone treatment of insulin-resistant mice increased LPL mRNA in white AT but not in skeletal muscle [83]. Interestingly, such specificity extends to the level of AT depot, as treatment of rats with a non-thiazolidinedione PPARγ agonist upregulated LPL mRNA and activity in sc (inguinal) but not visceral (retroperitoneal) AT [84]. Such a preferential increase in substrate delivery to sc fat could contribute to the AT remodeling that occurs with TZD treatment [85]. The data suggests a synergistic action of Sp-1 and SREBP-1 on LPL transcription; this would represent a convergence of signaling from the pathways of cholesterol and triglyceride metabolism.

3.2.2. *Fatty acid transporters*

While diffusion of free fatty acids (FFA) across the lipid bilayer of the plasma membrane is rapid [86], at physiological FFA: albumin ratios the uptake of long chain FA (LCFA) into adipocytes is a saturable process and multiple lines of evidence support the concept that at least a portion of FFA uptake is protein mediated (reviewed in [87]). Several different proteins are involved in this process including plasma membrane fatty acid-binding protein (FABPpm), fatty acid transport protein (FATP) and fatty acid translocase (FAT). FABPpm is totally extracellular and is thought to serve as a temporary reservoir of circulating FFA, passing them off to transport proteins. There are six members of the FATP family, FATP-1 being the most abundant in AT, both adipocytes and macrophages, while FATP-4 is also present in adipocytes [87]. FATP-1 possesses Acyl-CoA synthase activity [88], which permits the transported FA to be trapped within the cell and directed toward TG synthesis. FAT is identical to CD36, the class B scavenger receptor which in macrophages serves as the oxidized LDL receptor [87].

A PPRE has been identified in the FATP-1 promoter [89]. The nature of the PPAR involved in FATP-1 gene expression is cell-type specific. In rodents and cultured cell systems, PPARα activators (fibrates) increase FATP-1 mRNA in liver but have little or no effect in adipocytes, while TZDs alter FATP-1 mRNA only in adipocytes [90,91]. The data in humans are mixed, as brief rosiglitazone treatment (4 h) of isolated adipocytes had no effect on FATP-1 mRNA [92], while *in vivo* treatment (2 months) showed an increase [93]. There is similar tissue selectivity for the control of FAT gene expression, responses in liver occurring through PPARα and those in AT induced by PPARγ ligands [90,94]. The ability of *in vivo* lipid infusion and oxidized LDL to upregulate FAT expression are also mediated by PPARγ [95]. However, it has been suggested that the upstream FAT promoter lacks a classic PPRE and the effects of PPARγ ligands are indirect, by influencing SREBP-1c binding [94].

3.2.3. *Fatty acid-binding proteins*

Subsequent to diffusion and transport, cytosolic FFA are complexed with intracellular FABPs. FABPs increase the solubility of FFAs, augment FFA uptake by increasing the FFA concentration gradient and serve to direct intracellular FFAs to specific fates (reviewed in [96]). Nine members of the FABP subfamily of lipid-binding proteins have been identified. The major form in adipocytes and macrophages is A-FABP (adipocyte-type-FABP, Fabp4 or aP2). Adipocytes also contain E-FABP (epidermal-type-FABP, Fabp5) [97]. Tissue-specific expression of FABPs is driven by enhancers present in their promoters; for A-FABP it is an AP-1 site [96]. Other regulation of A-FABP is provided by C/EBP sites, as well as a PPRE [96]. The PPRE drives fatty acid-mediated regulation of A-FABP expression. It is interesting to note that A-FABP directly interacts with PPARγ in 3T3-L1 adipocytes [96]. This could represent a mechanism by which FAs and other PPAR ligands are directed to their targets in the nucleus.

3.2.4. *Phosphoenolpyruvate carboxykinase*

Efficient storage of FA requires esterification to TG. The backbone for TG formation is provided by glycerol-3-phosphate (G3P), arising from glucose uptake into the cell during the fed state. In the fasting state, this adipocyte G3P can be generated by glyceroneogenesis from substrates such as lactate or pyruvate, as there is usually little glycerol kinase activity to permit reutilization of glycerol generated from lipolysis. The key enzyme in the glyceroneogenesis pathway is the cytosolic form of phosphoenolpyruvate carboxykinase (PEPCK). Adipose-specific deletion of PEPCK results in a failure to re-esterify glycerol resulting in a lean phenotype, while over-expression of PEPCK in AT increased triglyceride storage in transgenic animals (reviewed in [96a]).

There is strong tissue specificity in control of PEPCK expression, reflecting the different roles of the enzyme; controlling gluconeogenesis in liver and glyceroneogenesis in AT [98,99]. Much of the tissue selectivity is provided by the two PPREs found in the PEPCK promoter [99]. Designated PCK2 and gAFI/PCK1, the former mediates PEPCK induction during adipogenesis and upregulation in response to TZDs [99]. This response is specific for PPARγ, as PPARα and -β selective agonists are without effect [99]. The other PPRE, gAF1/PCK1, influences the tissue-specific responses to glucocorticoids. In adipocytes, glucorticoids suppress PEPCK expression, which involves binding of PPARγ/RXRα and COUP-TFII, while in liver the response is an induction, mediated by COUP-TFI and HNF4 [98].

3.2.5. *Perilipin*

Properly stored TG does not exist as lipid micelles. Rather, the lipid droplet is coated by members of the family of lipid droplet-associated proteins. In adipocytes, this role is filled by the perilipin family of lipid-binding proteins, including perilipin, Adipophilyn and TIP47(reviewed in [100]). Alternative splicing of the perilipin gene results in two products, perilipin A and -B; perilipin A is the hormone sensitive form (see below) [101]. Perlipin serves two purposes, to protect the lipid droplet from hydrolysis in the basal state, and to augment stimulated lipolysis. Protein kinase A-mediated phosphorylation of HSL initiates translocation of HSL from the cytoplasm to the surface of the lipid droplet [102]. Perilpin A is phosphorylated at the same time, which both permits docking of HSL and disrupts the protein coat of the lipid droplet [101,102]. Data on the expression of the perilipin gene in human AT depots are variable. There are several reports that the content of perilipin mRNA is greater in sc AT compared to om tissue, but such differences are not seen at the level of protein expression [103,104]. Such variability would not be surprising given that the perilipin protein is stabilized by the presence of FA [101].

Two putative PPREs have been identified in the upstream promoter of the perilipin gene [105]. A PPARγ/RXRα complex is necessary for full activity of the promoter, as neither C/EBPα, SREBP-1a nor LXRα were capable of activating a reporter gene containing the promoter [105]. The PPREs are highly selective for PPARγ2. This organization of the promoter would explain the upregulation of perilipin expression that occurs during adipocyte differentiation [101] and with TZD treatment [105].

3.2.6. *Hormone-sensitive lipase*

Fulfillment of the role of AT as the major storage site for energy-producing substrate requires mobilization of the lipid stores, with release of FFA to the circulation for delivery to other tissues. TG are hydrolyzed, for the greatest part, by HSL (reviewed in [106]). Three isoforms of HSL have been identified [107]. Proteins of 84–88 kDa are expressed in multiple tissues, including adipocytes, while a 130 kDa form is expressed exclusively in testes [108]. The use of alternative promoters is responsible for the production of the two forms from a single gene [106]. While the predominant regulation of HSL activity occurs through phosphorylation and translocation, gene expression in the adipocyte is upregulated by glucose. A glucose response element (GRE) has been identified in the human adipocyte HSL promoter that binds both upstream stimulatory factor-1 (USF1) and USF-2; the glucose response also requires binding of Sp1 and Sp3 to an E-box [109].

3.2.7. *Glucose transporters*

While AT represents a secondary site for glucose utilization, adipocyte glucose transport often reflects that of the whole body and influences other adipocyte behaviors. Glucose transport into adipocytes is mediated by two members of the family of facilitated glucose carriers (reviewed in [110]); GLUT1 and GLUT4. GLUT1 is constitutively expressed and predominately localized to the plasma membrane and is primarily responsible for basal transport. Meanwhile, GLUT4 is responsible for insulin-stimulated increases in cellular transport in cardiac and skeletal muscle and adipocytes, rapidly translocating from intracellular pools to the cell surface.

Transcriptional regulation of GLUT4 expression must be considered in two contexts, during adipocyte differentiation and in mature adipocytes. The GLUT4 promoter contains a repressor element (G4RE) that is active only in preadipocytes as the factors binding to G4RE are present only in non-differentiated cells [111]. While canonical PPAR and C/EBP-binding sites have not been identified in the adipocyte GLUT4 promoter [112], this does not rule out atypical PPREs and CREs. This supposition is supported by the requirement for PPARγ and C/EBPβ or C/EBPδ to support GLUT4 expression during differentiation [113]. While C/EBPα is not essential for GLUT4 expression during adipogenesis [113], it mediates glucocorticoid regulation of GLUT4 in differentiated cells [114]. GLUT4 transcription is induced by LXR activation under the same circumstances where the genes involved in gluconeogenesis are downregulated in liver [115], an example of coordinated regulation of glucose metabolism. While insulin is an important factor driving adipogenesis and GLUT4 induction, in mature adipocytes it represses GLUT4 transcription [116]. This response involves phosphorylation of nuclear factor-1 (NF1). Increased binding of NF1 to the GLUT4 promoter also mediates repression of GLUT4 transcription in response to elevations of cAMP [117].

3.2.8. *Transcriptional regulation of adipokine production*
One of the most exciting developments in the field of adipocyte biology has been the identification of AT as an endocrine organ, secreting a number of factors that act to influence multiple tissues (reviewed in [118,119]). Table 1 lists some of these factors. While such factors are collectively described as "adipokines," recognizing their production in AT, they can differ in their cell of origin. Production can also vary between AT depots, both features are described in Table 1. For secreted factors it is especially true that factors acting at the transcriptional level is only one level of regulation, especially since post-translational modifications are important for a number of adipokines [120,121].

3.2.9. *Adiponectin*
The appearance of adiponectin mRNA is one of the markers of late stage adipocyte differentiation [122]. As with other adipocyte genes, the binding of PPARγ, C/EBPα and SREBP-1c are all needed for the differentiation-related induction of adiponectin expression [123]; SREBP-1c also maintains basal expression. Thiazolidinediones can also upregulate adiponectin expression in mature adipocytes, through binding of a PPARγ/RXR heterodimer to the PPRE in the promoter [123,124]. The response to TZDs in differentiated cells does not require C/EBPα [125]. However, C/EBP is needed to mediate the upregulation of adiponectin that occurs in response to elevated glucose levels [125].

Table 1
Factors secreted from adipose tissue and their cells of origin

Factor	Source
Adiponectin	Ad (sc > v)
Leptin	Ad (sc > v)
Resistin	Mp > Ad (Om > sc)
Angiotensin II	Mast cells > Ad (v > sc)
Adpsin/ASP (acylation stimulating protein)	Ad > Mp
IL-6	Ad (v > sc)
MCP-1 (monocyte chemoattractant protein)	svf > Ad
PAI-1 (plasminogen activator inhibitor-1)	svf > Ad (v > sc)
TNF-α (tumor necrosis factor alpha)	svf > Ad (v > sc)

Notes: Abbreviations: Ad – adipocyte, sc – subcutaneous AT depot, v – visceral AT, Om – omental AT, svf – stromal vascular fraction, Mp – macrophage.

3.2.10. *Leptin*
Transcription of the leptin gene *in vitro* is stimulated by exposure to glucose and/or insulin, mimicking feeding *in vivo* [126]. This response is mediated by SREBP1 binding [126]. C/EBPα can also maintain leptin expression [127], and TZDs act to block this effect, while having little independent influence.

3.2.11. *Resistin*
An Sp1-binding site has been identified in the promoter to the human resistin gene [128]. Sp1 binding to the site increases during adipocyte differentiation, in parallel with resistin expression [128]. The same transcription factor is involved in the induction of resistin in response to high-glucose levels. Both SREBP1c and C/EBPα have been shown to bind to the human resistin promoter and to increase resistin mRNA [129]. In humans, resistin is primarily expressed in macrophages [130] and downregulated by TZD treatment. As expected, the promoter contains several putative PPREs, at least one of which binds PPARγ [131].

3.2.12. *MCP-1*
Basal expression of MCP-1 appears to require Sp1 [132]. Sp1 is also necessary, along with NF-κB, for TNF-α activation of the MCP-1 gene [132,133]. Other stimulatory responses to IL-6 and phorbol esters, require NF-κB as well [133].

3.2.13. *IL-6*
As with the genes for other inflammatory factors, NF-κB is required for IL-6 expression, especially in response to other interleukins [134]. Binding of C/EBP to a site just upstream of NF-κB augments activation of the IL-6 gene.

3.2.14. *PAI-1*
The transcription factors responsible for regulation of PAI-1 expression are stimulus specific. As was the case for MCP-1, binding of NF-κB is needed to mediate the response to TNF-α [135]. Meanwhile, the ability of elevated FFA to increase PAI-1 expression has been mapped to a region of the promoter similar to an Sp1-binding site [136]. FKHR, a member of the Forkhead/winged helix family of transcription factors, is required for insulin-stimulated PAI-1 transcription [137]; Smad3 and Smad4 play a similar role for the response to TGFβ [138].

Several organizing features become apparent for the transcriptional regulation of the functions of AT concerning fatty acid metabolism and adipokine secretion. For those genes directly involved in mediating or influencing fatty acid metabolism, a common factor is PPARγ. Since fatty acids or their metabolites are the native ligands for PPARγ, the involvement of PPARγ completes a metabolic-sensing loop for activating metabolic processes. In the case of inflammatory responses mediated by the adipocyte production of cytokines, the key factor is NF-κB. Since NF-κB function can also be influenced by products of lipid metabolism [139], the possibility is that increased lipid metabolism may control multiple transcriptional programs to drive adipokine expression and production.

4. Impact of PPAR agonists on adipokines in disease states

As already discussed in the preceding sections, AT is no longer considered just an inert storage depot for lipids, but is an active endocrine organ secreting several hormones termed adipokines which not only influence energy homeostasis, but also have significant effects on other metabolic functions including insulin sensitivity, vascular inflammation and endothelial function. In this section, we will review the role of various adipokines in specific disease states characterized by insulin resistance.

4.1. *Insulin resistance*

The metabolic syndrome is a cluster of interrelated common clinical disorders, including obesity, insulin resistance, glucose intolerance, hypertension and dyslipidemia (hypertriglyceridemia and low HDL cholesterol levels). According to recently defined criteria, the metabolic syndrome is associated with a greater risk of atherosclerotic cardiovascular disease than any of its individual components. Primary defects in energy balance that produce obesity (and visceral adiposity in particular) are sufficient to drive all aspects of the syndrome. Obesity also leads to a proinflammatory and prothrombotic state that potentiates atherosclerosis.

Insulin resistance is of major clinical importance because of the key role it plays in the development of type 2 diabetes. However, there is growing evidence that insulin resistance is intricately involved in the development of not only hyperglycemia, but also dyslipidemia, hypertension, hypercoagulation, vasculopathy and, ultimately, premature atherosclerotic cardiovascular disease [140]. This cluster of metabolic abnormalities has been variously termed the "Insulin Resistance Syndrome," the "Cardiovascular Dysmetabolic syndrome," or simply the "Metabolic Syndrome". AT and adipokines appear to play a key role in the development of insulin resistance and the metabolic syndrome [141]. An increase in AT mass is associated with increases in circulating FFAs and alterations in adipokine production, with overexpression of TNF-α, interleukin-6 (IL-6), PAI-1 and resistin and underexpression of adiponectin in AT. All of these abnormalities have the potential to contribute to the worsening of insulin sensitivity [118].

It is well known that elevated FFAs result in peripheral insulin resistance in both humans and animal models [142]. TNF-α also is a major proinflammatory cytokine secreted by adipocytes and stromovascular cells and implicated in the development of insulin resistance. AT TNF-α exerts its deleterious effects in an autocrine and paracrine fashion. It is important to note that the role of TNF-α in the development of insulin resistance in humans is not conclusive and treatment with TNF-α neutralizing antibodies improves insulin sensitivity in rodents but not in patients with type 2 diabetes [143].

IL-6 is a circulating pleiotropic cytokine, which is secreted by several cell types in addition to AT and acts both in a local and systemic manner to modulate insulin sensitivity [118]. Visceral AT is the source for most of the circulating IL-6, which may be derived not from adipocytes, *per se*, but from stromal immune cells. Plasma IL-6 levels positively correlate with human obesity and insulin resistance in several studies

[144], and weight loss significantly decreases both serum and AT IL-6 levels. However, as with TNF-α, the role of IL-6 in worsening insulin resistance in humans (in contrast to animal studies) is not conclusive and in a recent study, acute IL-6 administration did not impair glucose homeostasis in healthy individuals [144].

Another recently discovered adipokine that has been implicated in the development of insulin resistance is resistin. Although initial data suggested that resistin levels were elevated in animal models of insulin resistance and decreased by insulin sensitizers, subsequent studies suggest that obesity and insulin resistance are associated with decreased resistin expression [118]. This may be explained by the fact that in some studies, insulin and TNF-α (both elevated in obesity) have been shown to inhibit resistin expression [118]. In humans, while some studies [145,146] have reported positive correlations of plasma resistin with obesity and insulin resistance, others have found no correlation at all between obesity, insulin resistance and resistin levels in normal, insulin-resistant or type 2 diabetic subjects [147,148]. Potential reasons for this could be population differences or relate to the sensitivity of individual assays [130]. However, it is clear from the data to date that elevated resistin levels do not play a major role in the insulin resistance associated with obesity [149].

In contrast to all the above adipokines, which decrease insulin sensitivity, leptin and adiponectin improve insulin sensitivity. Leptin is secreted mainly by SC adipocytes in proportion to AT mass and nutrition status. Subjects with generalized lipodystrophy with absence of AT have very low levels of leptin and manifest severe insulin resistance along with hyperglycemia, hepatic steatosis and hypertriglyceridemia. Leptin replacement therapy in these individuals has been shown to improve glucose, lower triglyceride levels and also improve hepatic and peripheral insulin sensitivity [150].

Of all the adipokines described above, the one, which has generated the most recent attention, is adiponectin. Adiponectin is the most abundant gene product in adipocytes and accounts for 0.01% of total plasma protein. It has been implicated with playing an important role not only in the pathogenesis of insulin resistance, but also in energy homeostasis, inflammation and atherosclerosis. Serum adiponectin levels are lower in patients with type 2 diabetes, obesity and CAD than in healthy subjects [151]. In some studies, adiponectin has been shown to decrease circulating FFAs by increasing fat oxidation in skeletal muscle [152]. Adiponectin also directly stimulates glucose uptake in adipocytes and muscle by activating AMP-activated protein kinase [153].

It is clear that there is growing evidence to implicate adipokines in the pathogenesis of insulin resistance which is known to be intricately involved in the development of disease states like the metabolic syndrome, type 2 diabetes, hypertension and premature atherosclerotic cardiovascular disease. The TZDs (rosiglitazone and pioglitazone) are a class of anti-diabetic agents that are well known to reduce insulin resistance. Treatment with TZDs in humans leads to an increased potential for subcutaneous fat deposition and a decrease in visceral fat tissue (which is known to be strongly associated with insulin resistance and increased cardiovascular risk) [67]. Thiazolidinedione treatment also leads to lower circulating FFA levels, due to decreased lipolysis and increased TG synthesis. In addition to effects on FFAs, TZD treatment *in vitro* has been shown to reduce adipocyte secretion of TNF-α and IL-6 and also prevent their inhibitory effects on adipocyte insulin-signaling mechanisms [154]. In humans, TZD therapy is associated with a decrease in TNF-α levels in both obese non-diabetic and diabetic subjects [155] but no change in IL-6 levels in patients with type 2 diabetes [156]. The effects of TZDs on resistin are still unclear. In animal studies, AT resistin expression is increased after treatment with several different classes of PPARγ agonists [157]. However, in a study with human abdominal sc adipocytes [158], rosiglitazone blocked insulin-mediated release of resistin secretion *in vitro*.

The TZDs are well known to favor an increase in body fat mass and although leptin levels are strongly correlated with body fat concentration, in recent human studies there was no change in either plasma leptin or sc adipocyte leptin mRNA concentrations after pioglitazone treatment [155,159], despite significant increases in body fat mass.

Of all the adipokines, the induction of AT adiponectin expression and consequent increases in circulating adiponectin levels probably represents one of the most important potential mechanisms for PPARγ-mediated enhancement of whole-body insulin sensitivity [160]. *In vivo* treatment of type 2 diabetic patients with TZDs markedly increases circulating concentrations of adiponectin [66].

4.2. *Obesity and disorders of appetite regulation/energy expenditure*

The adipokines play a significant role in the pathogenesis and development of obesity through the regulation of appetite and energy expenditure in the body [161]. Among the adipokines, leptin is the hormone, which plays a primary role in body weight regulation and, along with insulin, functions as a critical signal to the brain in the long-term regulation of energy homeostasis and body adiposity. Although initially viewed as an anti-obesity hormone, leptin's primary role is to serve as a metabolic signal of energy sufficiency rather than excess [118]. Thus, the major function of leptin appears to be to adapt to low-energy intake rather than to restrain overeating and obesity. Leptin levels rapidly decrease with caloric restriction and weight loss and this is associated with an adaptive physiological response that includes hyperphagia and decreased energy expenditure. Similar responses are observed in leptin-deficient mice and humans, despite marked obesity. The administration of low doses of leptin in these individuals diminishes appetite and induces weight loss [118]. On the other hand, individuals with more common forms of obesity have higher circulating leptin levels and treatment with exogenous leptin is without effect. The mechanism for this leptin resistance is unknown but may result from defects in leptin signaling or transport across the blood–brain barrier [118].

The role of the PPARγ agonists in modulating the effects of leptin and the other adipokines on energy regulation is not well defined. In human studies, treatment with TZDs in patients with type 2 diabetes does not result in any significant changes in either serum leptin or AT leptin mRNA concentrations [155,159]. In patients with lipodystrophy, although in most studies there is an improvement in fat distribution, improvements in metabolic parameters have been variable [162].

4.3. *Atherosclerosis*

There is growing evidence that adipokines play an important role in the development of atherosclerosis and further that the TZDs as PPARγ agonists modify this risk of atherosclerosis progression [163]. The adipokines implicated in the induction of a pro-inflammatory state and oxidative damage leading to the initiation and progression of atherosclerosis include angiotensin-II, PAI-1, TNF-α, leptin and IL-6 [119]. These adipokines enhance the attachment and migration of monocytes into the vessel wall and their conversion into macrophages. Importantly, TNF-α activates NF-κB and sets off a series of vascular inflammatory changes, including the expression of vascular adhesion molecules and the activation of a pro-inflammatory macrophage state. Leptin and IL-6 also have pro-atherogenic effects and IL-6 in particular stimulates hepatic production of CRP, which is an important marker of vascular inflammation and predictor of clinical atherosclerosis. The proteins of the renin angiotensin system (RAS) and PAI-1 are also produced in AT and play a role in the promotion of atherosclerosis. Angiotensin II enhances foam cell formation, stimulates intracellular and vascular adhesion molecule production and enhances the metabolism of NO into oxygen free radicals, which damage the vascular tissue. PAI-1 inhibits the breakdown of fibrin clots and plays a key role in promoting thrombus formation upon rupture of unstable atherosclerotic plaques. Adiponectin, in contrast to the above adipokines, is anti-atherogenic. Among other effects, it inhibits TNF-α expression in macrophages and AT, as well as TNF-α induced pro-atherogenic effects. Adenovirus-expressed adiponectin has been shown to reduce atherosclerotic lesions in a mouse model of atherosclerosis, and adiponectin-deficient mice exhibit an excessive vascular remodeling response to injury. Clinically, high-adiponectin levels are associated with a lower risk for myocardial infarction among healthy men [164] and a moderately decreased CAD risk (mediated in part by effects of adiponectin on HDL cholesterol levels) even in diabetic men [165].

Thus, it is clear that the adipokines have multiple effects to modulate atherosclerosis. These effects are influenced by PPARγ agonists – the TZDs, which have been shown to have significant effects in negatively regulating macrophage activation; inhibiting the production of inflammatory cytokines (TNF α, IL-6); and inhibiting the proliferation and migration of vascular SMC and improving the stability of the atherosclerotic plaque [166]. These TZD effects on the vascular endothelium may be mediated, at least in part, through their effects to increase adiponectin production.

4.4. *Polycystic ovary syndrome*

Polycystic ovary syndrome (PCOS) is one of the most common endocrine-metabolic diseases, affecting up to 10% of women of reproductive age and characterized by hyperandrogenism and insulin resistance [167]. Most women with PCOS have central obesity and there is growing evidence that the adipokines (mainly adiponectin) play a role in the metabolic abnormalities of the syndrome and possibly contribute to the development and/or maintenance of insulin resistance, independent from adiposity. Adipokine levels have been measured in several studies of women with PCOS and the results have been variable. In these studies, women with PCOS had normal leptin levels; lower (or normal) adiponectin levels; and elevated to normal resistin levels as compared to weight matched controls [168]. In some studies, there appears to be a strong relationship to body mass for leptin and adiponectin, but not for resistin, and in controls but not in PCOS, there appears to be significant correlations between leptin and adiponectin and leptin with resistin. In one study, in normal controls all adipocytokines correlated with markers of insulin resistance, while in the PCOS subjects there was no such relationship. However, in other studies, serum adiponectin levels have been shown to be significantly correlated with measures of insulin sensitivity in both normal weight and obese PCOS subjects [169,170]. The varying results in these studies may be attributed, at least in part, to heterogeneous patient populations.

Since insulin resistance is a cardinal feature of PCOS, one therapeutic approach is to use drugs to improve insulin sensitivity and ovarian function. The TZDs appear to be ideally suited to this task and studies have demonstrated that the use of pioglitazone and rosiglitazone result in improving insulin sensitivity and hyperandrogenism, despite associated increases in adiposity [171].

4.5. *Lipodystrophy (including hiv-associated lipodystrophy)*

Although obesity causes insulin resistance, it is paradoxical that the absence of AT also causes insulin resistance and diabetes in humans and genetically engineered animal models. Lipoatrophy and lipodystrophy are features of a group of heterogeneous syndromes caused by genetic (e.g Dunnigan-type familial partial lipodystrophy), immune or infectious/drug-associated conditions (HIV-associated lipodystrophy) and characterized by a paucity of fat, insulin resistance and hypertriglyceridemia [172,173]. Owing to a lack of AT, limited quantities of TG can be stored in fat and excess TGs then tend to accumulate in the liver and skeletal muscles, contributing to insulin resistance. If patients develop diabetes, the syndrome is referred to as lipoatrophic diabetes. Severe lipodystrophy is characterized by low levels of several of the adipokines including leptin, adiponectin and resistin [174].

Since activation of PPARγ promotes adipocyte differentiation, it would be expected that dominant-negative mutations of PPARγ would result in lipodystrophy. Indeed, a syndrome of lipodystrophy, hypoadiponectinemia, severe hyperinsulinemia, early onset hypertension and response to TZD therapy has been described in three patients with dominant-negative mutations [175]. Thiazolidinedione treatment has also been found to improve metabolic control and increase body fat in patients with lipoatrophic diabetes [162]. The other logical treatment for non-HIV lipodystrophies is the administration of recombinant leptin, which improves glycemia, reduces hepatic steatosis, decreases intramyocellular lipid levels and improves insulin sensitivity in patients with severe lipodystrophies and hypoleptinemia [172].

It is well known that HIV-1-infected patients on antiretroviral therapy frequently develop a lipodystrophy syndrome, characterized by peripheral lipoatrophy and visceral fat redistribution associated with metabolic alterations including dyslipidemia and insulin resistance. Although the pathophysiology of this disorder remains unclear, it is now being increasingly recognized that both direct drug toxicity due to anti-retroviral treatment with protease inhibitors (PIs) and nucleoside analogue inhibitors of the viral reverse transcriptase (NRTIs) [176], as well as abnormal fat distribution play major roles [177]. *In vitro*, both PIs and NRTIs have been shown to inhibit adipocyte differentiation and induce insulin resistance and apoptosis in adipose cells and also to increase the expression and secretion of pro-inflammatory cytokines like TNF-α and IL-6, as well as decrease adiponectin levels. Similar changes are observed in fat and serum from HIV-1-infected lipodystrophic patients under antiviral treatment with PIs and NRTIs. Resistin has also been shown to play a role in HIV associated lipodystrophy. In a recent study among 24 HIV-infected subjects with insulin resistance and lipoatrophy, resistin levels were found to be elevated at baseline (compared to matched controls) and subsequently decreased after treatment with a TZD [178]. Thus, altered adipokine secretion may lead to altered adipocyte differentiation, apoptosis, lipoatrophy and insulin resistance [176]. Thus, the PPARs, especially PPARγ, are at the center of a complex system by which the cell types in AT sense and respond to the circulating lipid environment to regulate multiple aspects of metabolism.

References

[1] C. Toldt, Contribution to the histology and physiology of adipose tissue, Sitzber. Akad. Wiss. Wien. Math. Naturwiss. Kl. 62 (1870) 445.

[2] W. Flemming, On the formation and regression of fat cells in connective tissue with comment on the structure of the latter, Arch. R. Mikr. Anat. 7 (1871) 32.

[3] F. Wassermann, The development of adipose tissue, in: A.E. Reynold, G.F. Cahill (Eds.), Handbook of Physiology: Adipose Tissue, American Physical Society, Washington, DC, 1965, pp. 87–100.

[4] A.A. Maximow, W. Bloom, A Textbook on Histology, W. B. Saunders and Co., Philadelphia, 1948.

[5] G.J. Hausman, D.R. Campion, R.J. Martin, Search for the adipocyte precursor cell and factors that promote its differentiation, J. Lipid Res. 21 (1980) 657–670.

[6] C.M. Poissonnet, A.R. Burdi, F.L. Bookstein, Growth and development of human adipose tissue during early gestation, Early Hum. Dev. 8 (1983) 1–11.

[7] M. Morimura, O. Ishiko, T. Sumi, H. Yoshida, S. Ogita, Angiogenesis in adipose tissues and skeletal muscles with rebound weight-gain after diet-restriction in rabbits, Int. J. Mol. Med. 8 (2001) 499–503.

[8] M.A. Rupnick, D. Panigrahy, C.Y. Zhang, S.M. Dallabrida, B.B. Lowell, R. Langer, M.J. Folkman, Adipose tissue mass can be regulated through the vasculature, Proc. Natl. Acad. Sci. USA 99 (2002) 10730–10735.

[9] A.R. Burdi, C.M. Poissonnet, S.M. Garn, M. Lavelle, M.D. Sabet, P. Bridges, Adipose tissue growth patterns during human gestation: a histometric comparison of buccal and gluteal fat depots, Int. J. Obes. 9 (1985) 247–256.

[10] C.M. Poissonnet, M. LaVelle, A.R. Burdi, Growth and development of adipose tissue, J. Pediatr. 113 (1988) 1–9.

[11] A. Margeli, G. Kouraklis, S. Theocharis, Peroxisome proliferator activated receptor-gamma (PPAR-gamma) ligands and angiogenesis, Angiogenesis 6 (2003) 165–169.

[12] X. Xin, S. Yang, J. Kowalski, M.E. Gerritsen, Peroxisome proliferator-activated receptor gamma ligands are potent inhibitors of angiogenesis *in vitro* and *in vivo*, J. Biol. Chem. 274 (1999) 9116–9121.

[13] S. Cinti, M. Cigolini, M. Morroni, M.C. Zingaretti, S-100 protein in white preadipocytes: an immunoelectronmicroscopic study, Anat. Rec. 224 (1989) 466–472.

[14] R. Aubert, J.P. Suquet, D. Lemonnier, Long-term morphological and metabolic effects of early under- and over-nutrition in mice, J. Nutr. 110 (1980) 649–661.

[15] D.S. Lewis, H.A. Bertrand, C.A. McMahan, H.C. McGill, K.D. Carey Jr., E.J. Masoro, Influence of preweaning food intake on body composition of young adult baboons, Am. J. Physiol. 257 (1989) R1128–R1135.

[16] C.G. Brook, J.K. Lloyd, O.H. Wolf, Relation between age of onset of obesity and size and number of adipose cells, Br. Med. J. 2 (1972) 25–27.

[17] J. Hirsch, J.L. Knittle, Cellularity of obese and nonobese human adipose tissue, Fed. Proc. 29 (1970) 1516–1521.

[18] M. Dunlop, J.M. Court, J.B. Hobbs, T.J. Boulton, Identification of small cells in fetal and infant adipose tissue, Pediatr. Res. 12 (1978) 905–907.

[19] G.P. Ravelli, Z.A. Stein, M.W. Susser, Obesity in young men after famine exposure in utero and early infancy, N. Engl. J. Med. 295 (1976) 349–353.

[20] I.M. Faust, P.R. Johnson, J.S. Stern, J. Hirsch, Diet-induced adipocyte number increase in adult rats: a new model of obesity, Am. J. Physiol. 235 (1978) E279–E286.

[21] K.A. Larson, D.B. Anderson, The effects of lipectomy on remaining adipose tissue depots in the Sprague Dawley rat, Growth 42 (1978) 469–477.

[22] H. Hauner, M. Wabitsch, E.F. Pfeiffer, Differentiation of adipocyte precursor cells from obese and nonobese adult women and from different adipose tissue sites, Horm. Metab. Res. 19 (Suppl) (1988) 35–39.

[23] V. van Harmelen, T. Skurk, K. Rohrig, Y.M. Lee, M. Halbleib, I. Aprath-Husmann, H. Hauner, Effect of BMI and age on adipose tissue cellularity and differentiation capacity in women, Int. J. Obes. Relat. Metab. Disord. 27 (2003) 889–895.

[24] J.A. Levine, M.D. Jensen, N.L. Eberhardt, T. O'Brien, Adipocyte macrophage colony-stimulating factor is a mediator of adipose tissue growth, J. Clin. Invest. 101 (1998) 1557–1564.

[25] M. Rodbell, Metabolism of isolated fat cells. I. Effects of hormones on glucose metabolism and lipolysis, J. Biol. Chem. 239 (1964) 375–380.

[26] L.B. Salans, J.L. Knittle, J. Hirsch, The role of adipose cell size and adipose tissue insulin sensitivity in the carbohydrate intolerance of human obesity, J. Clin. Invest. 47 (1968) 153–165.

[27] S.C. Jamdar, L.J. Osborne, Glycerolipid biosynthesis in rat adipose tissue: VIII. Effect of obesity and cell size on [14C] acetate incorporation into lipids, Lipids 16 (1981) 830–834.

[28] V. Hill, N. Baker, Heterogeneous labeling of adipocytes during *in vivo–in vitro* incubation of epididymal fat pads of aging mice with [1-14C] palmitate, Lipids 18 (1983) 25–31.

[29] J.M. Friedman, Obesity in the new millennium, Nature 404 (2000) 632–634.

[30] T. Yamauchi, J. Kamon, H. Waki, K. Murakami, K. Motojima, K. Komeda, T. Ide, N. Kubota, Y. Terauchi, K. Tobe, H. Miki, A. Tsuchida, Y. Akaruma, R. Nagai, S. Kimura, T. Kadowaki, The mechanisms by which both heterozygous peroxisome proliferator-activated receptor gamma (PPARgamma) deficiency and PPARgamma agonist improve insulin resistance, J. Biol. Chem. 276 (2001) 41245–41254.

[31] V.R. Sopasakis, M. Sandqvist, B. Gustafson, A. Hammarstedt, M. Schmelz, X. Yang, P.A. Jansson, U. Smith, High local concentrations and effects on differentiation implicate interleukin-6 as a paracrine regulator, Obes. Res. 12 (2004) 454–460.

[32] G.S. Hotamisligil, N.S. Shargill, B.M. Spiegelman, Adipose expression of tumor necrosis factor-alpha: direct role in obesity-linked insulin resistance, Science 259 (1993) 87–91.

[33] C. Farnier, S. Krief, M. Blache, F. Diot-Dupuy, G. Mory, P. Ferre, R. Bazin, Adipocyte functions are modulated by cell size change: potential involvement of an integrin/ERK signalling pathway, Int. J. Obes. Relat. Metab. Disord. 27 (2003) 1178–1186.

[34] C. Knouff, J. Auwerx, Peroxisome proliferator-activated receptor-gamma calls for activation in moderation: lessons from genetics and pharmacology, Endocr. Rev. 25 (2004) 899–918.

[35] W.S. Yang, C.Y. Jeng, T.J. Wu, S. Tanaka, Y. Funahashi, Y. Matsuzawa, J.P. Wang, C.L. Chen, T.Y. Tai, L.M. Chuang, Synthetic peroxisome proliferator-activated receptor-gamma agonist, rosiglitazone increases plasma levels of adiponectin in type 2 diabetic patients, Diabetes Care 25 (2002) 376–380.

[36] B. Desvergne, L. Michalik, W. Wahli, Be fit or be sick: peroxisome proliferator-activated receptors are down the road, Mol. Endocrinol. 18 (2004) 1321–1332.

[37] M. Takahashi, Y. Kamei, O. Ezaki, Mest/Peg1 imprinted gene enlarges adipocytes and is a marker of adipocyte size, Am. J. Physiol. Endocrinol. Metab. 288 (2005) E117–E124.

[38] C.J. de Souza, M. Eckhardt, K. Gagen, M. Dong, W. Chen, D. Laurent, B.F. Burkey, Effects of pioglitazone on adipose tissue remodeling within the setting of obesity and insulin resistance, Diabetes 50 (2001) 1863–1871.

[39] G. Boden, P. Cheung, M. Mozzoli, S.K. Fried, Effect of thiazolidinediones on glucose and fatty acid metabolism in patients with type 2 diabetes, Metabolism 52 (2003) 753–759.

[40] F.D. DeMartinis, Very small fat cell populations determined by a modified osmium tetroxide-urea method, Am. J. Physiol. 249 (1985) C89–C96.

[41] P. Julien, J.P. Despres, A. Angel, Scanning electron microscopy of very small fat cells and mature fat cells in human obesity, J. Lipid Res. 30 (1989) 293–299.

[42] D.L. Crandall, M. DiGirolamo, Hemodynamic and metabolic correlates in adipose tissue: pathophysiologic considerations, FASEB J. 4 (1990) 141–147.

[43] H.-L. Vikman, J.J. Ohisalo, Regulation of adenylate cyclase in plasma membranes of human intraabdominal and abdominal subcutaneous adipocytes, Metabolism 42 (1993) 739–742.

[44] P. Mauriege, J.P. Despres, M. Marcotte, M. Ferland, A. Tremblay, A. Nadeau, S. Moorjani, P.J. Lupien, G. Theriault, C. Bouchard, Abdominal fat cell lipolysis, body fat distribution, and metabolic variables in premenopausal women, J. Clin. Endocrinol. Metab. 71 (1990) 1028–1035.

[45] C. Bouchard, J.P. Despres, P. Mauriege, Genetic and nongenetic determinants of regional fat distribution, Endocr. Rev. 14 (1993) 72–93.

[46] J. Hellmer, C. Marcus, T. Sonnenfeld, P. Arner, Mechanisms for differences in lipolysis between human subcutaneous and omental fat cells, J. Clin. Endocrinol. Metab. 75 (1992) 15–20.

[47] P. Engfeldt, J. Hellmer, H. Wahrenberg, P. Arner, Effects of insulin on adrenoceptor binding and rate of catrecholamine-induced lipolysis in isolated human fat cells, J. Biol. Chem. 263 (1988) 15553–15560.

[48] S.K. Fried, C.D. Russell, N.L. Grauso, R.E. Brolin, Lipoprotein lipase regulation by insulin and glucocorticoid in subcutaneous and omental adipose tissues of obese women and men, J. Clin. Invest. 92 (1993) 2191–2198.

[49] P. Bjorntorp, Hormonal control of regional fat distribution, Hum. Reprod. 12 (Suppl. 1) (1997) 21–25.

[50] I.J. Bujalska, S. Kumar, P.M. Stewart, Does central obesity reflect "Cushing's disease of the omentum"?, Lancet 349 (1997) 1210–1213.

[51] G.L. Stiles, M.G. Caron, R.J. Lefkowitz, Beta-adrenergic receptors: biochemical mechanisms of physiological regulation, Physiol. Rev. 64 (1984) 661–743.

[52] M. Cigolini, U. Smith, Human adipose tissue in culture. VIII. Studies on the insulin-antagonistic effect of glucocorticoids, Metabolism 28 (1979) 502–510.

[53] M. Lundgren, J. Buren, T. Ruge, T. Myrnas, J.W. Eriksson, Glucocorticoids down-regulate glucose uptake capacity and insulin-signaling proteins in omental but not subcutaneous human adipocytes, J. Clin. Endocrinol. Metab. 89 (2004) 2989–2997.

[54] G. De Pergola, The adipose tissue metabolism: role of testosterone and dehydroepiandrosterone, Int. J. Obes. Relat. Metab. Disord. 24 (Suppl. 2) (2000) S59–S63.

[55] A. Dicker, M. Ryden, E. Naslund, I.E. Muehlen, M. Wiren, M. Lafontan, P. Arner, Effect of testosterone on lipolysis in human pre-adipocytes from different fat depots, Diabetologia 47 (2004) 420–428.

[56] P. Marin, B. Oden, P. Bjorntorp, Assimilation and mobilization of triglycerides in subcutaneous abdominal and femoral adipose tissue *in vivo* in men: effects of androgens, J. Clin. Endocrinol. Metab. 80 (1995) 239–243.

[57] S.B. Pedersen, J.M. Bruun, F. Hube, K. Kristensen, H. Hauner, B. Richelsen, Demonstration of estrogen receptor subtypes alpha and beta in human adipose tissue: influences of adipose cell differentiation and fat depot localization, Mol. Cell Endocrinol. 182 (2001) 27–37.

[58] G. Grichting, L.K. Levy, H.M. Goodman, Relationship between binding and biological effects of human growth hormone in rat adipocytes, Endocrinology 113 (1983) 1111–1120.

[59] M. Rosenbaum, J.M. Gertner, N. Gidfar, J. Hirsch, R.L. Leibel, Effects of systemic growth hormone (GH) administration on regional adipose tissue in children with non-GH-deficient short stature, J. Clin. Endocrinol. Metab. 75 (1992) 151–156.

[60] H. Hauner, G. Entenmann, Regional variation of adipose differentiation in cultured stromal-vascular cells from the abdominal and femoral adipose tissue of obese women, Int. J. Obes. 15 (1991) 121–126.

[61] V. Van Harmelen, K. Rohrig, H. Hauner, Comparison of proliferation and differentiation capacity of human adipocyte precursor cells from the omental and subcutaneous adipose tissue depot of obese subjects, Metabolism 53 (2004) 632–637.

[62] T. Tchkonia, Y.D. Tchoukalova, N. Giorgadze, T. Poirtskhalava, I. Karagiannides, R.A. Forse, A. Koo, M. Stevenson, D. Chinnnappan, A. Cartwright, M.D. Jensen, J.L. Kirkland, Abundance of two human preadipocyte subtypes with distinct capacities for replication, adipogenesis, and apoptosis varies among fat depots, Am. J. Physiol. Endocrinol. Metab. 288 (2004) E267–E277.

[63] C.U. Niesler, K. Siddle, J.B. Prins, Human preadipocytes display a depot-specific susceptibility to apoptosis, Diabetes 47 (1998) 1365–1368.

[64] L. Dorstyn, S. Kumar, Differential inhibitory effects of CrmA, P35, IAP and three mammalian IAP homologues on apoptosis in NIH3T3 cells following various death stimuli, Cell. Death Differ. 4 (1997) 570–579.

[65] C.U. Niesler, J.B. Prins, S. O'Rahilly, K. Siddle, C.T. Montague, Adipose depot-specific expression of cIAP2 in human preadipocytes and modulation of expression by serum factors and TNF alpha, Int. J. Obes. Relat. Metab. Disord. 25 (2001) 1027–1033.

[66] H. Yki-Jarvinen, Thiazolidinediones, New Eng. J. Med. 351 (2004) 1106–1118.

[67] Y. Miyazaki, A. Mahankali, M. Matsuda, S. Mahankali, J. Hardies, K. Cusi, L.J. Mandarino, R.A. DeFronzo, Effect of pioglitazone on abdominal fat distribution and insulin sensitivity in type 2 diabetic patients, J. Clin. Endocrinol. Metab. 87 (2002) 2784–2791.

[68] D.G. Carey, G.J. Cowin, G.J. Galloway, N.P. Jones, J.C. Richards, N. Biswas, D.M. Doddrell, Effect of rosiglitazone on insulin sensitivity and body composition in type 2 diabetic patients, Obes. Res. 10 (2002) 1008–1015.

[69] M. Adams, C.T. Montague, J.B. Prins, J.C. Holder, S.A. Smith, L. Sanders, J.E. Digby, C.P. Sewter, M.A. Lazar, V.K. Chatterjee, S. O'Rahilly, Activators of peroxisome proliferator-activated receptor gamma have depot specific effects on human preadipocyte differentiation, J. Clin. Invest. 100 (1997) 3149–3153.

[70] P. Ferre, The biology of peroxisome proliferator-activated receptors: relationship with lipid metabolism and insulin sensitivity, Diabetes 53 (2004) S43–S50.

[71] R. Mukherjee, L. Jow, D. Noonan, D.P. McDonnell, Human and rat peroxisome proliferator activated receptors (PPARs) demonstrate similar tissue distribution but different responsiveness to PPAR activators, J. Steroid Biochem. Mol. Biol. 51 (1994) 157–166.

[72] R. Mukherjee, L. Jow, G.E. Croston, J.R. Paterniti, Identification, characterization, and tissue distribution of human peroxisome proliferator-activated receptor (PPAR) isoforms PPARγ2 versus PPARγ1 and activation with retinoid X receptor agonists and antagonists, J. Biol. Chem. 272 (1997) 8071–8076.

[73] I. Inoue, K. Shino, S. Noji, T. Awata, S. Katayama, Expression of peroxisome proliferator-activated receptor alpha (PPARα) in primary cultures of human vascular endothelial cells, Biochem. Biophys. Res. Comm. 246 (1998) 370–374.

[74] S.-L. Su, C.J. Simmons, B. Wisley, B. Ellis, D.A. Winegar, Monitoring of PPAR alpha protein expression in human tissue by use of PPAR alpha-specific MAbs, Hybridoma 17 (1998) 47–53.

[75] M. Loviscach, N. Rehman, L. Carter, S. Mudaliar, P. Mohadeen, T.P. Ciaraldi, J.H. Veerkamp, R.R. Henry, Distribution of peroxisome proliferator-activated receptors (PPARs) in human skeletal muscle and adipose tissue: relation to insulin action, Diabetologia 43 (2000) 304–311.

[76] A. Elbrecht, Y. Chen, C.A. Cullinan, N. Hayes, M.D. Leibowitz, D.E. Moller, J. Berger, Molecular cloning, expression and characterization of human peroxisome proliferator activated receptors gamma1 and gamma2, Biochem. Biophys. Res. Comm. 224 (1996) 431–437.

[77] L. Fajas, J.-C. Fruchart, J. Auwerx, PPARgamma3 mRNA: a distinct PPARgamma mRNA subtype transcribed from an independent promoter, FEBS Lett. 438 (1998) 55–60.

[78] L. Fajas, D. Auboeuf, E. Raspe, K. Schoonjans, A.-M. Lefebvre, R. Saladin, J. Najib, M. Laville, J.-C. Fruchart, S. Deeb, A. Vidal-puig, J. Flier, M.R. Briggs, B. Staels, H. Vidal, J. Auwert, The organization, promoter analysis, and expression of the human PPARgamma gene, J. Biol. Chem. 272 (1997) 18779–18789.

[79] R.H. Unger, L. Orci, Lipotoxic diseases of nonadipose tissues in obesity, Int. J. Obes. Relat. Metab. Disord. 24 (2000) S28–S32.

[80] Y. Schutz, Concept of fat balance in human obesity revisited with particular reference to de novo lipogenesis, Intl. J. Obes. 28 (2004) S3–S11.

[81] M. Merkel, R.H. Eckel, I.J. Goldberg, Lipoprotein lipase: genetics, lipid uptake, and regulation, J. Lipid Res. 43 (2002) 1997–2006.

[82] S. Enrback, B.G. Ohlsson, L. Samuelsson, G. Bjursell, Characterization of the human lipoprotein lipase (LPL) promoter: evidence of two cis-regulatory regions, LP-alpha and LP-beta, of importance for the differentiation-linked induction of the LPL gene during adipogenesis, Mol. Cell. Biol. 12 (1992) 4622–4633.

[83] H. Kageyama, T. Hirano, K. Okada, T. Ebara, A. Kageyama, T. Murakami, S. Shioda, M. Adachi, Lipoprotein lipase mRNA in white adipose tissue but not in skeletal muscle is increased by pioglitazone through PPAR-γ, Biochem. Biophys. Res. Comm. 305 (2003) 22–27.

[84] M. Laplante, H. Sell, K.L. MacNaul, D. Richard, J.P. Berger, Y. Deshaies, PPAR-gamma activation mediates adipose depot-specific effects on gene expression and lipoprotein lipase activity: mechanisms for modulation of postprandial lipemia and differential adipose accretion, Diabetes 52 (2003) 291–299.

[85] T. Kawai, I. Takei, Y. Oguma, N. Ohashi, S. Oguchi, F. Katsukawa, H. Hirose, A. Shiumada, K. Watanabe, T. Saruta, Effects of troglitazone on fat distribution in the treatment of male type 2 diabetics, Metabolism 49 (1999) 1102–1107.

[86] J.A. Hamilton, W. Guo, F. Kamp, Mechanism of cellular uptake of long-chain fatty acids: Do we need cellular proteins?, Mol. Cell Biochem. 239 (2002) 17–23.

[87] A. Stahl, A current review of fatty acid transport proteins (SLC27), Pflugers Arch. – Eur. J. Physiol. 447 (2004) 722–727.

[88] A.M. Hall, A.J. Smith, D.A. Bernlohr, Characterization of the Acyl-CoA synthase activity of purified murine fatty acid transport protein 1, J. Biol. Chem. 278 (2003) 43008–43013.

[89] B.I. Frohnert, T.Y. Hui, D.A. Bernlohr, Identification of a functional peroxisome proliferator-responsive element in the murine fatty acid transport gene, J. Biol. Chem. 274 (1999) 3970–3977.

[90] K. Motojima, P. Passilly, J.M. Peters, F.J. Gonzalez, N. Latruffe, Expression of putative fatty acid transporter genes are regulated by peroxisome proliferator-activated receptor alpha and gamma activators in a tissue- and inducer-specific manner, J. Biol. Chem. 273 (1998) 16710–16714.

[91] G. Martin, K. Schoonjans, A.-M. Lefebvre, B. Staels, J. Auwerx, Coordinate regulation of the expression of the fatty acid transport protein and acyl-Coa synthase genes by PPARalpha and PPARgamma activators, J. Biol. Chem. 272 (1997) 28210–28217.

[92] H. Rieusset, J. Auwerx, H. Vidal, Regulation of gene expression by activation of the peroxisome proliferator-activated receptor γ with rosiglitazone (BRL49653) in human adipocytes, Biochem. Biophys. Res. Comm. 265 (1999) 265–271.

[93] G. Boden, C. Homko, M. Mozzoli, L.C. Scowe, C. Nichols, P. Cheung, Thiazolidinediones upregulate fatty acid uptake and oxidation in adipose tissue of diabetic patients, Diabetes 54 (2005) 880–885.

[94] O. Sato, C. Kuriki, Y. Fukui, K. Motojima, Dual promoter structure of mouse and human fatty acid translocase/CD36 genes and unique transcriptional activation by peroxisome proliferator-activated receptor alpha and gamma ligands, J. Biol. Chem. 277 (2002) 15703–15711.

[95] J. Feng, J. Han, S.F. Pearce, R.L. Silverstein, A.M.J. Gotto, D.P. Hajjar, A.C. Nicholson, Induction of CD36 expression by oxidised LDL and IL-4 by a common signaling pathway dependent on protein kinase C and PPAR-gamma, J. Lipid Res. 41 (2000) 688–696.

[96] N.H. Haunerland, F. Spener, Fatty acid-binding proteins—insights from genetic manipulations, Prog. Lipid Res. 43 (2004) 328–349;

[96a] L. Reshef, Y. Olswang, H. Cassuto, B. Blum, C.M. Croniger, S.C. Kalhan, S.M. Tilghman, R.W. Hanson, Glyceroneogenesis and the triglyceride/fatty acid cycle, J. Biol. Chem. 78 (2003) 30413–30416.

[97] J.F.C. Glatz, J. Storch, Unravelling the significance of cellular fatty acid-binding proteins, Curr. Op. Lipid 12 (2001) 267–274.

[98] E.G. Beale, C. Forest, R.E. Hammer, Regulation of cytosolic phosphoenolpyruvate carboxykinase gene expression in adipocytes, Biochimie 85 (2003) 1207–1211.

[99] M. Glorian, E. Duplus, E.G. Beale, D.K. Scott, D.K. Granner, C. Forest, A single element in the phosphoenolpyruvate carboxykinase gene mediates thiazolidinedione action specifically in adipocytes, Biochimie 83 (2001) 933–943.

[100] C. Londos, D.L. Brasaemle, C.J. Schultz, J.P. Segrest, A.R. Kimmel, Perilipins, ADRP, and other proteins that associate with intracellular neutral lipid droplets in animal cells, Sem. Cell Develop. Biol. 10 (1999) 51–58.

[101] J.T. Tansey, C. Sztalryd, E.M. Hlavin, A.R. Kimmel, C. Londos, The central role of perilipin A in lipid metabolism and adipocyte lipolysis, Life 56 (2004) 379–385.

[102] C. Sztalryd, G. Xu, H. Dorward, J.T. Tansey, J.A. Contreras, A.R. Kimmel, C. Londos, Perilipin A is essential for the translocation of hormone-sensitive lipase during lipolytic activation, J. Cell. Biol. 161 (2003) 1093–1103

[103] Y. Wang, S. Sullivan, M. Trujillo, M.-J. Lee, S. Schneider, R.E. Brolin, Y.H. Kang, Y. Werber, A.S. Greenberg, S.K. Fried, Perilipin expression in human adipose tissues: effects of obesity, gender and depot, Obes. Res. 288 (2003) 930–936.

[104] E. Arvidsson, L. Blomqvist, M. Ryden, Depot-specific differences in perilipion mRNA but not protein expression in obesity, J. Intern. Med. 255 (2004) 595–601.

[105] N. Arimura, T. Horiba, M. Imagawa, M. Shimizu, R. Sato, The peroxisome proliferator-activated receptor γ regulates expression of the perilipin gene in adipocytes, J. Biol. Chem. 279 (2004) 10070–10076.

[106] C. Holm, Molecular mechanisms regulating hormone-sensitive lipase and lipolysis, Biochem. Soc. Trans. 31 (2003) 1120–1124.

[107] S.J. Yeaman, Hormone-sensitive lipase – new roles for an old enzyme, Biochem. J. 379 (2004) 11–22.

[108] R. Blaise, J. Grober, P. Rouet, G. Tavernier, D. Daegelen, D. Langin, Testis expression of hormone-sensitive lipase is conferred by a specific promoter that contains four regions binding testicular nuclear proteins, J. Biol. Chem. 274 (1999) 9327–9334.

[109] F. Smih, P. Rouet, S. Lucas, A. Mairal, C. Sengenes, M. Lafontan, S. Vaulont, M. Casado, D. Langin, Transcriptional regulation of adipocyte hormone-sensitive lipase by glucose, Diabetes 51 (2002) 293–300.

[110] M. Uldry, B. Thorens, The SLC2 family of facilitated hexose and polyol transporters, Pflugers Arch-Eur. J. Physiol. 447 (2004) 480–489.

[111] N. Yokomori, M. Tawata, T. Onaya, A transcriptional repressor regulates mouse GLUT4 gene expression during the differentiation of 3T3-L1 cells, Diabetes 48 (1999) 2471–2474.

[112] O. Ezaki, Regulatory elements in the insulin-responsive glucose transporter 4 gene, Biochem. Biophys, Res. Commun. 241 (1997) 1–6.

[113]. Z. Wu, Y. Xie, R.F. Morrison, N.L.R. Bucher, S.R. Farmer, PPARgamma induces the insulin-dependent glucose transporter GLUT4 in the absence of C/EBPalpha during the conversion of 3T3 fibroblasts into adipocytes, J. Clin. Invest. 101 (1998) 22–32.

[114] K.H. Kaestner, R.J. Christy, M.D. Lane, Mouse insulin-responsive glucose transporter gene: characterization of the gene and transactivation by the CCAAT/enhancer binding protein, Proc. Natl. Acad. Sci. USA 87 (1990) 251–255.

[115] W.S. Yang, S.S. Deeb, Sp1 and Sp3 transactivate the human lipoprotein lipase gene promoter through binding to a CT element: synergy with the sterol regulatory element binding protein and reduced transactivation of a naturally occurring promoter variant, J. Lipid Res. 39 (1998) 2054–2064.

[116] D.W. Cooke, M.D. Lane, A sequence element in the GLUT4 gene that mediates repression by insulin, J. Biol. Chem. 273 (1998) 6210–6217.

[117] D.W. Cooke, M.D. Lane, Transcription factor NF1 mediates repression of the GLUT4 promoter by cyclic-AMP, Biochem. Biophys. Res. Comm. 260 (1999) 600–604.

[118] E.E. Kershaw, J.S. Flier, Adipose tissue as an endocrine organ, J. Clin. Endocrinol. Metab. 89 (2004) 2548–2556.

[119] M.W. Rajala, P.E. Scherer, Minireview: the adipocyte-at the crossroads of energy homeostasis, inflammation, and atherosclerosis, Endocrinology 144 (2003) 3765–3773.

[120] R. Rea, R. Donnelly, resistin: an adipocyte-derived hormone. Has it a role in diabetes and obesity?, Diab. Obes. Metab. 6 (2004) 163–170.

[121] U.B. Pajvani, X. Du, T.P. Combs, A.H. Berg, M.W. Rajala, T. Schulthess, J. Engel, M. Brownlee, P.E. Scherer, Structure–function studies of the adipocyte-secreted hormone Acrp30/adiponectin, Implications for metabolic regulation and bioactivity. J. Biol. Chem. 278 (2003) 9073–9085.

[122] A.H. Berg, T.P. Combs, P.E. Scherer, ACRP30/adiponectin: an adipokine regulating glucose and lipid metabolism, Trends Endocrinol. Metab. 13 (2002) 84–89.

[123] B. Gustafson, M.M. Jack, S.W. Cushman, U. Smith, Adiponectin gene activation by thiazolidinediones requires PPAR gamma 2, but not C/EBP alpha-evidence for differential regulation of the aP2 and adiponectin genes, Biochem. Biophys. Res. Comm. 308 (2003) 933–939.

[124] M. Iwaki, M. Matsuda, N. Maeda, T. Funahashi, Y. Matsuzawa, M. Makishima, I. Shimomura, Induction of adiponectin, a fat-derived antidiabetic and antiatherogenic factor, by nuclear receptors, Diabetes 52 (2003) 1655–1663.

[125] S.K. Park, S.Y. Oh, M.Y. Lee, S. Yoon, K.S. Kim, J.W. Kim, CCAAT/enhancer binding protein and nuclear factor-Y regulate adiponectin gene expression in adipose tissue, Diabetes 53 (2004) 2757–2766.

[126] J.B. Kim, P. Sarraf, M. Wright, K.M. Yao, E. Mueller, G. Solanes, B.B. Lowell, B.M. Spiegelman, Nutritional and insulin regulation of fatty acid synthase and leptin gene expression through ADD1/SREBP1, J. Clin. Invest. 101 (1998) 1–9.

[127] A.N. Hollenberg, V.S. Susulic, J.P. Madura, B. Zhang, D.E. Moller, P. Tontonoz, P. Sarraf, B.M. Spiegelan, B.B. Lowell, Functional antagonism between CCAAT/Enhancer binding protein-alpha and peroxisome proliferator-activated receptor-gamma on the leptin receptor, J. Biol. Chem. 272 (1997) 5283–5290.

[128] S.S. Chung, H.H. Choi, K.W. Kim, Y.M. Cho, H.K. Lee, K.S. Park, regulation of human resistin gene expression in cell systems: an important role of stimulatory protein 1 interaction with a common promoter polymorphic site, Diabetologia 48 (2005) 1150–1158.

[129] J.B. Seo, M.J. Noh, E.J. Yoo, S.Y. Park, J. Park, I.K. Lee, S.D. Park, J.B. Kim, Functional characterization of the human resistin promoter with adipocyte determination- and differentiation-dependent factor 1/sterol regulatory element binding protein 1c and CCAAT enhancer binding protein-alpha, Mol. Endocrinol. 17 (2003) 1522–1533.

[130] C.M. Steppan, M.A. Lazar, The current biology of resistin, J. Intl. Med. 255 (2004) 439–447.

[131] L. Patel, A.C. Buckels, I.J. Kinghorn, P.R. Murdock, J.D. Holbrook, C. Plimpton, C.H. Macphee, S.A. Smith, resistin is expressed in human macrophages and directly regulated by PPAR gamma activators, Biochem. Biophys. Res. Comm. 300 (2003) 472–476.

[132] D. Ping, G. Boekhoudt, F. Zhang, A. Morris, S. Philpsen, S.T. Warren, J.M. Boss, Sp1 binding is critical for promoter assembly and activation of the MCP-1 gene by tumor necrosis factor, J. Biol. Chem. 275 (2000) 1708–1714.

[133] A. Ueda, K. Okuda, S. Ohno, A. Shirai, T. Igarashi, K. Matsunaga, J. Fukushima, S. Kawamoto, Y. Ishigatsubo, T. Okubo, NF-kappa B and Sp1 regulate transcription of the human monocyte chemoattractant protein-1 gene, J. Immunol. 153 (1994) 2052–2063.

[134] L.D. Vales, E.M. Friedel, Binding of C/EBP and RBP (CBF1) to overlapping sites regulates interlukin-6 gene expression, J. Biol. Chem. 277 (2002) 43438–43446.

[135] G. Wolf, Insulin resistance and obesity: resistin, a hormone secreted by adipose tissue, Nutr. Rev. 62 (2004) 389–399.

[136] Y. Chen, J.J. Billadello, D.J. Schneider, Identification and localization of a fatty acid response region in the human plasminogen activator inhibitor-1 gene, Arterioscler Thromb. Vasc. Biol. 20 (2000) 2696–2701.

[137] A.I. Vulin, F.M. Stanley, A Forkhead/winged helix-related transcription factor mediates insulin-increased plasminigen activator inhibitor-1 gene transcription, J. Biol. Chem. 277 (2002) 20169–20176.

[138] S.L. Stroschein, W. Wang, K. Luo, Cooperative binding of Smad proteins to two adjacent DNA elements in the plasminogen activator inhibitor-1 promoter mediates transforming growth factor beta-induced smad-dependent transcriptional activation, J. Biol. Chem. 274 (1999) 9431–9441.

[139] S. Sinha, G. Perdomo, N.F. Brown, R.M. O'Doherty, Fatty acid-induced insulin resistance in L6 myotubes is prevented by inhibition of activation and nuclear localization of nuclear factor kB, J. Biol. Chem. 279 (2004) 41294–41301.

[140] T.C. Fagan, P.C. Deedwania, The cardiovascular dysmetabolic syndrome, Am. J. Med. 105 (1998) 77S–82S.

[141] G.E. Sonnenberg, G.R. Krakower, A.H. Kissebah, A novel pathway to the manifestations of metabolic syndrome, Obes. Res. 12 (2004) 180–186.

[142] G. Boden, M. Laakso, Lipids and glucose in type 2 diabetes: what is the cause and effect?, Diabetes Care 27 (2004) 2253–2259.

[143] F. Ofei, S. Hurel, J. Newkirk, M. Sopwith, R Taylor, Effects of an engineered human anti-TNF-alpha antibody (CDP571) on insulin sensitivity and glycemic control in patients with NIDDM, Diabetes 45 (1996) 881–885.

[144] A.G. Pittas, N.A. Joseph, A S Greenberg, Adipocytokines and insulin resistance, J. Clin. Endocrinol. Metab. 89 (2004) 447–452.

[145] J.V. Silha, M. Krsek, V. Hana, J. Marek, J. Jezkova, V. Weiss, L.J. Murphy, Perturbations in adiponectin, leptin and resistin levels in acromegaly: lack of correlation with insulin resistance, Clin. Endocrinol. 58 (2003) 736–742.

[146] M. Degawa-Yamauchi, J.E. Bovenkerk, B.E. Juliar, W. Watson, K. Kerr, R. Jones, Q. Zhu, R.V. Considine, Serum resistin (FIZZ3) protein is increased in obese humans, J. Clin. Endocrinol. Metab. 88 (2003) 5452–5455.

[147] J.H. Lee, J.L. Chan, N. Yiannakouris, M. Kontogianni, E. Estrada, R. Seip, C. Orlova, C.S. Mantzoros, Circulating resistin levels are not associated with obesity or insulin resistance in humans and are not regulated by fasting or leptin administration: cross-sectional and interventional studies in normal, insulin-resistant, and diabetic subjects, J. Clin. Endocrinol. Metab. 88 (2003) 4848–4856.

[148] O. Ukkola, M. Santaniemi, Adiponectin: a link between excess adiposity and associated comorbidities?, J. Mol. Med. 80 (2002) 696–702.

[149] P. Arner, The adipocyte in insulin resistance: key molecules and the impact of the thiazolidinediones, Trends Endocrinol. Metab. 14 (2003) 137–145.

[150] K.F. Petersen, E.A. Oral, S. Dufour, D. Befroy, C. Ariyan, C. Yu, G.W. Cline, A.M. DePaoli, S.I. Taylor, P. Gorden, G.I. Shulman, Leptin reverses insulin resistance and hepatic steatosis in patients with severe lipodystrophy, J. Clin. Invest. 109 (2002) 1345–1350.

[151] C. Weyer, T. Funahashi, S. Tanaka, K. Hotta, Y. Matsuzawa, R.E. Pratley, P.A. Tataranni, Hypoadiponectinemia in obesity and type 2 diabetes: close association with insulin resistance and hyperinsulinemia, J. Clin. Endocrinol. Metab. 86 (2001) 1930–1935.

[152] J. Fruebis, T.-S. Tsao, S. Javorschi, D. Ebberts-Reed, M.R.S. Erickson, F.T. Yen, B.E. Bihain, H.F. Lodish, Proteolytic cleavage product of 30-kDa adipocyte complement-related protein increases fatty acid oxidation in muscle and causes weight loss in mice, Proc. Natl. Acad. Sci. USA 98 (2001) 2005–2010.

[153] T. Yamauchi, J. Kamon, Y. Minokoshi, Y. Ito, H. Waki, S. Uchida, S. Yamashita, M. Noda, S. Kita, K. Ueki, K. Eto, Y. Akanuma, P. Froguel, F. Foufelle, P. Ferre, D. Carling, S. Kimura, R. Nagai, B.B. Kahn, T. Kadowaki, Adiponectin stimulates glucose utilization and fatty acid oxidation by activating AMP-activated protein kinase, Nat. Med. 8 (2002) 1288–1295.

[154] C. Lagathu, J.P. Bastard, M. Auclair, M. Maachi, J. Capeau, M. Caron, Chronic interleukin-6 (IL-6) treatment increased IL-6 secretion and induced insulin resistance in adipocyte: prevention by rosiglitazone, Biochem. Biophys. Res. Comm. 311 (2003) 372–379.

[155] Y. Miyazaki, A. Mahankali, E. Wajcberg, M. Bajaj, L.J. Mandarino, R.A. DeFronzo, Effect of pioglitazone on circulating adiponectin levels and insulin sensitivity in type 2 diabetic patients, J. Clin. Endocrinol. Metab. 89 (2004) 4312–4319.

[156] S.M. Haffner, A.S. Greenberg, W.M. Weston, H. Chen, K. Williams, M.I. Freed, Effect of rosiglitazone treatment on nontraditional markers of cardiovascular disease in patients with type 2 diabetes mellitus, Circulation 106 (2002) 679–684.

[157] J.M. Way, C.Z. Gorgun, Q. Tong, K.T. Uysal, K.K. Brown, W.W. Harrington, W.R. Oliver Jr., T.M. Willson, S.A. Kliewer, G.S. Hotamisligil, Adipose tissue resistin expression is severely suppressed in obesity and stimulated by peroxisome proliferator-activated receptor gamma agonists, J. Biol. Chem. 276 (2001) 25651–25653.

[158] P.G. McTernan, F.M. Fisher, G. Valsamakis, R. Chetty, A. Harte, C.L. McTernan, P.M. Clark, S.A. Smith, A.H. Barnett, S. Kumar, Resistin and type 2 diabetes: regulation of resistin expression by insulin and rosiglitazone and the effects of recombinant resistin on lipid and glucose metabolism in human differentiated adipocytes, J. Clin. Endocrinol. Metab. 88 (2003) 6098–6106.

[159] I. Bogacka, X. Hui, G.A. Bray, S.A. Smith, The effect of pioglitazone on peroxisome proliferator-activated receptor-g target genes related to lipid storage *in vivo*, Diabetes Care 27 (2004) 1660–1667.

[160] T.P. Combs, J.A. Wagner, J. Berger, T. Doebber, W.-J. Wang, B.B. Zhang, M. Tanen, A.H. Berg, S. O'Rahilly, D.B. Savage, et al., Induction of adipocyte complement-related protein of 20 kDa by PPARgamma agonists: a potential mechanism of insulin sensitization, Endocrinology 143 (2002) 998–1007.

[161] J.M. Friedman, J.L. Halaas, Leptin and the regulation of body weight in mammals, Nature 395 (1998) 763–770.

[162] E. Arioglu, J. Duncan-Morin, N. Sebring, K.I. Rother, N. Gottlieb, J. Lieberman, D. Herion, D.E. Kleiner, J. Reynolds, A. Premkumar, A.E. Sumner, J. Hoofnagle, M.L. Reitman, S.I. Taylor, Efficacy and safety of troglitazone in the treatment of lipodystrophy syndromes [see comment]. Ann. Inter. Med. 133 (2000) 263–274.

[163] C.J. Lyon, R.E. Law, W.A. Hsueh, Minireview: adiposity, inflammation, and atherogenesis, Endocrinology 144 (2003) 2195–2200.

[164] T. Pischon, C.J. Girman, G.S. Hotamisligil, N. Rifai, F.B. Hu, E.B. Rimm, Plasma adiponectin levels and risk of myocardial infarction in men, J. Am. Med. Assn. 291 (2004) 1730–1737.

[165] M.B. Schulze, I. Shai, E.B. Rimm, T. Li, N. Rifai, F.B. Hu, Adiponectin and future coronary heart disease events among men with type 2 diabetes, Diabetes 54 (2005) 534–539.

[166] S. Mudaliar, R.R. Henry, PPAR agonists in health and disease: a pathophysiologic and clinical overview, Curr. Opin. Endocrinol. Diabetes 9 (2002) 285–302.

[167] R.S. Legro, Polycystic ovary syndrome: the new millennium, Mol. Cell. Endocrinol. 184 (2001) 87–93.

[168] F. Orio, S. Palomba, T. Cascella, G. Milan, R. Mioni, C. Pagano, F. Zullo, A. Colao, G. Lombardi, R. Vettor, Adiponectin levels in women with polycystic ovary syndrome, J. Clin. Endocrinol. Metab. 88 (2003) 2619–2623.

[169] J. Spranger, J. Mohlig, U. Wegewitz, M. Ristow, A.F.H. Pfeiffer, T. Schill, H.W. Schlosser, G. Brabant, C. Schofl, Adiponectin is independently associated with insulin sensitivity in women with polycystic ovary syndrome, Clin. Endocrinol. 61 (2004) 738–746.

[170] V. Seplilian, M. Nagamani, Adiponectin levels in women with polycystic ovary syndrome and severe insulin resistance, J. Soc. Gynecol. Invest. 12 (2005) 129–134.

[171] C. Ortega-Gonzalez, S. Luna, L. Hernandez, G. Crespo, P. Aguayo, Arteaga-G. Troncoso, A. Parra, Responses of serum androgen and insulin resistance to metformin and pioglitazone in obese, insulin-resistant women with polycystic ovary syndrome, J. Clin. Endocrinol. Metab. 90 (2005) 1360–1365.

[172] A. Garg, Acquired and inherited lipodystrophies, New Eng. J. Med. 350 (2004) 1220–1234.

[173] E.A. Oral, V. Simha, E. Ruiz, A. Andewelt, A. Premkumar, P. Snell, A.J. Wagner, A.M. DePaoli, M.L. Reitman, S.I. Taylor, P. Gorden, A. Garg, Leptin-replacement therapy for lipodystrophy, New Eng. J. Med. 346 (2002) 570–578.

[174] M.L. Reitman, E. Arioglu, O. Gavrilova, S.I. Taylor, Lipoatrophy revisited. Trends Endocrinol, Metab 11 (2000) 410–416.

[175] D.B. Savage, G.D. Tan, C.L. Acerini, S.A. Jebb, M. Agostini, M. Gurnell, R.L. Williams, A.M. Umpleby, E.L. Thomas, J.D. Bell, A.K. Dixon, F. Dunne, R. Boianai, S. Cinti, A. Vidol-Puig,

F. Karpe, V.K. Chatterjee, S. O'Rahilly, Human metabolic syndrome resulting from dominant-negative mutations in the nuclear receptor peroxisome proliferator-activated receptor-γ, Diabetes 52 (2003) 910–917.

[176] C. Lagathu, M. Kim, M. Maachi, C. Vigouroux, P. Cervera, J. Capeau, M. Caron, J.P. Bastard, HIV antiretroviral treatment alters adipokine expression and insulin sensitivity of adipose tissue *in vitro* and *in vivo*, Biochimie 87 (2005) 65–71.

[177] D.C. Mynarcik, T. Combs, M.A. McNurlan, P.E. Scherer, E. Komaroff, M.C. Gelato, Adiponectin and leptin levels in HIV-infected subjects with insulin resistance and body fat redistribution, J. AIDS 31 (2002) 514–520.

[178] D. Kamin, C. Hadigan, M. Lehrke, S. Mazza, M.A. Lazar, S. Grinspoon, Resistin levels in HIV-infected patients with lipoatrophy decrease in response to rosiglitazone, J. Clin. Endocrinol. Metab. 90 (2005) 3423–3426.

Chapter 7

FOXC2 in the adipocyte

Sven Enerbäck

Medical Genetics, Dept of Medical Biochemistry, Göteborg University, Medicinareg. 9A, Box 440, SE 405 30 Göteborg, Sweden

Abstract

The adipocyte is equipped to handle fatty acids and its potentially toxic metabolites, enabling efficient use of triglycerides (TGs) as the major vehicle for storing superfluous energy. For the first time in history, large human populations are subjected to a wealth of cheap, accessible and palatable calories. This has created a large-scale situation not previously encountered, in which the capacity to store TGs in adipocytes is an important determinant of human health. Too few adipocytes (e.g., lipodystrophia) or a situation in which all adipocytes are filled, to their maximum capacity (e.g., severe obesity), will create very similar and unfavorable metabolic situations in which ectopic TG stores will appear in tissues like liver and muscle – a situation in which the adipocyte has lost its fat-storing monopoly [1]. This chapter sets out to discuss the role of the *forkhead* transcription factor FOXC2 as a regulator of adipocyte metabolism emphasizing on its capacity to protect against diet-induced insulin resistance and possibly overt type 2 diabetes through enhancing dissipation of energy, and thus maintaining ample TG storage capacity in adipose tissue.

1. Introduction

Until recently, not much was known about the postnatal function of FOXC2, a winged-helix transcription factor expressed in adipocytes. Studies using gene-targeted mice demonstrate a crucial role for *Foxc2* during early embryogenesis and establish *Foxc2* as an important factor for proper development of facial mesenchyme, vertebrates and aortic arch [2,3]. Other studies show that mutations in the *FOXC2* locus are associated with a rare disorder, Lymphedema–Distichiasis Syndrome (LDS; OMIM #153400), displaying many symptoms, albeit in a milder form, in common with the phenotype of mice lacking *Foxc2* [2,3]. Hence, this condition could be regarded as a disease caused by hampered *FOXC2* function during a critical early developmental decision and is distinct from its postnatal function. Since LDS patients have not been examined with regard to other

ADVANCES IN MOLECULAR AND CELLULAR ENDOCRINOLOGY
VOLUME 5 ISSN 1569-2566/DOI 10.1016/S1569-2566(06)05007-1

possible phenotypes and mice with a null mutation in the *Foxc2* locus die embryonically or perinatally [2,3], little was known about the function of *FOXC2* during postnatal life. In a previous publication, we demonstrated a previously unknown role for *FOXC2* – as a key regulator of adipocyte metabolism [4]. We have since, in collaboration with others, shown an intricate regulation of Foxc2 steady-state mRNA levels in 3T3-L1 adipocytes [5] as well as an association of high-plasma triglyceride (TG) levels and decreased-insulin sensitivity in individuals with a certain single nucleotide polymorphism (SNP) in their *FOXC2* 5′-flanking region [6]. Recently, a family was described in which an insertional mutation in the *FOXC2* locus segregates not only with LDS but also with type 2 diabetes [7]. Thus, supporting the view that FOXC2 is potentially an important factor in metabolism and type 2 diabetes [4,6]. In the following, FOXC2 will be discussed as a metabolic regulator in adipocytes with consequences for systemic lipid and glucose metabolism. Furthermore, a role for FOXC2 as modulator of the adipocyte's intrinsic sensitivity to adrenergic stimuli is discussed and put into a broader perspective in which the sympathetic nervous system (SNS) could prove to be of great importance. Finally, I speculate about the implications of altered adrenergic sensitivity in adipocytes, with regard to white versus brown adipogenesis and energy expenditure. This may shed light on new ways to treat obesity, insulin resistance and ultimately type 2 diabetes.

2. The gene and its expression profile

Interest in the forkhead family of genes stems from an early observation made when studying transcriptional activation of the human lipoprotein lipase (LPL) promoter [8]. Here, two *cis*-elements, LP-α and LP-β, were shown to interact with a transcription factor displaying a binding specificity similar to what, at the time, had been described for HNF3α, β and γ [9]. We could also show that this factor contributed to the adipocyte differentiation-linked induction of the *LPL* gene. The finding of a hypothetical forkhead protein interacting with the human *LPL* promoter prompted us to initiate a screen for forkhead genes using the highly conserved DNA-binding domain from *HNF3α, β* and *γ* as a probe mixture. Under low-stringency conditions, both cDNA and genomic libraries of human and mouse origins were screened. This enabled us to isolate some 12 previously unknown winged-helix genes [10–13], including *FOXC2*. In order to identify the forkhead gene(s) responsible for the interactions with the LPL promoter, we screened several human adipocyte cDNA libraries. In this screen, we identified *FOXC2* as an adipocyte-expressed forkhead gene. Others and we have since shown that FOXC2, in the adult organism, is expressed not only in adipocytes but also in lymphatic vessels, eyelid tissue, kidney glomeruli and striated-skeletal muscle [4,6,14].

3. Function in metabolism

In transgenic mice over-expressing FOXC2 in adipocytes, we demonstrated a pleiotropic effect on gene expression, which leads to a lean and insulin-sensitive phenotype [4].

FOXC2 affected adipocyte metabolism by increasing the sensitivity of the β-adrenergic-cAMP-protein kinase A (PKA) signaling pathway through alteration of adipocyte PKA holoenzyme composition.

FOXC2 upregulates the level of the PKA regulatory subunit $RI\alpha$, normally not expressed in adipocytes, while expression of the regulatory subunit $RII\beta$ that is normally expressed in adipocytes, remained unaffected (Fig. 1). This leads to an increased PKA sensitivity since $RI\alpha$ has a higher affinity for cAMP as compared with $RII\beta$. Thus, adipocytes from *FOXC2* tg mice had a lower threshold for PKA activation by adrenergic stimuli compared to wt littermates due to a PKA isozyme switch. This is in accordance with what has been reported for mice with targeted disruption of the $RII\beta$ gene [15].

For a given increase in intracellular cAMP concentration, adipocytes with higher FOXC2 expression transgenic mice increase their PKA dependent phospho-kinase activity more than the controls. Thus, cellular events like mitochondrogenesis and uncoupling protein-1 (UCP-1) induction, both elicited by PKA signaling, contribute to a lean and insulin-sensitive phenotype. In this way, excess energy is dissipated as heat rather than stored as TGs. This will ensure ample TG storage capacity in the adipocyte, hence ectopic lipid deposits in organs like skeletal muscle and liver may be prevented. Evidence from cell transfection experiments using a human $RI\alpha$ promoter reporter construct demonstrated that FOXC2 co-transfection induced the $RI\alpha$ promoter approximately 3-fold [4]. In adipose tissue from FOXC2 tg mice, there was also an induction of $RI\alpha$ transcription measured as steady-state mRNA levels [4]. In 3T3-L1 adipocytes, transfection and electromobility gel-shift experiments indicate that FOXC2 expression promotes the release of a potential repressor form an upstream region of the $RI\alpha$ promoter [16]. Apart from effects on PKA, FOXC2 also affects adipocyte metabolism directly through activation of target genes in white adipose tissue (WAT) and

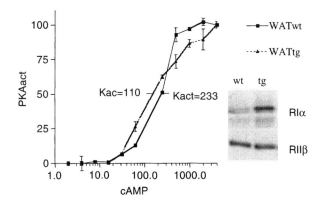

Fig. 1. Kinase activities toward the artifical PKA substrate Kemptide measured in WAT homogenates from tg and wt littermate mice incubated with increasing concentrations of cAMP. Total cAMP-inducible activity was set to 100%. Right panel, immunoblot demonstrating WAT levels of $RI\alpha$ and $RII\beta$. The altered PKA holoenzyme composition in tg adipocyte with a higher level of $RI\alpha$ renders these adipocytes more sensitive to adrenergic stimuli, reflected by a lower Kact value 110 nM as compared with 233 nM for wt adipocytes.

brown adipose tissue (BAT), which are involved in (i) insulin action, e.g., insulin receptor (ii) adipogenesis, e.g., PPARγ (iii) glucose metabolism, e.g., GLUT4 [4]. With a combined approach, using both administration of labeled metabolites and hyperinsulinemic–euglycemic clamp assays to assess insulin action *in vivo*, we demonstrated that FOXC2 tg mice were completely protected from diet-induced insulin resistance. FOXC2 tg mice did not increase their intramuscular fatty acyl CoA levels in response to a high fat diet nor did they have the expected reduced-insulin mediated suppression of hepatic glucose production [17]. This suggests that adipose-specific over-expression of FOXC2 in WAT affects whole body insulin sensitivity and protected the liver from fat-induced insulin resistance.

4. Regulation of FOXC2

After 2–6 h, 3T3-L1 adipocytes upregulate Foxc2 steady-state mRNA levels, approximately 3-fold in response to 100 ng/ml of insulin as an immediate early response [5]. In human adipocytes, steady-state levels of FOXC2 mRNA display a 3-fold induction when cells are exposed to 1 nM insulin, with a significant induction observed after 3 h followed by a peak at 6 h [6]. Thus, it appears that insulin regulates FOXC2 mRNA levels both in human and rodent fat cells. Adipocytes of 3T3-L1 origin double their FOXC2 mRNA levels after treatment with murine TNFα (50 ng/ml) for 2 h [5]. Furthermore, it was shown that a cAMP agonist such as 8-CPTcAMP (100 μM) upregulates FOXC2 mRNA levels 3-fold after 2 h. The cAMP induction was abolished in the presence of the PKA inhibitor KT5720, but not the insulin- and TNF α-induction [5], suggesting that regulation of FOXC2 involves stimuli other than those mediated through PKA. In this way, FOXC2 will respond both to increased sympathetic outflow – closely related to obesity-induced resistance of leptin feed back – as well as to hormonal patterns seen in many cases of insulin resistance, e.g., high levels of insulin and TNFα·

5. WAT versus BAT

One of the most striking features of mice over-expressing FOXC2 in their adipocytes is the increase of BAT and decrease of WAT (Fig. 2). We do not know if these mechanisms are direct effects of FOXC2 action on target genes or indirect effects mediated through PKA. In mice lacking the PKA subunit RIIβ, WAT is scarce whereas BAT is increased in size [15]. Thus, altered PKA composition has been shown to affect the WAT versus BAT ratio. Farmer and coworkers have shown that FOXC2 inhibits adipocyte differentiation in 3T3-L1 cells [18]. The authors speculate that this might be part of a regulatory mechanism, which favors differentiation of brown adipocytes as opposed to white adipocytes. When applying the protocols used in this paper for 3T3-L1 adipocyte differentiation, usually only white adipocytes will form. This opens an interesting question of whether inhibition of white adipogenesis *per se* enough to "passively" allow for the expansion of BAT are specific signals required? In another model, also addressing

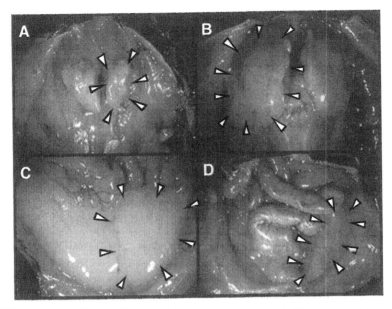

Fig. 2. Wild-type mouse (A, C) with normal interscapular BAT depot (A) and intraabdominal WAT depots (C). In aP2 FOXC2, tg mice there is a dramatic increase in BAT depot size (B) and a reduction in intraabdominal WAT depots. See Plate 3 in Colour Plate Section.

WAT/BAT differentiation, Kristiansen et al. showed that functional inactivation of the retinoblastoma protein (pRb) in mouse embryonic fibroblasts (MEFs) and 3T3-L1 cells leads to differentiation of adipocytes with gene expression profiles, such as induction of UCP-1 and mitochondrial content that is typical of a brown adipocyte [19]. In this system, one of the first changes noted was an induction of FOXC2 and its target gene cAMP-dependent protein kinase regulatory subunit $RI\alpha$. This induction precedes that of UCP-1 [19].

6. Protection against diet-induced insulin resistance

Apart from altered adipocyte PKA holoenzyme composition, FOXC2 also induces a decrease in phosphodiesterase activity (preliminary data) and an upregulation of β-adrenergic receptors [4]. In this way, sympathetic signaling through the β-adrenergic/ PKA pathway will be enhanced on at least three separate levels (Fig. 3).

These processes will lead to an increased-UCP-1 expression, hyperplasia of BAT and an increase in mitochondrial activity and biogenesis [4]. Furthermore, several genes of importance for metabolism such as *IR*, *IRS1*, *IRS2* and *GLUT4* are up-regulated as a consequence of increased-FOXC2 expression. Thus, direct-target gene activation will also contribute to the lean and insulin-sensitive phenotype seen in mice with increased expression of FOXC2 in adipocytes. This will lead to an ability

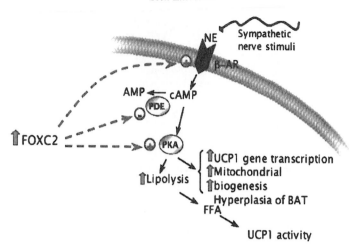

Fig. 3. FOXC2 induces increased sensitivity in the β-adrenergic pathway by acting at three different levels. See Plate 4 in Colour Plate Section.

to dissipate excess energy through adaptive thermogenesis, which together with other factors will favor a lean and insulin-sensitive phenotype [4]. The fact that, obesity, diet-induced insulin resistance and overt type 2 diabetes are associated with chronically elevated levels of TNFα and insulin would argue that under these circumstances FOXC2 levels are induced, perhaps as part of protective mechanism.

7. Human data

In a first study on human populations, with regard to the *FOXC2* locus and possible implications for metabolism, a common C/T *FOXC2* polymorphism was described, upstream of the *FOXC2* ORF (open reading frame). The *T-allele* was shown to be associated with enhanced-insulin sensitivity and lower TG levels [6]. In other population association studies, investigators have found evidence for an association between makers in the FOXC2 locus and metabolic parameters while others have failed [20–24]. In an interesting paper regarding familial combined hyperlipidemia (FCHL), Pajukanta et al. report a combined analysis of two genomewide scans performed on Finish and Dutch populations. Here, they suggest that FOXC2, at 16q24.1, is a good candidate for FCHL. Furthermore, evidence for association with polymorphic markers at the *FOXC2* locus ($p = 0.005$) was obtained with regard to TG levels and/or heavy density lipoprotein-C (HDL-C) suggesting that allelic variants of *FOXC2* may regulate TG and/or HDL-C levels in humans and hence be a causative factor in FCHL [25]. Recently, a novel frameshift mutation in *FOXC2* has been shown to be associated with type 2 diabetes in a fairly large family over three generations [7]. In a recent study of non-obese individuals with and without insulin resistance, FOXC2 mRNA levels were significantly lower ($p < 0.03$) among insulin-resistant subjects [26]. Taken together there is a substantial amount of information that links *FOXC2* to human lipid and glucose metabolism.

8. The autonomic nervous system

Using fluorescent dyes, Wirsén demonstrated for the first time that cate-cholaminergic innervation included WAT and BAT [27]. Initially, it was reported that only WAT vasculature was supplied by catecholaminergic innervation and not the adipocytes *per se* [28]. Using electron microscopy, Slavin and Ballard could show that white adipocytes indeed received direct innervation of the SNS [29]. Injection of the retrograde fluorescent neural tracer fluorogold into epididymal or inguinal WAT fat pads revealed a more rostral position of neurons, in the sympathetic chain, that innervate the epididymal pad as compared with those innervating inguinal adipose tissue [30]. This interesting finding points out the possibility that different fat pads could be selectively regulated by the SNS. Whether this diversity is also found in the brain was addressed using pseudorabies virus (PRV) as a transneuronal tract tracer. PRV is taken up by neurons and transported to higher CNS levels transsynaptically. Initial studies performed using PRV tracer failed to identify a specific WAT "signature" in the CNS pattern of PRV positive cells [31]. Thus, no specific groups of cells in CNS seemed to be responsible for WAT SNS innervation. It rather appeared as if SNS innervation of WAT was part of a more general SNS outflow from the brain. However, in a more recent study from the same laboratory, the authors analyzed the pattern of PRV positive neurons, which were immunocytochemically labeled to reveal their content of specific neurotransmitters. They identified that there was a specific neurochemical identity of SNS outflow from brain to WAT [32]. FOXC2's role in relation to selective, depot specific, innervation of adipose tissue would be one where it modulates the intracellular sensitivity of the PKA pathway.

Another interesting question is whether alterations in sympathetic outflow can affect WAT versus BAT partitioning. It is possible that either a precursor cell population is selected for the BAT cell lineage due to a high endogenous sensitivity in the PKA pathway conceivably under FOXC2 regulation or that a depot specific increase in sympathetic outflow selects depots that will develop into BAT. The rich innervation of the interscapular BAT depot in mice would be consistent with the latter hypothesis. In cases of human cathecholamine-producing tumors (pheochromocytomas), an increase of UCP-1 expressing BAT has been demonstrated at several different anatomical locations, e.g., perirenal and along major blood vessels [33,34]. The fact that adipose tissue cells in a general, non-depot specific, way respond to increased catecholamine levels by promoting the occurrence of BAT or BAT-like cells interspersed within WAT, might indicate an inherent difference in intrinsic sensitivity of the PKA pathway among adipocytes. It is also possible that a combination of these factors is what determines the BAT/WAT ratio. A consequence of this hypothesis is the intriguing possibility that only one type of adipocyte might exist and that this cell can appear in an array of different phenotypes, the extremes being a monloclular WAT- and a multilocular BAT-cell.

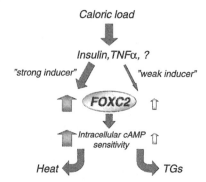

Fig. 4. FOXC2 as a regulator of metabolic efficency. According to this hypothesis a strong induction of FOXC2 in response to a caloric load leads to a metabolic situation in which a large portion of the ingested calories would be dissipated as heat, due to increased sensitivity of the β-adrenergic/PKA pathway, whereas a weaker induction induces conservation of the caloric load as triglycerides. (Reproduced with permission from *Cell*, copyright Elsevier Science.) See Plate 5 in Colour Plate Section.

9. Future

In Fig. 4, our hypothesis regarding FOXC2 and its role as a regulator of metabolism has been depicted. Furthermore, FOXC2 is mechanistically interesting since it holds the promise of finding a drug target that would regulate, in a rather tissue-specific manner, intracellular PKA sensitivity by altering PKA holoenzyme composition. This may prove to have a beneficial effect on diet-induced insulin resistance and type 2 diabetes. To find such candidate drugs, new and innovative ways to screen substance libraries for FOXC2-linked effects are clearly needed.

Acknowledgment

This work was made possible with support from: The Swedish Research Council (K2002-99BI-14383-01A, K2002-31X-12186-06A), EU-grants QLK3-CT-2002-02149 and LSHM-CT-2003-503041 (SE), The Swedish Cancer Society, The Arne and IngaBritt Lundberg Foundation and The Söderberg Foundation.

References

[1] A. Cederberg, S. Enerback, Insulin resistance and type 2 diabetes – an adipocentric view, Curr. Mol. Med. 3 (2003) 107–125.

[2] G.E. Winnier, L. Hargett, B.L. Hogan, The winged helix transcription factor MFH1 is required for proliferation and patterning of paraxial mesoderm in the mouse embryo, Genes. Dev. 11 (1997) 926–940.

[3] K. Iida, H. Koseki, H. Kakinuma, N. Kato, Y. Mizutani-Koseki, H. Ohuchi, H. Yoshioka, S. Noji, K. Kawamura, Y. Kataoka, F. Ueno, M. Taniguchi, N. Yoshida, T. Sugiyama, N. Miura, Essential

roles of the winged helix transcription factor MFH-1 in aortic arch patterning and skeletogenesis, Development 124 (22) (1997) 4627–4638.

[4] A. Cederberg, L.M. Gronning, B. Ahren, K. Tasken, P. Carlsson, S. Enerback, FOXC2 is a winged helix gene that counteracts obesity, hypertriglyceridemia, and diet-induced insulin resistance, Cell 106 (2001) 563–573.

[5] L.M. Gronning, A. Cederberg, N. Miura, S. Enerback, K. Tasken, Insulin and TNF alpha induce expression of the forkhead transcription factor gene Foxc2 in 3T3-L1 adipocytes via PI3 K and ERK 1/2-dependent pathways, Mol. Endocrinol. 16 (2002) 873–883.

[6] M. Ridderstrale, E. Carlsson, M. Klannemark, A. Cederberg, C. Kosters, H. Tornqvist, H. Storgaard, A. Vaag, S. Enerback, L. Groop, FOXC2 mRNA Expression and a 5′ untranslated region polymorphism of the gene are associated with insulin resistance, Diabetes 51 (2002) 3554–3560.

[7] C. Yildirim-Toruner, K. Subramanian, L. El Manjra, E. Chen, S. Goldstein, E. Vitale, A novel frameshift mutation of FOXC2 gene in a family with hereditary lymphedema–distichiasis syndrome associated with renal disease and diabetes mellitus, Am. J. Med. Genet. 131A (2004) 281–286.

[8] S. Enerback, B.G. Ohlsson, L. Samuelsson, G. Bjursell, Characterization of the human lipoprotein lipase (LPL) promoter: evidence of two *cis*-regulatory regions, LP-alpha and LP-beta, of importance for the differentiation-linked induction of the LPL gene during adipogenesis, Mol. Cell. Biol. 12 (1992) 4622–4633.

[9] E. Lai, V.R. Prezioso, W.F. Tao, W.S. Chen, J.E. Darnell Jr., Hepatocyte nuclear factor 3 alpha belongs to a gene family in mammals that is homologous to the Drosophila homeotic gene forkhead, Genes Dev. 5 (1991) 416–427.

[10] A. Cederberg, R. Betz, S. Lagercrantz, C. Larsson, M. Hulander, P. Carlsson, S. Enerback, Chromosome localization, sequence analysis, and expression pattern identify FKHL 18 as a novel human forkhead gene, Genomics 44 (1997) 344–346.

[11] S. Ernstsson, S. Pierrou, M. Hulander, A. Cederberg, M. Hellqvist, P. Carlsson, S. Enerback, Characterization of the human forkhead gene FREAC-4. Evidence for regulation by Wilms' tumor suppressor gene (WT-1) and p53, J. Biol. Chem. 271 (1996) 21094–21099.

[12] S. Ernstsson, R. Betz, S. Lagercrantz, C. Larsson, S. Ericksson, A. Cederberg, P. Carlsson, S. Enerback, Cloning and characterization of freac-9 (FKHL17), a novel kidney-expressed human forkhead gene that maps to chromosome 1p32-p34, Genomics 46 (1997) 78–85.

[13] S. Pierrou, M. Hellqvist, L. Samuelsson, S. Enerback, P. Carlsson, Cloning and characterization of seven human forkhead proteins: binding site specificity and DNA bending, Embo. J. 1354 (1994) 5002–5012.

[14] S.L. Dagenais, R.L. Hartsough, R.P. Erickson, M.H. Witte, M.G. Butler, T.W. Glover, Foxc2 is expressed in developing lymphatic vessels and other tissues associated with lymphedema-distichiasis syndrome, Gene Expression Patterns 4 (2004) 611–619.

[15] D.E. Cummings, E.P. Brandon, J.V. Planas, K. Motamed, R.L. Idzerda, G.S. McKnight, Genetically lean mice result from targeted disruption of the RII beta subunit of protein kinase A, Nature 382 (1996) 622–626.

[16] M.K. Dahle, L.M. Gronning, A. Cederberg, H.K. Blomhoff, N. Miura, S. Enerback, K.A. Tasken, K. Tasken, Mechanisms of FOXC2- and FOXD1-mediated regulation of the RI alpha subunit of cAMP-dependent protein kinase include release of transcriptional repression and activation by protein kinase B alpha and cAMP, J. Biol. Chem. 277 (2002) 22902–22908.

[17] J.K. Kim, H.-J. Kim, S.-Y. Park, A. Cederberg, R. Westergren, D. Nilsson, T. Higashimori, Y.-R. Cho, Z.-X. Liu, J. Dong, G.W. Cline, S. Enerback, G.I. Shulman, Adipocyte-specific overexpression of FOXC2 prevents diet-induced increase in intramuscular fatty acyl CoA and insulin resistance, Diabetes 54(6) (2005) 1657–1663.

[18] K.E. Davis, M. Moldes, S.R. Farmer, The forkhead transcription factor FoxC2 inhibits white adipocyte differentiation, J. Biol. Chem. 279 (2004) 42453–42461.

[19] J.B. Hansen, C. Jorgensen, R.K. Petersen, P. Hallenborg, R. De Matteis, H.A. Boye, N. Petrovic, S. Enerback, J. Nedergaard, S. Cinti, H. te Riele, K. Kristiansen, Retinoblastoma protein functions as a molecular switch determining white versus brown adipocyte differentiation, Proc. Natl. Acad. Sci.

USA 101(12) (2004) 4112–4117. Epub 2004 Mar 15. Erratum in: Proc. Natl. Acad. Sci. USA 101(17) (2004) 6833.

[20] A. Fritsche, F. Machicao, H. Staiger, H.U. Haring, M. Stumvoll, Lack of association between metabolic traits and the -512 polymorphism in FOXC2 in german people with normal glucose tolerance, Diabetologia 47 (2004) 756–757.

[21] G.B. Di Gregorio, R. Westergren, S. Enerback, T. Lu, P.A. Kern, Expression of FOXC2 in adipose and muscle and its association with whole body insulin sensitivity, Am. J. Physiol. Endocrinol. Metab. 287 (2004) E799–E803.

[22] K. Yanagisawa, L. Hingstrup Larsen, G. Andersen, T. Drivsholm, A. Cederberg, R. Westergren, K. Borch-Johnsen, O. Pedersen, S. Enerback, T. Hansen, The FOXC2 -512C > T variant is associated with hypertriglyceridaemia and increased serum C-peptide in Danish Caucasian glucose-tolerant subjects, Diabetologia 46 (2003) 1576–1580.

[23] P. Kovacs, A. Lehn-Stefan, M. Stumvoll, C. Bogardus, L.J. Baier, Genetic variation in the human winged helix/forkhead transcription factor gene FOXC2 in Pima Indians, Diabetes 52 (2003) 1292–1295.

[24] H. Osawa, H. Onuma, A. Murakami, M. Ochi, T. Nishimiya, K. Kato, I. Shimizu, Y. Fujii, J. Ohashi, H. Makino, Systematic search for single nucleotide polymorphisms in the FOXC2 gene: the absence of evidence for the association of three frequent single nucleotide polymorphisms and four common haplotypes with Japanese type 2 diabetes, Diabetes. 52(2) (2003) 562–567.

[25] P. Pajukanta, H. Allayee, K.L. Krass, A. Kuraishy, A. Soro, H.E. Lilja, R. Mar, M.R. Taskinen, I. Nuotio, M. Laakso, J.I. Rotter, T.W. de Bruin, R.M. Cantor, A.J. Lusis, L. Peltonen, Combined analysis of genome scans of Dutch and Finnish families reveals a susceptibility locus for high-density lipoprotein cholesterol on chromosome 16q, Am. J. Hum. Genet. 72(4) (2003) 903–917.

[26] X. Yang, S. Enerback, U. Smith, Reduced expression of FOXC2 and brown adipogenic genes in human subjects with insulin resistance, Obes. Res. 11 (2003) 1182–1191.

[27] C. Wirsén, Studies in lipid mobilization with special reference to morphological and histochemical aspects, Acta Physiol. Scand 65 (1965) 146.

[28] C. Wirsén, Adrenergic innervation of adipose tissue examined by flourescence microscopy, Nature 202 (1964) 913.

[29] B.G. Slavin, K.W. Ballard, Morphological studies on the adrenergic innervation of white adipose tissue, Anat. Rec. 191(3) (1978) 377–389.

[30] T.G. Youngstrom, T.J. Bartness, Catecholaminergic innervation of white adipose tissue in the Siberian hamster, Am. J. Physiol. 37 (1995) R744–R751.

[31] M. Bamshad, V.T. Aoki, M.G. Adkinson, W.S. Warren, T.J. Bartness, Central nervous system origins of the sympathetic nervous system outflow to white adipose tissue, Am. J. Physiol. 275 (1998) R291–R299.

[32] H. Shi, T.J. Bartness, Neurochemical phenotype of sympathetic nervous system outflow from brain to white fat, Brain Res. Bull. 54 (2001) 375–385.

[33] G. Garruti, D. Ricquier, Analysis of uncoupling protein and its mRNA in adipose tissue deposits of adult humans, Int. J. Obes. Relat. Metab. Disord. 16 (1992) 383–390.

[34] F. Bouillaud, F. Villarroya, E. Hentz, S. Raimbault, A.M. Cassard, D. Ricquier, Detection of brown adipose tissue uncoupling protein mRNA in adult patients by a human genomic probe. Clin. Sci. (Lond.) 75 (1988) 21–27.

Chapter 8

Regulation of adipocyte differentiation and metabolism by Wnt signaling and C/EBP transcription factors

Isabelle Gerin[1,2], Hyuk C. Cha[1], Ormond A. MacDougald[1]

[1]*Department of Molecular and Integrative Physiology, University of Michigan Medical School, Ann Arbor, MI, USA;*
[2]*Laboratoire de Chimie Physiologique, Université Catholique de Louvain, B-1200 Brussels, Belgium*

Summary

Obesity is associated with insulin resistance, dyslipidemia and other risk factors for type 2 diabetes. The recognition that adipose tissues are not just passive storage vessels for energy, but are endocrine organs that influence glucose tolerance and insulin sensitivity has spurred investigations into the development, metabolism, and endocrine properties of adipocytes. In this chapter, we discuss Wnt signaling as an important endogenous inhibitor of adipogenesis. Recent work *in vivo* has highlighted the potential for Wnt molecules to impair adipose tissue development and influence insulin sensitivity and glucose tolerance. The program of adipogenesis has been extensively studied, and integral roles for PPARγ, C/EBPα, and C/EBPβ have been established. While the importance of PPARγ to diabetes will be covered in another chapter, herein we review structure and functions of C/EBP family members, as well as mechanisms whereby these transcription factors regulate adipocyte differentiation, metabolism, and hepatic glucose homeostasis.

1. Introduction

Adipocytes were classically considered to be passive fat depots for energy storage. However, it is now known that adipose tissues are important endocrine organs, which secrete hormones that influence glucose tolerance and insulin sensitivity. These secreted factors include leptin [1], adiponectin [2,3], resistin [4], and inflammatory cytokines such as TNFα and IL-6 [5]. Because of the relationship between adipose

ADVANCES IN MOLECULAR AND CELLULAR ENDOCRINOLOGY
VOLUME 5 ISSN 1569-2566/DOI 10.1016/S1569-2566(06)05008-3

tissue and whole body energy metabolism, investigations into the development, metabolism, and endocrine properties of adipose tissues are important for our understanding of type 2 diabetes.

The importance of adipose tissue for metabolic homeostasis is underscored by the consequences of an excess or deficiency of this tissue. For example, obesity is associated with insulin resistance, hyperglycemia, dyslipidemia, and hypertension, all of which are part of the metabolic syndrome and are risk factors for type 2 diabetes and cardiovascular disease [6]. An insufficiency of adipose tissue is also associated with type 2 diabetes [7–9]. Because of the dramatic rise in the incidence of obesity and type 2 diabetes, considerable research has focused on understanding the development and metabolism of adipocytes, with the hope of providing targets for treatment of type 2 diabetes.

Adipocytes develop from pluripotent mesenchymal stem cells that can also give rise to myocytes, osteoblasts, and chondrocytes [10,11]. Factors that stimulate differentiation to one lineage often suppress progression to other lineages. For example, Wnt signaling inhibits adipogenesis, but promotes osteoblastogenesis as well as myogenesis [12–15]. Transgenic mice in which adipose tissue development is impaired by Wnt10b have improved glucose tolerance and insulin sensitivity, providing evidence that Wnt signaling can influence whole body energy metabolism [16]. One focus for this chapter will be the regulation of adipogenesis and energy homeostasis by Wnt signaling.

During preadipocyte commitment, mesenchymal precursors lose their pluripotency, and cells become restricted to the adipocyte lineage. The development of immortalized preadipocyte lines in the 1970s by Green and colleagues [17,18] has been essential for elucidating the program of adipogenesis (Fig. 1). The cascade of genetic

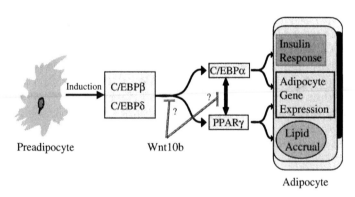

Fig. 1. Program of Adipogenesis. Inducers of preadipocyte differentiation stimulate expression of C/EBP*β* and C/EBP*δ*, which then activate transcription of both C/EBP*α* and PPAR*γ*. The master adipogenic transcription factors, C/EBP*α* and PPAR*γ*, enforce each other's expression through a positive feedback loop. During adipogenesis, C/EBP*α* is required for acquisition of insulin sensitivity, while PPAR*γ* is necessary for accumulation of lipid. Although not fully characterized, both transcription factors play key roles in expression of a subset of adipocyte genes. Together, C/EBP*α* and PPAR*γ* stimulate the full complement of genes required to create the adipocyte phenotype. Wnt signaling inhibits differentiation by blocking expression of these master adipogenic transcription factors. See Plate 6 in Colour Plate Section.

events that occurs during preadipocyte differentiation is initiated by the addition of inducers of adipogenesis, which often include methylisobutylxanthine, dexamethasone, insulin, and fetal bovine serum (reviewed in [19–21]). During differentiation, preadipocytes synchronously reenter the cell cycle for one or two rounds of mitosis [21], and then acquire the morphological and molecular characteristics of adipocytes. Stimulation of preadipocyte differentiation rapidly increases expression of CAAT/ enhancer-binding protein (C/EBP)β and C/EBPδ, which then activate transcription of both C/EBPα and peroxisome proliferator-activated receptor (PPAR)γ. C/EBPα increases expression of PPARγ, and *vice versa*. Thus, these master regulators of adipogenesis are maintained at high levels through a positive feedback loop [22]. Both transcription factors make important and independent contributions to adipocyte development (Fig. 1). For example, C/EBPα is required for acquisition of insulin sensitivity, and PPARγ is necessary for accumulation of lipid [23]. Although not fully characterized, each transcription factor is required for expression of a subset of adipocyte genes. Together, C/EBPα and PPARγ stimulate the full complement of genes required to create the adipocyte phenotype.

Roles for PPARγ in energy homeostasis have been the subject of intense scrutiny following the discovery that PPARγ ligands decrease blood glucose of patients with type 2 diabetes [24,25]. In adipose tissue, synthetic PPARγ ligands alter metabolism (e.g. decreased free fatty acid levels) and secretion of adipokines (increased adiponectin, decreased resistin), leading to improved insulin sensitivity in liver and muscle [25]. The central role of C/EBPα in adipocyte differentiation and metabolism, as well as adipokine gene expression, suggests that this transcription factor may also play a role in glucose homeostasis. This idea is supported by research indicating that C/EBPα is required for development of insulin sensitivity during adipogenesis [26–28]. Thus, the C/EBP family of transcription factors, and their roles in adipogenesis and whole body metabolism will be another focus of this chapter.

2. Roles for Wnt signaling in adipogenesis and glucose homeostasis

The Wnt family of secreted lipid-modified glycoproteins was named as an amalgamation of wingless and Int-1 [29]. Wingless mutations in *Drosophila* lead to development of flies without wings [30,31]. The mammalian homolog of wingless, Int-1, was subsequently identified as a locus activated by insertion of mouse mammary tumor virus [32]. The 19 Wnt proteins act through autocrine and paracrine mechanisms to have profound effects on most if not all aspects of cell fate, including differentiation and apoptosis. In addition, dysregulation of Wnt expression and/or Wnt signaling is commonly associated with cancer [33]. Signaling by Wnts can be through pathways that are independent of β-catenin (Fig. 2) [34]. However, the most fully characterized signaling pathway is through β-catenin, in which Wnt proteins bind to frizzled receptors and low density lipoprotein receptor-related protein (LRP) coreceptors to inhibit activity of glycogen synthase kinase 3 (GSK3) through a mechanism involving disheveled and axin (Fig. 2) [34]. In the absence of Wnt signaling, phosphorylation of β-catenin by GSK3 targets β-catenin for proteasome-mediated

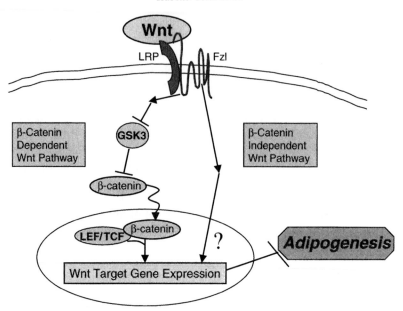

Fig. 2. Wnt signaling inhibits adipogenesis through β-catenin dependent and independent pathways. Wnt acts through Frizzled receptors and LRP coreceptors to inhibit activity of glycogen synthase kinase 3, thus resulting in hypophosphorylation and stabilization of β-catenin. After translocation to the nucleus, β-catenin acts through TCF/LEF transcription factors to ultimately inhibit expression of C/EBPα and PPARγ, and thereby block preadipocyte differentiation. In addition, Wnt may inhibit adipocyte conversion through a Wnt signaling pathway independent of β-catenin. See Plate 7 in Colour Plate Section.

turnover. However, in the presence of Wnt signaling, the hypophosphorylated β-catenin accumulates in cytoplasm, and translocates to the nucleus where it stimulates gene expression after binding to transcription factors, including members of T-cell factor/lymphoid-enhancer factor (TCF/LEF) family (Fig. 2).

Based upon our experiments on GSK3 as a C/EBPα kinase [35], and the knowledge that Wnt signaling plays broad roles in development, including in fate of mesenchymal progenitors [33], we investigated whether Wnt signaling regulates adipogenesis. Inhibition of Wnt signaling with dominant-negative TCF4, overexpression of axin, or addition of purified recombinant Wnt inhibitors to preadipocyte media all result in adipogenesis in the absence of standard inducing agents [12,36]. These data indicate that endogenous Wnt signaling in preadipocytes represses adipogenesis and that Wnt signaling is mediated, at least in part, through the canonical Wnt pathway. Furthermore, ectopic expression of Wnt1, Wnt10b, or a dominant stable β-catenin in 3T3-L1 preadipocytes blocks adipocyte differentiation [12,37,38], as do pharmacological inhibitors of GSK3 [12,36]. Although these results provide compelling evidence that the β-catenin dependent pathway inhibits adipogenesis, we have also observed that activation of a β-catenin-independent pathway with a constitutively activated frizzled2 protein also impairs adipogenesis (Kennell and MacDougald, unpublished data). Of the 19 Wnt ligands, Wnt10b is a promising candidate for the endogenous Wnt because it is expressed in 3T3-L1 preadipocytes, and expression of Wnt10b declines during differentiation. This pattern of expression is supported by the fact that Wnt10b mRNA is expressed in the stromal–vascular fraction of white adipose tissue, which is enriched for preadipocytes, but not in the adipocyte fraction [36].

Although the specific mechanism whereby Wnt signaling inhibits adipogenesis is not fully characterized, it is well established that Wnt signaling does not influence the rapid and transient expression of C/EBPβ and C/EBPδ, but totally blocks expression of the two master adipogenic transcription factors, C/EBPα and PPARγ [12,36] (Fig. 1). Consistent with this mechanism, expression of either C/EBPα or PPARγ is sufficient to rescue differentiation of Wnt-expressing preadipocytes. Expression of Wnt10b may also inhibit adipogenesis at least in part through dysregulation of mitotic clonal expansion [39]. For instance, induction of cell cycle genes is largely blunted at 16 h, and this is correlated with decreased expression of E2F4, hypo-phosphorylation of p130, and impaired induction of the cyclin-dependent kinase inhibitor, p21 [39]. These mechanisms are further supported by our experiments in which we treated differentiating preadipocytes with small molecule activators of Wnt signaling and found that exposure during the first four days of adipogenesis was sufficient to completely block conversion to adipocytes [36]. These data suggest that one of the early events during the process of adipocyte differentiation is the decline of Wnt10b, which allows for correct mitotic clonal expansion and expression of essential adipocyte transcription factors. Of the agents used to induce differentiation, it is the increase in cAMP stimulated by the phosphodiesterase inhibitor, methy-lisobutylxanthine, which is sufficient to suppress expression of Wnt10b [36].

To establish the effects of Wnt10b on adipose tissue development, we created transgenic mice in which Wnt10b is expressed from the FABP4 promoter [16]. As expected, FABP4-Wnt10b mice have impaired development of adipose tissue throughout the body with a reduction of 50% in adipose tissue depots and total body lipid. Consistent with the established relationship between the amount of adipose tissue and insulin resistance, these transgenic mice have increased glucose tolerance, and increased insulin sensitivity. In addition, these mice are resistant to high fat diet-induced obesity and are even more glucose-tolerant than wild-type mice fed a low fat diet. Although these data suggest that Wnt10b may play a role in glucose homeostasis, whether these effects are direct or indirect remain to be established. Interestingly, inhibition by Wnt10b of white adipose tissue development results in lean mice without lipodystrophic diabetes, perhaps because of the maintenance of leptin levels in FABP4-Wnt10b mice [16].

While white adipose tissue plays an important role in energy storage and home-ostasis, brown adipose tissue releases energy in the form of heat, and thus plays an important role in adaptive thermogenesis [40–42]. Brown adipocytes are also derived from mesenchymal stem cells, and development of brown fat occurs late during embryonic life [40]. Although the program of brown adipogenesis has not been as extensively studied as that of white, the process of differentiating into brown or white adipocytes appears to share many common features [43]. Furthermore, regulation of adipogenesis by Wnt signaling also appears to be shared. For example, we recently observed that activation of Wnt signaling inhibits brown adipogenesis in two *in vitro* models [44]. While enforced expression of C/EBPα or PPARγ rescues the adipogenic program, rescue of the thermogenic program requires expression of PPARγ and PPARγ coactivator-1α (PGC-1α). This important transcriptional coactivator is sufficient to increase mitochondrial biogenesis and expression of uncoupling protein 1 in preadipocytes, and can play an important regulatory role for energy metabolism in a number of tissues, including liver and muscle [45,46]. Expression of Wnt10b from the FABP4 promoter profoundly inhibits development of brown adipose tissue, and these transgenic mice are insensitive to adrenergic induction of uncoupling protein 1 and thermogenesis [44].

In addition to blocking development of brown adipocytes, Wnt signaling also influences metabolism after differentiation has occurred. For example, exposure of differentiated brown adipocytes to activators of Wnt signaling causes a decline in brown adipocyte genes, without influencing expression of common adipocyte markers. Suppression of PGC-1α appears to play an intermediary role in repression of uncoupling protein 1 by Wnt [44]. Consistent with these *in vitro* observations, expression of Wnt10b from the uncoupling protein 1 promoter results in interscapular tissue with the histological and molecular characteristics of white adipose tissue, suggesting that Wnt signaling transdifferentiates brown adipocytes into white [44]. Finally, the inverse relationship between expression of Wnt10b, and expression of PGC-1α and uncoupling protein 1 in cold challenged or genetically obese mice suggests a role for Wnt signaling in plasticity of white and brown adipocytes *in vivo*.

Although effects of Wnt signaling on glucose homeostasis may be mediated in part through effects on adipose tissue development and metabolism, the widespread expression of Wnts in other tissues important for energy homeostasis suggests that other mechanisms are plausible. For example, the Wnt coreceptor, LRP5, is expressed in pancreatic β cells where it modulates glucose-induced insulin secretion. While LRP5−/−mice are glucose intolerant, their insulin sensitivity is similar to control mice [47]. Wnt3a and Wnt5a interact with glucose to potentiate insulin secretion from isolated islets, and these effects of Wnt are dependent upon expression of LRP5. Thus, Wnt signaling modulates glucose-induced insulin secretion and plays a role in normal glucose metabolism. Findings such as these suggest that understanding Wnt signaling pathways could lead to novel therapeutic strategies for the treatment of type 2 diabetes.

Further evidence for a role of Wnt signaling in normal glucose metabolism and type 2 diabetes comes from linkage analysis in humans. In examining the association of Wnt genes with type 2 diabetes in the Japanese population, Kanazawa et al. [48] report that a single-nucleotide polymorphism locus in the Wnt5b gene is strongly associated with type 2 diabetes. Although Wnt5b may provide susceptibility to diabetes through mechanisms in a number of tissues (e.g. pancreas, liver), they propose a model in which Wnt5b influences adipocyte function. During adipogenesis of preadipocytes, Wnt5b is transiently induced, coincident with expression of C/EBPβ. Furthermore, ectopic expression of Wnt5b appears to slightly increase adipogenesis and expression of adipocyte genes [48]. Although the signaling pathway and mechanism remain uncharacterized, these data provide further evidence that Wnt signaling plays a role in adipose tissue development, glucose homeostasis, and type 2 diabetes.

3. Role of C/EBPS in hepatocyte differentiation and liver metabolism

The potential for C/EBPs to influence diabetes is not restricted to their role in adipocyte differentiation and metabolism. For example, C/EBPα is required for hepatic expression of enzymes involved in carbohydrate metabolism, including glycogen synthase, glucose-6-phosphatase, and phosphoenolpyruvate carboxykinase ([49], Table 1). Indeed, mice lacking C/EBPα die of hypoglycemia soon after birth. Interestingly, replacement of C/EBPα with C/EBPβ completely restores hepatic gene expression and phenotype [50], underscoring the overlap in activity of these factors, at least in liver. Not surprisingly, C/EBPβ is also involved in hepatic gene expression and glucose metabolism (Table 1). In this case, C/EBPβ−/− mice have fasting hypoglycemia because of reduced hepatic glucose production [51,52]; however, glucose-6-phosphatase and phosphoenolpyruvate carboxykinase is expressed normally [51]. Croniger et al. [53] suggest that the aberrant glucose production is due to impaired cAMP production and decrease activity of protein kinase A. The role of C/EBPs in liver function and diabetes will also be covered in detail elsewhere within this text (J. Friedman Chapter).

Table 1
White adipose tissue and liver phenotypes in mice lacking C/EBP transcription factors, or in which C/EBPβ replaces C/EBPα

Mutation	White adipose tissue	Liver
C/EBPα −/−	No lipid accumulation	Early postpartum death No lipid accumulation Hypoglycemia due to decreased PEPCK and G6Pase expression Lack of glycogen storage due to decreased expression of glycogen synthase
C/EBPβ in C/EBPα locus	Reduced lipid accumulation Decreased expression of leptin and adipsin but PPARγ, Glut4, FAS normal	Function normal
C/EBPβ −/−	Reduced gonadal fat pad weight	Reduced glucose production
	Normal expression of C/EBPα and PPARγ	Impaired production of cAMP
	Lower levels of leptin	Decreased protein kinase A activity
C/EBPβ and δ−/−	Reduction of epididymal fat mass	Not determined
	Normal expression of C/EBPα and PPARγ	

4. Roles for C/EBPs in adipocyte differentiation and metabolism

C/EBPs are a family of transcription factors that contain a region rich in basic amino acids, which mediates DNA binding, and a leucine zipper, which allows dimer formation (bZIP). The six C/EBP members, C/EBPα, C/EBPβ, C/EBPγ, C/EBPδ, C/EBPε, and CHOP (C/EBP homologous protein; C/EBPξ), all share sequence identity (>90%) in the C-terminal 55–65 amino-acid residues, which contains the bZIP domain. C/EBPα was the first member of the family to be purified and cloned [54]. C/EBPα was originally cloned from rat liver tissue as a protein that bound the albumin promoter. This protein was found to bind CCAAT *cis*-regulatory sequences common to many RNA polymerase II transcribed promoters as well as the enhancer core elements found in several viruses [55]. Soon thereafter, C/EBPβ and C/EBPδ were also cloned [56–58], giving birth to the C/EBP gene family, which is part of a larger bZIP family of transcription factors that includes c-fos, c-jun, and CREB [59].

Adipose tissue expresses C/EBPα, C/EBPβ, C/EBPδ, C/EBPγ, and CHOP. Although C/EBPα, C/EBPβ, and C/EBPδ are well established as important stimulators of adipogenesis and will be discussed in the following sections, CHOP also regulates preadipocyte differentiation but as a suppressor [60]. As is typical of adipocyte repressors, CHOP is expressed in preadipocytes and declines early during the differentiation process. Furthermore, enforced expression of CHOP inhibits the induction of C/EBPβ and C/EBPα [60]. Work from the Lane laboratory suggests that endogenous CHOP interacts with C/EBPβ, delaying the acquisition of DNA-binding activity and activation of C/EBPα gene expression [61]. Inhibition of adipogenesis by CHOP is mediated early during differentiation as overexpression of C/EBPα rescues adipogenesis [60]. Consistent with this mechanism, expression of endogenous CHOP increases late during adipogenesis where its role in adipocyte biology remains unknown. Although not yet characterized, C/EBPγ may also influence adipogenesis. This member of the C/EBP family contains a basic region and leucine zipper but not a transactivation domain, and expression of C/EBPγ is transiently induced during adipogenesis. C/EBPγ inhibits C/EBPβ activity in certain cell types [62], raising the possibility that this member of the C/EBP family might also modulate preadipocyte differentiation. In summary, for adipogenesis to progress, the differentiating preadipocyte must carefully regulate levels and activities of stimulatory and inhibitory C/EBP family members.

4.1. C/EBPβ

C/EBPβ mRNA is translated from internal initiation sites resulting in three forms, all of which share the C-terminal bZIP domain. The different forms of C/EBPβ are Liver Activator Proteins (LAP) 1 and 2, which are 38 and 34 kDa [63], also termed LAP* and LAP, and a dominant-negative form called Liver Inhibitory Protein (LIP), which is 20 kDa [64]. LAP1 is identical to LAP2 except that the mouse protein contains an additional 21 amino acids at the N-terminus. LAP1 specifically interacts with a chromatin-modifying protein complex to influence gene expression in myeloid and other cell types [65,66].

During adipogenesis, C/EBPβ and C/EBPδ are rapidly and transiently induced in response to a cAMP-elevating agent and glucocorticoid, respectively. Inducers of differentiation cause confluent, growth-arrested preadipocytes to reenter the cell cycle and to undergo one to two rounds of cell division. The importance of 'mitotic clonal expansion' has been controversial. Although the hypothesis that mitosis is required for activation of adipocyte gene expression during differentiation is supported by a considerable body of literature [67–71], some reports suggest that 3T3-L1 and human preadipocytes can differentiate into adipocytes without further mitosis [72,73]. In addition, while expression of C/EBPβ rises dramatically following induction of adipogenesis, the activity is repressed by a number of mechanisms until after mitotic clonal expansion has been initiated.

Mechanisms whereby the activity of C/EBPβ is regulated include repression of DNA binding activity by CHOP [60], and inhibition of transcriptional activity by ETO/MTG8 [74]. This transcriptional repressor is found in preadipocytes and expression declines rapidly during adipogenesis. Binding of ETO/MTG8 to C/EBPβ inhibits transactivation of the C/EBPα promoter, and enforced expression of ETO/MTG8 inhibits adipogenesis.

C/EBPβ activity may also be regulated by posttranslational modifications including SUMOylation and phosphorylation [75–77]. For example, a recent study from the farmer laboratory suggests that phosphorylation of C/EBPβ at a consensus ERK/GSK3 site is required for expression of C/EBPα, and subsequent expression of adiponectin [78]. Once activated, the fully competent C/EBPβ then induces transcription of C/EBPα, which blocks further cell division through effects on p21 and other cell cycle regulators [79,80].

A critical role for C/EBPβ in adipogenesis has been uniformly observed in experiments utilizing immortalized preadipocyte lines [81,82]. However less consistent results have been observed in primary mouse embryonic fibroblasts lacking C/EBPβ. Although Tang et al. [68] found that mitotic clonal expansion and adipocyte differentiation do not occur in C/EBPβ−/− embryonic fibroblasts, Tanaka et al. [83] found that differentiation did occur, but with reduced frequency. In our hands, C/EBPβ−/− embryonic fibroblasts undergo robust differentiation when induced to differentiate in the presence of a PPARγ ligand such as troglitazone (Gerin and MacDougald, unpublished data). Thus the apparent requirement for C/EBPβ in adipogenesis of primary embryonic fibroblasts may be influenced by differentiation protocol, although other factors such as genetic background or method of isolation cannot be excluded.

A preponderance of evidence from *in vitro* experiments indicates a stimulatory role for C/EBPβ in adipogenesis, and this is partially supported by *in vivo* findings (Table 1). Although Tanaka et al. [83] observed only a trend toward reduced adipocity in mice lacking C/EBPβ, more extensive experimentation from the Friedman laboratory [51,52] revealed that gonadal and periuterine fat pad weights are reduced by 40% and 50%, respectively. The decreased adipose tissue mass found in these mice is associated with reduced plasma leptin [52], as well as reduced fasting plasma glucose, insulin and FFA levels [52,53], which may contribute to increased skeletal muscle insulin sensitivity (Table 1). The adipose tissue that develops in C/EBPβ−/− mice expresses C/EBPα, PPARγ, FABP4, and lipoprotein lipase at normal levels; however, size of adipocytes is decreased by ~50%, suggesting that reduced adipose tissue of C/EBPβ−/− mice is largely due to altered lipid accumulation rather than adipogenesis *per se* (Friedman – this book). Thus, it is clear that C/EBPβ is not strictly required for development of adipocytes. A compensatory role for C/EBPδ is possible, as mice lacking both C/EBPβ and C/EBPδ have a further decline in mass of epididymal adipose tissue [83].

4.2. C/EBPα

4.2.1. *Structure and mechanism of action*
As with other members of the C/EBP family, the C-terminus of C/EBPα contains the bZIP domain. The basic region binds to a consensus DNA sequence of (A/G)TTGCG(T/C)AA(T/C), based upon interactions with random oligonucleotides *in vitro* [84]. Nuclear localization sequences are embedded within the basic DNA-binding domain [85], and C/EBPα appears to be constitutively nuclear [86]. Within the nucleus, C/EBPα is largely bound to pericentromeric AT-rich regions. The leucine zipper forms dimers through an alpha helical coiled-coil [87–90]. C/EBPα can form homodimers, heterodimers with other members of the C/EBP family [58,59,91], and heterodimers with other bZIP proteins, including ATF2 [92]. Although not rigorously tested in cells, the formation of dimers *in vitro* is mainly regulated by the relative concentration of each isoform.

Translational control of C/EBPα is similar to that described above for C/EBPβ, with leaky scanning translation predominantly from the first and third start codons, giving rise to C/EBPα isoforms of 42 and 30 kDa [93,94]. p42C/EBPα stimulates adipogenesis, blocks mitosis, and is a more potent transactivator than p30C/EBPα [94,95]. Indeed, p30C/EBPα inhibits the transactivation and DNA-binding activities of the p42 isoform by competing for bindings sites and by forming a heterodimer with the full-length protein [94]. The cellular ratio of p42C/EBPα to p30C/EBPα is important for control of cell division, as a mutation that increases the relative synthesis of p30C/EBPα is associated with secondary acute myelogenous leukemia [96].

The N-terminus of C/EBPα has multiple transactivation domains, including several highly conserved regions separated by strings of glycines and prolines [97]. Our group found that chimeric proteins between certain conserved regions and the bZIP domain are sufficient to transactivate the leptin promoter [97]. A number of laboratories have also analyzed the transactivation domains of C/EBPα [97–99], and the activities of N-terminal regions were originally defined by McKnight [98]. Analysis of structure–function relationships indicates that cooperativity between transactivation domains of C/EBPα is necessary for transcriptional activity and induction of adipogenesis [97,100], thus providing hints as to the complexity of protein–protein interactions required for this process.

The coactivators and corepressors utilized by C/EBPα during adipocyte differentiation and metabolism have not been well studied. However, physical and functional interactions have been described between C/EBPα and p300, a nuclear coactivator [97], p21, a cyclin-dependent kinase inhibitor [79], Cdk2 and Cdk4, which are cyclin-dependent kinases [101], and E2F/Rb complexes [80]. In addition, C/EBPα also directly represses activity of E2F, a key transcriptional regulator of cell cycle genes [102]. Further work needs to be performed to dissect the components of the transcriptional complexes formed by C/EBPα to mediate effects on adipogenesis.

Posttranslational modifications are a common mechanism for regulation of protein structure and protein–protein interactions, and modification of C/EBPα by SUMOylation and phosphorylation has been described [103–105]. In 3T3-L1 adipocytes, mobility shifts indicate that p30C/EBPα is rapidly dephosphorylated in response to insulin [105]. Three sites of phosphorylation were identified within this protein; T222, T226, and S230, two of which are regulated by insulin [35]. Upon treatment with insulin, T222 and T226 are dephosphorylated through inactivation of GSK3 and the actions of protein phosphatase 1 or 2A. Interestingly, S230 is not required as a priming site for phosphorylation of the GSK3 sites, as is often the case for GSK3 substrates [106]. Another site of phosphorylation, S193, also appears to be dephosphorylated in response to insulin. In this case, activation of the phosphatidylinositol-3-kinase pathway and Akt stimulates nuclear localization of protein phosphatase 2A and subsequent dephosphorylation of S193. Functional consequences of this posttranslational modification were characterized in liver tumors, where it was revealed that dephosphorylation of this site was required for interactions with E2F-Rb, cdk2, cdk4, and inhibition of cell-cycle progression [106].

Insulin also stimulates transient phosphorylation of S21, with activated ERK1/2 binding to a domain just C-terminal to the acceptor site. Although phosphorylation of S21 is not required for lipid accumulation, it does cause dynamic changes in the structure of C/EBPα [107], and phosphorylation may be required for certain aspects of the mature adipocyte phenotype (Cha and MacDougald, unpublished data). Phosphorylation of C/EBPα appears to be particularly important for regulation of granulopoiesis – with phosphorylation of S21 inhibiting granulopoiesis and phosphorylation of S248 promoting this process [107,108]. Regulation of the C/EBPs is not confined to only phosphorylation, as SUMOylation has been reported for both C/EBPα and C/EBPβ [75,103,104]. Further work is required to define the importance of SUMOylation in the ability of C/EBPs to influence differentiation and metabolism.

C/EBPα is also regulated at the transcriptional level. Although the C/EBPα gene is transcriptionally inactive in preadipocytes, expression of C/EBPβ and/or PPARγ is sufficient to activate this gene during adipogenesis. C/EBPα binds to and activates its own promoter through a positive feedback process [109,110]. Within fully differentiated adipocytes, transcription of multiple C/EBP family members, including C/EBPα is regulated by insulin and glucocorticoids, potentially mediating effects of these hormones on metabolic processes [111,112].

4.2.2. *Roles in adipogenesis*
The role of C/EBPα in development and metabolism of a number of cell types has been extensively studied, including hepatocytes, hematopoietic lineages, and type II pneumocytes [113,114]. However, here we review the role of C/EBPα as one of the master transcription factors during adipogenesis. Following induction of C/EBPβ,

and C/EBPδ, C/EBPα, along with PPARγ, is thought to promote expression of genes essential for developing and maintaining the differentiated adipocyte state [115]. Specifically, C/EBPα regulates a broad range of cellular functions by transactivating promoters for many adipocyte genes, including PPARγ, FABP4, leptin, insulin receptor, stearoyl-CoA desaturase I, acetyl-CoA carboxylase, and GLUT4 [115,116]. Evidence also suggests that C/EBPα is required during adipogenesis for development of insulin-stimulated glucose uptake in fully differentiated adipocytes [26,28].

In vivo studies in which the C/EBPα gene is knocked out in mice further illuminate the importance of this molecule in adipocyte development, with absence of C/EBPα resulting in a lack of white adipose tissue development [49] (Table 1). Analysis of the white adipose tissue phenotype in C/EBPα−/− mice was complicated by profound hypoglycemia and perinatal fatality. To overcome this technical issue, these mice were crossed to transgenic mouse expressing C/EBPα from a liver-specific promoter. C/EBPα−/− mice with expression of C/EBPα in liver from the albumin promoter have normal hepatic function, and yet are devoid of adipose tissue in many depots [117].

The roles of specific C/EBPs have been complicated by coexpression of family members in cells throughout the body. To help delineate independent functions of C/EBPs, the C/EBPα locus was replaced with C/EBPβ [50]. While C/EBPβ compensated for the lack of C/EBPα function in lung and liver, it could not fully substitute for C/EBPα in white adipose tissues (Table 1). The development of this mouse model was crucial for establishing the critical and specific role of C/EBPα in adipose development because fatal lung and liver phenotypes precluded analysis of other tissues.

A large body of research has elucidated roles for C/EBPα in adipocyte differentiation and development; however, there is very little knowledge related to the importance of C/EBPα in adipocytes after differentiation has occurred. One hypothesis is that removal of C/EBPα could result in dedifferentiation of adipocytes characterized by loss of lipid accumulation and reduced expression of adipocyte genes. Insight could be gained from studies performed on PPARγ, the other major regulator of adipogenesis, but these results are controversial. For example, adenoviral vector-based expression of a dominant negative form of PPARγ in adipocytes suggests that absence of PPARγ activity results in dedifferentiation of adipocytes [118], with reduced expression of key enzymes that contribute to lipid synthesis. In contrast, Camp et al. [119] found that while a PPARγ antagonist, PD068235, blocked adipogenesis of 3T3-L1 preadipocytes, this agent did not alter adipocyte morphology or expression of downstream targets such as PPARγ, FABP4, and Cbl-associated protein [119]. Notably, C/EBPα was reduced in adipocytes expressing dominant negative PPARγ, suggesting a possible explanation for the different results. Further studies, perhaps using RNAi or other methods to suppress expression of C/EBPα after adipogenesis has occurred, will be required to determine the roles of this transcription factor in maintaining the adipocyte phenotype.

4.2.3. *Role in insulin sensitivity*
A number of studies have pointed to a role for C/EBPα in the establishment of insulin-stimulated glucose uptake in adipocytes. In C/EBPα-deficient embryonic fibroblasts, overexpression of PPARγ is sufficient to induce lipid accumulation

and expression of some adipocyte genes, including GLUT4 [26]. However, these 'adipocytes' do not transport glucose in response to insulin. Further analyses revealed that these cells have reduced expression of insulin receptor and insulin receptor substrate-1, and impaired phosphorylation of these factors in response to insulin [26]. Additional studies suggest that basal glucose transport is far higher in C/EBPα$-$/$-$ embryonic fibroblasts because C/EBPα is required to suppress the fast basal exocytosis of GLUT4-associated vesicles [27]. Thus, C/EBPα is required, in this model, for the early steps in insulin signaling, as well as cytoplasmic retention of GLUT4 in the absence of insulin.

Studies performed on NIH-3T3 fibroblasts, which do not express endogenous C/EBPα, support some of these findings [28]. Although induction of differentiation in these cells by expression and activation of ectopic PPARγ results in adipocytes with accumulation of lipid and expression of FABP4, like C/EBPα$-$/$-$ embryonic fibroblasts, these cells also do not transport glucose in response to insulin [28]. The mechanism proposed for lack of insulin sensitivity is an absence of GLUT4 expression, presumably because of a lack of C/EBPα. Consistent with this hypothesis, expression of C/EBPα in NIH-3T3 cells induces spontaneous adipogenesis and the full adipogenic program, including GLUT4 expression and insulin-stimulated glucose uptake [28]. Further mechanistic analysis in PPARγ-expressing NIH-3T3 cells reveals that GLUT4 vesicle trafficking appears normal, and that it is only lack of GLUT4 expression that precludes development of insulin-stimulated glucose uptake [120]. Together, these studies indicate that C/EBPα plays a critical role in establishing insulin signaling mechanisms and insulin-stimulated glucose uptake in adipocytes.

The C/EBP transcription factors are potentially important for our understanding of diabetes. Given that polymorphisms in PPARγ [121] are associated with obesity and diabetes, and mutations in C/EBPα are also related to disease [122–124], it is possible that sequence variations in C/EBPα influence insulin sensitivity and other metabolic functions of hepatocytes and adipocytes. Their essential role in adipogenesis, and in the case of C/EBPα, insulin sensitivity, suggests that understanding C/EBP transcription factors will be important for treatment and/or prevention of certain aspects of the diabetes pathophysiology.

Acknowledgments

This work was supported by grants from the National Institutes of Health to O.A.M. (DK51563 and DK62876). Fellowships were from the Center for Organogenesis and the Belgian Fonds National de la Recherche Scientifique (I.G. is Chargé de Recherches).

References

[1] Y. Zhang, R. Proenca, M. Maffei, M. Barone, L. Leopold, J.M. Friedman, Positional cloning of the mouse *obese* gene and its human homologue, Nature 372 (1994) 425–432.
[2] P.E. Scherer, S. Williams, M. Fogliano, G. Baldini, H.F. Lodish, A novel serum protein similar to C1q, produced exclusively in adipocytes, J. Biol. Chem. 270 (1995) 26746–26749.

[3] E. Hu, P. Liang, B.M. Spiegelman, AdipoQ is a novel adipose-specific gene dysregulated in obesity, J. Biol. Chem. 271 (1996) 10697–10703.

[4] C.M. Steppan, S.T. Bailey, S. Bhat, E.J. Brown, R.R. Banerjee, C.M. Wright, H.R. Patel, R.S. Ahima, M.A. Lazar, The hormone resistin links obesity to diabetes, Nature 409 (2001) 307–312.

[5] G.S. Hotamisligil, N.S. Shargill, B.M. Spiegelman, Adipose expression of tumor necrosis factor-alpha: direct role in obesity-linked insulin resistance, Science 259 (1993) 87–91.

[6] B.B. Kahn, J.S. Flier, Obesity and insulin resistance, J. Clin. Invest. 106 (2000) 473–481.

[7] E. Arioglu, K.I. Rother, M.L. Reitman, A. Premkumar, S.I. Taylor, Lipoatrophy syndromes: when 'too little fat' is a clinical problem, Pediatr. Diabetes 1 (2000) 155–168.

[8] J. Moitra, M.M. Mason, M. Olive, D. Krylov, O. Gavrilova, B. Marcus-Samuels, L. Feigenbaum, E. Lee, T. Aoyama, M. Eckhaus, M.L. Reitman, C. Vinson, Life without white fat: a transgenic mouse, Genes Dev. 12 (1998) 3168–3181.

[9] I. Shimomura, R.E. Hammer, J.A. Richardson, S. Ikemoto, Y. Bashmakov, J.L. Goldstein, M.S. Brown, Insulin resistance and diabetes mellitus in transgenic mice expressing nuclear SREBP-1c in adipose tissue: model for congenital generalized lipodystrophy, Genes Dev. 12 (1998) 3182–3194.

[10] S.M. Taylor, P.A. Jones, Multiple new phenotypes induced in 10T1/2 and 3T3 cells treated with 5-azacytidine, Cell 17 (1979) 771–779.

[11] M.F. Pittenger, A.M. Mackay, S.C. Beck, R.K. Jaiswal, R. Douglas, J.D. Mosca, M.A. Moorman, D.W. Simonetti, S. Craig, D.R. Marshak, Multilineage potential of adult human mesenchymal stem cells, Science 284 (1999) 143–147.

[12] S.E. Ross, N. Hemati, K.A. Longo, C.N. Bennett, P.C. Lucas, R.L. Erickson, O.A. MacDougald, Inhibition of adipogenesis by Wnt signaling, Science 289 (2000) 950–953.

[13] M.E. Nuttall, J.M. Gimble, Controlling the balance between osteoblastogenesis and adipogenesis and the consequent therapeutic implications, Curr. Opin. Pharmacol 4 (2004) 290–294.

[14] H. Hu, M.J. Hilton, X. Tu, K. Yu, D.M. Ornitz, F. Long, Sequential roles of Hedgehog and Wnt signaling in osteoblast development, Development 132 (2004) 49–60.

[15] G. Cossu, U. Borello, Wnt signaling and the activation of myogenesis in mammals, EMBO J. 18 (1999) 6867–6872.

[16] K.A. Longo, W.S. Wright, S. Kang, I. Gerin, S.H. Chiang, P.C. Lucas, M.R. Opp, O.A. MacDougald, Wnt10b inhibits development of white and brown adipose tissues, J. Biol. Chem. 279 (2004) 35503–35509.

[17] H. Green, O. Kehinde, An established preadipose cell line and its differentiation in culture II. Factors affecting the adipose conversion, Cell 5 (1975) 19–27.

[18] H. Green, O. Kehinde, Spontaneous heritable changes leading to increased adipose conversion in 3T3 cells, Cell 7 (1976) 105–113.

[19] E.D. Rosen, B.M. Spiegelman, Molecular regulation of adipogenesis, Ann. Rev. Cell. Dev. Biol. 16 (2000) 145–171.

[20] S.M. Rangwala, M.A. Lazar, Transcriptional control of adipogenesis, Ann. Rev. Nutr. 20 (2000) 535–559.

[21] O.A. MacDougald, M.D. Lane, Transcriptional regulation of gene expression during adipocyte differentiation, Ann. Rev. Biochem. 64 (1995) 345–373.

[22] E.D. Rosen, C.H. Hsu, X. Wang, S. Sakai, M.W. Freeman, F.J. Gonzalez, B.M. Spiegelman, C/EBPalpha induces adipogenesis through PPARgamma: a unified pathway, Genes Dev. 16 (2002) 22–26.

[23] E.D. Rosen, P. Sarraf, A.E. Troy, G. Bradwin, K. Moore, D.S. Milstone, B.M. Spiegelman, R.M. Mortensen, PPARγ is required for differentiation of adipose tissue *in vivo* and *in vitro*, Mol. Cell 4 (1999) 611–617.

[24] H. Yki-Jarvinen, Thiazolidinediones, N. Engl. J. Med. 351 (2004) 1106–1118.

[25] S.M. Rangwala, M.A. Lazar, Peroxisome proliferator-activated receptor gamma in diabetes and metabolism, Trends Pharmacol. Sci. 25 (2004) 331–336.

[26] Z. Wu, E.D. Rosen, R. Brun, S. Hauser, G. Adelmant, A.E. Troy, C. McKeon, G.J. Darlington, B.M. Spiegelman, Cross-regulation of C/EBPα and PPARγ controls the transcriptional pathway of adipogenesis and insulin sensitivity, Mol. Cell 3 (1999) 151–158.

[27] N. Wertheim, Z. Cai, T.E. McGraw, The transcription factor CCAAT/enhancer-binding protein alpha is required for the intracellular retention of GLUT4, J. Biol. Chem. 279 (2004) 41468–41476.

[28] A.K. El-Jack, J.K. Hamm, P.F. Pilch, S.R. Farmer, Reconstitution of insulin-sensitive glucose transport in fibroblasts requires expression of both PPARγ and C/EBPα, J. Biol. Chem. 274 (1999) 7946–7951.

[29] R. Nusse, A. Brown, J. Papkoff, P. Scambler, G. Shackleford, A. McMahon, R. Moon, H. Varmus, A new nomenclature for int-1 and related genes: the Wnt gene family, Cell 64 (1991) 231.

[30] F. Rijsewijk, M. Schuermann, E. Wagenaar, P. Parren, D. Weigel, R. Nusse, The Drosophila homolog of the mouse mammary oncogene int-1 is identical to the segment polarity gene wingless, Cell 50 (1987) 649–657.

[31] C.V. Cabrera, M.C. Alonso, P. Johnston, R.G. Phillips, P.A. Lawrence, Phenocopies induced with antisense RNA identify the wingless gene, Cell 50 (1987) 659–663.

[32] R. Nusse, H.E. Varmus, Many tumors induced by the mouse mammary tumor virus contain a provirus integrated in the same region of the host genome, Cell 31 (1982) 99–109.

[33] K.M. Cadigan, R. Nusse, Wnt signaling: a common theme in animal development, Genes Dev. 11 (1997) 3286–3305.

[34] R.T. Moon, B. Bowerman, M. Boutros, N. Perrimon, The promise and perils of Wnt signaling through beta-catenin, Science 296 (2002) 1644–1646.

[35] S.E. Ross, R.L. Erickson, N. Hemati, O.A. MacDougald, Glycogen synthase kinase 3 is an insulin-regulated C/EBPα kinase, Mol. Cell. Biol. 19 (1999) 8433–8441.

[36] C.N. Bennett, S.E. Ross, K.A. Longo, L. Bajnok, N. Hemati, K.W. Johnson, S.D. Harrison, O.A. MacDougald, Regulation of Wnt signaling during adipogenesis, J. Biol. Chem. 277 (2002) 30998–31004.

[37] M. Moldes, Y. Zuo, R.F. Morrison, D. Silva, B.H. Park, J. Liu, S.R. Farmer, Peroxisome-proliferator-activated receptor gamma suppresses Wnt/beta-catenin signalling during adipogenesis, Biochem. J. 376 (2003) 607–613.

[38] J.A. Kennell, E.E. O'Leary, B.M. Gummow, G.D. Hammer, O.A. MacDougald, T-cell factor 4N (TCF-4N), a novel isoform of mouse TCF-4, synergizes with beta-catenin to coactivate C/EBPalpha and steroidogenic factor 1 transcription factors, Mol. Cell. Biol. 23 (2003) 5366–5375.

[39] S.E. Ross, R.L. Erickson, I. Gerin, P.M. DeRose, L. Bajnok, K.A. Longo, D.E. Misek, R. Kuick, S.M. Hanash, K.B. Atkins, S.M. Andresen, H.I. Nebb, L. Madsen, K. Kristiansen, O.A. MacDougald, Microarray analyses during adipogenesis: understanding the effects of Wnt-signaling on adipogenesis and the roles of LXRa in adipocyte metabolism, Mol. Cell. Biol. 22 (2002) 5989–5999.

[40] B. Cannon, J. Nedergaard, Brown adipose tissue: function and physiological significance, Physiol. Rev. 84 (2004) 277–359.

[41] J. Himms-Hagen, Does brown adipose tissue (BAT) have a role in the physiology or treatment of human obesity?, Rev. Endocr. Metab. Disord. 2 (2001) 395–401.

[42] B.B. Lowell, B.M. Spiegelman, Towards a molecular understanding of adaptive thermogenesis, Nature 404 (2000) 652–660.

[43] E.D. Rosen, C.J. Walkey, P. Puigserver, B.M. Spiegelman, Transcriptional regulation of adipogenesis, Genes Dev. 14 (2000) 1293–1307.

[44] S. Kang, L. Bajnok, K.A. Longo, R.K. Petersen, J.B. Hansen, K. Kristiansen, O.A. MacDougald, Effects of Wnt signaling on brown adipocyte differentiation and metabolism mediated by PGC-1alpha, Mol. Cell. Biol. 25 (2005) 1272–1282.

[45] J. Lin, P.H. Wu, P.T. Tarr, K.S. Lindenberg, J. St-Pierre, C.Y. Zhang, V.K. Mootha, S. Jager, C.R. Vianna, R.M. Reznick, L. Cui, M. Manieri, M.X. Donovan, Z. Wu, M.P. Cooper, M.C. Fan, L.M. Rohas, A.M. Zavacki, S. Cinti, G.I. Shulman, B.B. Lowell, D. Krainc, B.M. Spiegelman, Defects in adaptive energy metabolism with CNS-linked hyperactivity in PGC-1alpha null mice, Cell 119 (2004) 121–135.

[46] P. Puigserver, B.M. Spiegelman, Peroxisome proliferator-activated receptor-gamma coactivator 1 alpha (PGC-1 alpha): transcriptional coactivator and metabolic regulator, Endocr. Rev. 24 (2003) 78–90.

[47] T. Fujino, H. Asaba, M.J. Kang, Y. Ikeda, H. Sone, S. Takada, D.H. Kim, R.X. Ioka, M. Ono, H. Tomoyori, M. Okubo, T. Murase, A. Kamataki, J. Yamamoto, K. Magoori, S. Takahashi, Y. Miyamoto, H. Oishi, M. Nose, M. Okazaki, S. Usui, K. Imaizumi, M. Yanagisawa, J. Sakai, T.T. Yamamoto, Low-density lipoprotein receptor-related protein 5 (LRP5) is essential for normal cholesterol metabolism and glucose-induced insulin secretion, Proc. Natl. Acad. Sci. USA 100 (2003) 229–234.

[48] A. Kanazawa, S. Tsukada, A. Sekine, T. Tsunoda, A. Takahashi, A. Kashiwagi, Y. Tanaka, T. Babazono, M. Matsuda, K. Kaku, Y. Iwamoto, R. Kawamori, R. Kikkawa, Y. Nakamura, S. Maeda, Association of the gene encoding wingless-type mammary tumor virus integration-site family member 5B (WNT5B) with type 2 diabetes, Am. J. Hum. Genet. 75 (2004) 832–843.

[49] N.D. Wang, M.J. Finegold, A. Bradley, C.N. Ou, S.V. Abdelsayed, M.D. Wilde, L.R. Taylor, D.R. Wilson, G.J. Darlington, Impaired energy homeostasis in C/EBPα knockout mice, Science 269 (1995) 1108–1112.

[50] S.S. Chen, J.F. Chen, P.F. Johnson, V. Muppala, Y.H. Lee, C/EBPbeta, when expressed from the C/ebpalpha gene locus, can functionally replace C/EBPalpha in liver but not in adipose tissue, Mol. Cell. Biol. 20 (2000) 7292–7299.

[51] S. Liu, C. Croniger, C. Arizmendi, M. Harada-Shiba, J. Ren, V. Poli, R.W. Hanson, J.E. Friedman, Hypoglycemia and impaired hepatic glucose production in mice with a deletion of the C/EBPbeta gene, J. Clin. Invest. 103 (1999) 207–213.

[52] L. Wang, J. Shao, P. Muhlenkamp, S. Liu, P. Klepcyk, J. Ren, J.E. Friedman, Increased insulin receptor substrate-1 and enhanced skeletal muscle insulin sensitivity in mice lacking CCAAT/enhancer-binding protein beta, J. Biol. Chem. 275 (2000) 14173–14181.

[53] C.M. Croniger, C. Millward, J. Yang, Y. Kawai, I.J. Arinze, S. Liu, M. Harada-Shiba, K. Chakravarty, J.E. Friedman, V. Poli, R.W. Hanson, Mice with a deletion in the gene for CCAAT/enhancer-binding protein beta have an attenuated response to cAMP and impaired carbohydrate metabolism, J. Biol. Chem. 276 (2001) 629–638.

[54] W.H. Landschulz, P.F. Johnson, E.Y. Adashi, B.J. Graves, S.L. McKnight, Isolation of a recombinant copy of the gene encoding C/EBP, Genes Dev. 2 (1988) 786–800.

[55] P.F. Johnson, W.H. Landschulz, B.J. Graves, S.L. McKnight, Identification of a rat liver nuclear protein that binds to the enhancer core element of three animal viruses, Genes Dev. 1 (1987) 133–146.

[56] C.-J. Chang, T.-T. Chen, H.-Y. Lei, D.-S. Chen, S.-C. Lee, Molecular cloning of a transcription factor, AGP/EBP, that belongs to members of the C/EBP family, Mol. Cell. Biol. 10 (1990) 6642–6653.

[57] V. Poli, F.P. Mancini, R. Cortese, IL-6DBP, a nuclear protein involved in interleukin-6 signal transduction, defines a new family of leucine zipper proteins related to C/EBP, Cell 63 (1990) 643–653.

[58] Z. Cao, R.M. Umek, S.L. McKnight, Regulated expression of three C/EBP isoforms during adipose conversion of 3T3-L1 cells, Genes Dev. 5 (1991) 1538–1552.

[59] S.C. Williams, C.A. Cantwell, P.F. Johnson, A family of C/EBP-related proteins capable of forming covalently linked leucine zipper dimers *in vitro*, Genes Dev. 5 (1991) 1553–1567.

[60] N. Batchvarova, X.-Z. Wang, D. Ron, Inhibition of adipogenesis by the stress-induced protein CHOP (Gadd 153), EMBO J. 14 (1995) 4654–4661.

[61] Q.Q. Tang, M.D. Lane, Role of C/EBP homologous protein (CHOP-10) in the programmed activation of CCAAT/enhancer-binding protein-beta during adipogenesis, Proc. Natl. Acad. Sci. USA 97 (2000) 12446–12450.

[62] S.E. Parkin, M. Baer, T.D. Copeland, R.C. Schwartz, P.F. Johnson, Regulation of CCAAT/enhancer-binding protein (C/EBP) activator proteins by heterodimerization with C/EBPgamma (Ig/EBP), J. Biol. Chem. 277 (2002) 23563–23572.

[63] P. Descombes, M. Chojkier, S. Lichtsteiner, E. Falvey, U. Schibler, LAP, a novel member of the C/EBP gene family, encodes a liver-enriched transcriptional activator protein, Genes Dev. 4 (1990) 1541–1551.

[64] P. Descombes, U. Schibler, A liver-enriched transcriptional activator protein, LAP, and a transcriptional inhibitory protein, LIP, are translated from the same mRNA, Cell 67 (1991) 569–579.

[65] V. Begay, J. Smink, A. Leutz, Essential requirement of CCAAT/enhancer binding proteins in embryogenesis, Mol. Cell. Biol. 24 (2004) 9744–9751.

[66] L.M. Bundy, L. Sealy, CCAAT/enhancer binding protein beta (C/EBPbeta)-2 transforms normal mammary epithelial cells and induces epithelial to mesenchymal transition in culture, Oncogene 22 (2003) 869–883.

[67] Q.-Q. Tang, M.D. Lane, Activation and centromeric localization of CCAAT/enhancer-binding proteins during the mitotic clonal expansion of adipocyte differentiation, Genes Dev. 13 (1999) 2231–2241.

[68] Q.Q. Tang, T.C. Otto, M.D. Lane, CCAAT/enhancer-binding protein beta is required for mitotic clonal expansion during adipogenesis, Proc. Natl. Acad. Sci. USA 100 (2003) 850–855.

[69] J.W. Zhang, Q.Q. Tang, C. Vinson, M.D. Lane, Dominant-negative C/EBP disrupts mitotic clonal expansion and differentiation of 3T3-L1 preadipocytes, Proc. Natl. Acad. Sci. USA 101 (2004) 43–47.

[70] Q.Q. Tang, T.C. Otto, M.D. Lane, Mitotic clonal expansion: a synchronous process required for adipogenesis, Proc. Natl. Acad. Sci. USA 100 (2003) 44–49.

[71] L. Fajas, Adipogenesis: a cross-talk between cell proliferation and cell differentiation, Ann. Med. 35 (2003) 79–85.

[72] Z. Qiu, Y. Wei, N. Chen, M. Jiang, J. Wu, K. Liao, DNA synthesis and mitotic clonal expansion is not a required step for 3T3-L1 preadipocyte differentiation into adipocytes, J. Biol. Chem. 276 (2001) 11988–11995.

[73] G. Entenmann, H. Hauner, Relationship between replication and differentiation in cultured human adipocyte precursor cells, Am. J. Physiol. 270 (1996) C1011–C1016.

[74] J.J. Rochford, R.K. Semple, M. Laudes, K.B. Boyle, C. Christodoulides, C. Mulligan, C.J. Lelliott, S. Schinner, D. Hadaschik, M. Mahadevan, J.K. Sethi, A. Vidal-Puig, S. O'Rahilly, ETO/MTG8 is an inhibitor of C/EBPbeta activity and a regulator of early adipogenesis, Mol. Cell. Biol. 24 (2004) 9863–9872.

[75] E.M. Eaton, L. Sealy, Modification of CCAAT/enhancer-binding protein-beta by the small ubiquitin-like modifier (SUMO) family members, SUMO-2 and SUMO-3, J. Biol. Chem. 278 (2003) 33416–33421.

[76] M. Wegner, Z. Cao, M. Rosenfeld, Calcium-regulated phosphorylation within the leucine zipper of C/EBPβ, Science 256 (1992) 370–373.

[77] H.-J. Tae, Z. Shaoying, K.-H. Kim, cAMP activation of CAAT enhancer-binding protein-βgene expression and promoter I of acetyl-CoA carboxylase, J. Biol. Chem. 270 (1995) 21487–21494.

[78] B.H. Park, L. Qiang, S.R. Farmer, Phosphorylation of C/EBPbeta at a consensus extracellular signal-regulated kinase/glycogen synthase kinase 3 site is required for the induction of adiponectin gene expression during the differentiation of mouse fibroblasts into adipocytes, Mol. Cell. Biol. 24 (2004) 8671–8680.

[79] N.A. Timchenko, M. Wilde, M. Nakanishi, J.R. Smith, G.J. Darlington, CCAAT/enhancer-binding protein α (C/EBPα) inhibits cell proliferation through the p21 (WAF-1/CIP-1/SCI-1) protein, Genes Dev. 10 (1996) 804–815.

[80] N.A. Timchenko, M. Wilde, P. Iakova, J.H. Albrecht, G.J. Darlington, E2F/p107 and E2F/p130 complexes are regulated by C/EBPα in 3T3-L1 adipocytes, Nucl. Acids Res. 17 (1999) 3621–3630.

[81] Z. Wu, Y. Xie, N.L.R. Bucher, S.R. Farmer, Conditional ectopic expression of C/EBPβ in NIH-3T3 cells induces PPARγ and stimulates adipogenesis, Genes Dev. 9 (1995) 2350–2363.

[82] W.-C. Yeh, Z. Cao, M. Classon, S.L. McKnight, Cascade regulation of terminal adipocyte differentiation by three members of the C/EBP family of leucine zipper proteins, Genes Dev. 9 (1995) 168–181.

[83] T. Tanaka, N. Yoshida, T. Kishimoto, S. Akira, Defective adipocyte differentiation in mice lacking the C/EBPβ and/or C/EBPδ gene, EMBO J. 16 (1997) 7432–7443.

[84] S. Osada, H. Yamamoto, T. Nishihara, M. Imagawa, DNA binding specificity of the CCAAT/enhancer-binding protein transcription factor family, J. Biol. Chem. 271 (1996) 3891–3896.

[85] S.C. Williams, N.D. Angerer, P.F. Johnson, C/EBP proteins contain nuclear localization signals imbedded in their basic regions, Gene Expression 6 (1997) 371–385.

[86] F. Schaufele, X. Wang, X. Liu, R.N. Day, Conformation of CCAAT/enhancer-binding protein alpha dimers varies with intranuclear location in living cells, J. Biol. Chem. 278 (2003) 10578–10587.

[87] W.H. Landschulz, P.F. Johnson, S.L. McKnight, The leucine zipper: a hypothetical structure common to a new class of DNA binding proteins, Science 240 (1988) 1759–1764.

[88] W.H. Landschulz, P.F. Johnson, S.L. McKnight, The DNA binding domain of the rat liver nuclear protein C/EBP is bipartite, Science 243 (1989) 1681–1688.

[89] C.R. Vinson, P.B. Sigler, S.L. McKnight, Scissor-grip model for DNA recognition by a family of leucine zipper proteins, Science 246 (1989) 911–916.

[90] H.C. Hurst, Transcription factors 1: bZIP proteins, Protein Profile 2 (1995) 101–168.

[91] D. Ron, J.F. Habener, CHOP, a novel developmentally regulated nuclear protein that dimerizes with transcription factors C/EBP and LAP and functions as a dominant-negative inhibitor of gene transcription, Genes Dev. 6 (1992) 439–453.

[92] J.D. Shuman, J. Cheong, J.E. Coligan, ATF-2 and C/EBPα can form a heterodimeric DNA binding complex *in vitro*, J. Biol. Chem. 272 (1997) 12793–12800.

[93] V. Ossipow, P. Descombes, U. Schibler, CCAAT/enhancer-binding protein mRNA is translated into multiple proteins with different transcription activation potentials, Proc. Natl. Acad. Sci. USA 90 (1993) 8219–8223.

[94] F.-T. Lin, O.A. MacDougald, A.M. Diehl, M.D. Lane, A 30 kilodalton alternative translation product of the CCAAT/enhancer binding protein a message: transcriptional activator lacking antimitotic activity, Proc. Natl. Acad. Sci. USA 90 (1993) 9606–9610.

[95] L.R. Hendricks-Taylor, G.J. Darlingtin, Inhibition of cell proliferation by C/EBPα occurs in many cell types, does not require the presence of p53 or Rb, and is not affected by large T-antigen, Nucl. Acids Res. 23 (1995) 4726–4732.

[96] T. Pabst, B.U. Mueller, P. Zhang, H.S. Radomska, S. Narravula, S. Schnittger, G. Behre, W. Hiddemann, D.G. Tenen, Dominant-negative mutations of CEBPA, encoding CCAAT/enhancer binding protein-alpha (C/EBPalpha), in acute myeloid leukemia, Nat. Genet. 27 (2001) 263–270.

[97] R.L. Erickson, N. Hemati, S.E. Ross, O.A. MacDougald, p300 coactivates the adipogenic transcription factor CCAAT/enhancer- binding protein alpha, J. Biol. Chem. 276 (2001) 16348–16355.

[98] A.D. Friedman, S.L. McKnight, Identification of two polypeptide segments of CCAAT/enhancer-binding protein required for transcriptional activation of the serum albumin gene, Genes Dev. 4 (1990) 1416–1426.

[99] C. Nerlov, E.B. Ziff, Three levels of functional interaction determine the activity of CCAAT/enhancer binding protein-α on the serum albumin promoter, Genes Dev. 8 (1994) 350–362.

[100] T.A. Pedersen, E. Kowenz-Leutz, A. Leutz, C. Nerlov, Cooperation between C/EBPalpha TBP/TFIIB and SWI/SNF recruiting domains is required for adipocyte differentiation, Genes Dev. 15 (2001) 3208–3216.

[101] H. Wang, P. Iakova, M. Wilde, A. Welm, T. Goode, W.J. Roesler, N.A. Timchenko, C/EBPalpha arrests cell proliferation through direct inhibition of Cdk2 and Cdk4, Mol. Cell 8 (2001) 817–828.

[102] B.T. Porse, T.A. Pedersen, X. Xu, B. Lindberg, U.M. Wewer, L. Friis-Hansen, C. Nerlov, E2F repression by C/EBPalpha is required for adipogenesis and granulopoiesis *in vivo*, Cell 107 (2001) 247–258.

[103] J. Kim, C.A. Cantwell, P.F. Johnson, C.M. Pfarr, S.C. Williams, Transcriptional activity of CCAAT/enhancer-binding proteins is controlled by a conserved inhibitory domain that is a target for sumoylation, J. Biol. Chem. 277 (2002) 38037–38044.

[104] L. Subramanian, M.D. Benson, J.A. Iniguez-Lluhi, A synergy control motif within the attenuator domain of CCAAT/enhancer-binding protein alpha inhibits transcriptional synergy through its PIASy-enhanced modification by SUMO-1 or SUMO-3, J. Biol. Chem. 278 (2003) 9134–9141.

[105] N. Hemati, S.E. Ross, R.L. Erickson, G.E. Groblewski, O.A. MacDougald, Signaling pathways through which insulin regulates CCAAT/enhancer binding protein α (C/EBPα) phosphorylation and gene expression in 3T3-L1 adipocytes: correlation with GLUT4 gene expression, J. Biol. Chem. 41 (1997) 25913–25919.

[106] G.L. Wang, P. Iakova, M. Wilde, S. Awad, N.A. Timchenko, Liver tumors escape negative control of proliferation via PI3K/Akt-mediated block of C/EBP alpha growth inhibitory activity, Genes Dev. 18 (2004) 912–925.

[107] O.C. Ross, H.S. Radomska, B. Wu, P. Zhang, J.N. Winnay, L. Bajnok, W.S. Wright, F. Schaufele, D.G. Tenen, O.A. MacDougald, Phosphorylation of C/EBPalpha inhibits granulopoiesis, Mol. Cell. Biol. 24 (2004) 675–686.

[108] G. Behre, S.M. Singh, H. Liu, L.T. Bortolin, M. Christopeit, H.S. Radomska, J. Rangatia, W. Hiddemann, A.D. Friedman, D.G. Tenen, Ras signaling enhances the activity of C/EBP alpha to induce granulocytic differentiation by phosphorylation of serine 248, J. Biol. Chem. 277 (2002) 26293–26299.

[109] R.J. Christy, K.H. Kaestner, D.E. Geiman, M.D. Lane, CCAAT/enhancer binding protein gene promoter: binding of nuclear factors during differentiation of 3T3-L1 preadipocytes, Proc. Natl. Acad. Sci. USA 88 (1991) 2593–2597.

[110] C. Legraverend, P. Antonson, P. Flodby, K.G. Xanthopoulos, High level activity of the mouse CCAAT/enhancer binding protein (C/EBPα) gene promoter involves autoregulation and several ubiquitous transcription factors, Nucl. Acids Res. 21 (1993) 1735–1742.

[111] O.A. MacDougald, P. Cornelius, F.-T. Lin, S.S. Chen, M.D. Lane, Glucocorticoids reciprocally regulate expression of the CCAAT/enhancer-binding protein α and δ genes in 3T3-L1 adipocytes and white adipose tissue, J. Biol. Chem. 269 (1994) 19041–19047.

[112] O.A. MacDougald, P. Cornelius, R. Liu, M.D. Lane, Insulin regulates transcription of the CCAAT/ enhancer binding protein (C/EBP) α, β, and δ genes in fully differentiated 3T3-L1 adipocytes, J. Biol. Chem. 270 (1995) 647 651.

[113] H.S. Radomska, H.C.S., P. Zhang, T. Cheng, S.D.T., T. D.G., CCAAT/Enhancer Binding Protein α is a regulatory switch sufficient for induction of granulocytic development from bipotential myeloid progenitors, Mol. Cell. Biol. 18 (1998) 4301–4314.

[114] P. Flodby, C. Barlow, H. Kylefjord, L. Ahrlund-Richter, K.G. Xanthopoulos, Increased hepatic cell proliferation and lung abnormalities in mice deficient in CCAAT/enhancer binding protein α, J. Biol. Chem. 271 (1996) 24753–24760.

[115] G.J. Darlington, S.E. Ross, O.A. MacDougald, The role of C/EBP genes in adipocyte differentiation, J. Biol. Chem. 273 (1998) 30057–30060.

[116] M.T. Travers, A.J. Vallance, H.T. Gourlay, C.A. Gill, I. Klein, C.B. Bottema, M.C. Barber, Promoter I of the ovine acetyl-CoA carboxylase-alpha gene: an E-box motif at -114 in the proximal promoter binds upstream stimulatory factor (USF)-1 and USF-2 and acts as an insulin-response sequence in differentiating adipocytes, Biochem. J. 359 (2001) 273–284.

[117] H.G. Linhart, K. Ishimura-Oka, F. DeMayo, T. Kibe, D. Repka, B. Poindexter, R.J. Bick, G.J. Darlington, C/EBPalpha is required for differentiation of white, but not brown, adipose tissue, Proc. Natl. Acad. Sci. USA 98 (2001) 12532–12537.

[118] Y. Tamori, J. Masugi, N. Nishino, M. Kasuga, Role of peroxisome proliferator-activated receptor-gamma in maintenance of the characteristics of mature 3T3-L1 adipocytes, Diabetes 51 (2002) 2045–2055.

[119] H.S. Camp, A. Chaudhry, T. Leff, A novel potent antagonist of peroxisome proliferator-activated receptor gamma blocks adipocyte differentiation but does not revert the phenotype of terminally differentiated adipocytes, Endocrinology 142 (2001) 3207–3213.

[120] D.N. Gross, S.R. Farmer, P.F. Pilch, Glut4 storage vesicles without Glut4: transcriptional regulation of insulin-dependent vesicular traffic, Mol. Cell. Biol. 24 (2004) 7151–7162.

[121] D. Altshuler, J.N. Hirschhorn, M. Klannemark, C.M. Lindgren, M.C. Vohl, J. Nemesh, C.R. Lane, S.F. Schaffner, S. Bolk, C. Brewer, T. Tuomi, D. Gaudet, T.J. Hudson, M. Daly, L. Groop, E.S. Lander, The common PPARgamma Pro12Ala polymorphism is associated with decreased risk of type 2 diabetes, Nat. Genet. 26 (2000) 76–80.

[122] H. Leroy, C. Roumier, P. Huyghe, V. Biggio, P. Fenaux, C. Preudhomme, CEBPA point mutations in hematological malignancies, Leukemia 19 (2005) 329–334.

[123] S. Frohling, H. Dohner, Disruption of C/EBPalpha function in acute myeloid leukemia, N. Engl. J. Med. 351 (2004) 2370–2372.

[124] A. Kaeferstein, U. Krug, J. Tiesmeier, M. Aivado, M. Faulhaber, M. Stadler, J. Krauter, U. Germing, W.K. Hofmann, H.P. Koeffler, A. Ganser, W. Verbeek, The emergence of a C/EBPalpha mutation in the clonal evolution of MDS towards secondary AML, Leukemia 17 (2003) 343–349.

Chapter 9

GATA proteins as molecular gatekeepers of adipogenesis

Judy Tsai[1], Qiang Tong[2], Gökhan S. Hotamisligil[1]

[1]*Department of Genetics and Complex Diseases, Harvard School of Public Health, Boston, MA, USA;*
[2]*USDA/ARS Children's Nutrition Research Center, Baylor College of Medicine, Houston, TX, USA*

Body weight regulation can be regarded as a finely tuned balance between energy storage and energy expenditure [1]. Energy storage has classically been associated with white adipose tissue which can accumulate energy in triglyceride-rich intracellular lipid droplets. However, the critical role of endocrine functions of adipocytes via production of bioactive lipids, cytokines, hormones, and other important signaling molecules has also become well established in recent years. As a tissue, white adipose accretion can be attributed to cell turnover (i.e., cell number) as well as increased lipid storage at the single-cell level (i.e., cell size). On the other hand, brown adipose tissue, a second adipose tissue type found only in mammals, is primarily involved in energy expenditure. Although brown adipocytes are also capable of lipid storage, albeit in much smaller lipid droplets than those found in white adipocytes, their function is principally associated with energy consumption. Brown adipose tissue protects the organism from cold exposure by initiating facultative thermogenesis in response to environmental changes. This tissue has also been demonstrated to hypertrophy in response to prolonged exposure to cold [2] as well as adrenergic stimulation [3]. Brown adipocytes uniquely express the founding member of the uncoupling protein family, mitochondrial membrane proteins whose dedicated function is to dissipate the proton gradient that would otherwise accumulate and become captured in ATP synthesis. Instead of generating energy-rich molecules of ATP, this "proton leak" results in futile cycling of electrons with the end product being heat production [4,5]. Uncoupling protein expression is induced when brown adipocytes in culture are adrenergically stimulated with reagents that elevate intracellular levels of cyclic AMP [6,7]. Given the opposite functions of these two adipose tissue types, it is tempting to speculate that shifting the balance in favor of energy expenditure either by increasing brown adipogenesis or by curbing white adipogenesis is a potential strategy to modulate adiposity.

ADVANCES IN MOLECULAR AND CELLULAR ENDOCRINOLOGY   © 2006 Elsevier B.V.
VOLUME 5 ISSN 1569-2566/DOI 10.1016/S1569-2566(06)05009-5   All rights reserved.

1. Transcriptional activators of adipogenesis

The transcriptional regulators that govern terminal differentiation of white and brown adipocytes have been elucidated through experiments in cultured cells and confirmed by many studies involving gene manipulation *in vivo*. Hormonal induction of preadipocytes in culture results in several rounds of cell division referred to as clonal expansion, followed by permanent growth arrest and terminal differentiation [8,9]. However, human preadipocytes presumably obviate this requirement [10], it is therefore, not clear whether clonal expansion is a universal requirement for proper adipocyte differentiation. At early stages of differentiation, there is a transient increase in expression of two members of the CCAAT/enhancer binding protein (C/EBP) family, C/EBPβ and δ, which is followed by an increased expression of peroxisome proliferator-activated receptor γ (PPARγ) [11,12]. In spite of their temporal expression pattern, it is unlikely that C/EBPβ and δ are solely responsible for the expression of PPARγ since C/EBPβ and δ double-knockout animals express normal levels of PPARγ in their white and brown adipose tissues [13]. PPARγ induces expression of a third C/EBP protein, C/EBPα, and these two factors subsequently autoregulate each other to elevate their expression levels to thus maintain the terminally differentiated state [14,15]. Following induction of PPARγ and C/EBPα, a gamut of adipogenic genes important for metabolic function and morphological changes are expressed. These include the adipocyte-specific fatty acid binding protein (aP2/FABP4), glucose transporter (Glut4), phosphoenolpyruvate carboxykinase (PEPCK), fatty acid synthase (FAS), hormone sensitive lipase (HSL), adipsin, leptin, and adiponectin, just to name a few [16]. In response to adrenergic stimulation, brown adipocytes express additional genes such as uncoupling protein-1 (UCP-1) [17,18], which is unique to this cell lineage, and PPARγ co-activator-1α (PGC-1α), which is preferentially expressed in brown adipose, but can also be found in muscle, liver and white adipose at low levels [19]. The roles of PPARγ and the C/EBP family during adipocyte differentiation as well as regulation of the late adipogenic markers, have been extensively reviewed previously [16,20].

2. Negative regulators of adipogenesis

In addition to these crucial transcription factors, which positively regulate adipogenesis, the identification of many factors that inhibit adipocyte differentiation clearly indicates that, in addition to transcriptional activation of key genes, repression of the adipogenic program is an equally vital component of adipocyte differentiation. Growth factors such as fibroblast growth factor (FGF), platelet-derived growth factor (PDGF), epidermal growth factor (EGF), and leukemia inhibitory factor (LIF) have all been documented to inhibit adipocyte differentiation in an autocrine fashion [21–24]. Although these factors can impede adipogenesis under certain experimental conditions, further studies are needed to define the appropriate physiological conditions for these events. Treatment of 3T3-L1 adipocytes with TGFβ, another growth factor, is coincidental with decreased gene expression of C/EBPα and PPARγ [25]. Recently, members of the Smad family in the TGFβ signaling pathway were implicated in regulating adipocyte differentiation through suppression of C/EBPα and PPARγ [26]. The anti-adipogenic effect of many of the growth factors mentioned above is thought to be mediated by mitogen-activated protein kinases (MAPK), which can phosphorylate PPARγ and result in decreased PPARγ transcriptional activity in response to mitogens [27].

In addition to growth factors, other soluble factors have been identified that negatively regulate adipogenesis. Soluble tumor necrosis factor-α (sTNFα) can prevent the differentiation of precursor cells, as well as stimulate lipolysis in differentiated adipocytes [28]. Interestingly, the transmembrane form of TNFα (mTNFα) can also inhibit differentiation in preadipocytes but not adipocytes [29] specifically through the TNFα receptor-1 (TNFR1) via its juxtamembrane (JM) and death domains. While deletion of the death domain results in decreased nuclear factor-κB (NF-κB) activation, this is not observed when the JM domain is deleted, which demonstrates that NF-κB activation may be dispensable for inhibition of adipogenesis [30]. Whereas MAPK has also been implicated in TNFα inhibition of adipogenesis, it appears not to be required under all experimental conditions [31,32]. Another soluble factor, Pref-1, is a transmembrane protein that belongs to a family of proteins containing EGF-like repeats, and was initially discovered to suppress adipogenesis when overexpressed in 3T3-L1 cells [33]. This finding was recently corroborated by *in vivo* expression of soluble Pref-1 in adipose tissue, which resulted in decreased adipose mass of several mesenteric fat pads, as well as decreased adipogenic gene expression and adipocyte size [34]. In addition to factors that can block differentiation by interfering with expression of transcription factors which initiate adipogenesis, such as PPARγ and C/EBP proteins, there exist other factors which can block differentiation at even earlier stages. For example, Wnt factors are glycoproteins secreted by adipocytes and contribute to the maintenance of the undifferentiated state of preadipocytes. Inhibition of the Wnt signaling pathway by perturbation of downstream effectors such as glycogen synthase kinase-3 (GSK3) activity or β-catenin phosphorylation results in spontaneous differentiation of 3T3-L1 preadipocytes [35,36].

These studies provide compelling evidence for the existence of regulatory pathways that either promote or counter adipocyte differentiation. It may be that active repression of negative regulatory pathways is a prerequisite for adipocyte differentiation, and exist so that the cell can respond to extracellular cues to either initiate or abstain from adipocyte differentiation. It is likely that repression of adipocyte differentiation can occur at any stage of a very long course of time, such as during lineage determination of a totipotent cell, or commitment of a pluripotent progenitor cell to the adipocyte lineage. Repressive mechanisms can also occur at later stages when a dedicated preadipocyte terminally differentiates to a mature adipocyte, including dedifferentiation and transdifferentiation events. This review will focus on regulators of early stages of adipogenesis. In particular, the role of GATA transcription factors in adipocyte differentiation and their possible role in determination of cell fate will be discussed. Owing to their expression pattern and unique function in both white and brown adipocyte precursors, GATA transcription factors are interesting molecular models to explore the poorly understood mechanisms controlling early stages of adipocyte differentiation.

3. Gata transcription factors

The GATA family of transcription factors is named for their ability to bind DNA at a cognate DNA sequence (A/T)GATA(A/G). They do so via two homologous zinc finger domains, each of which bears the signature sequence Cys-X_2-Cys-X_{17}-Cys-X_2-Cys [37]. Though similar in sequence, discrete functions have been ascribed to each zinc finger. The C-terminal zinc finger (known as Finger II) is indispensable for DNA binding [38], while the N-terminal zinc finger (known as Finger I) is required for transcriptional activation [39], presumably by stabilizing the DNA–protein complex [40]. GATA-1, the founding member of the GATA protein family, positively regulates transcription of most erythroid-specific genes by binding to the promoter regions of such genes [41]. Experiments conducted in chimeric mice derived from $GATA-1^{-/-}$ embryonic stem cells indicate that GATA-1 is necessary for full differentiation of the erythroid lineage [42], indicating a crucial role for GATA-1 as early as in the commitment of an unspecified erythroid precursor to the erythroid lineage. Since its discovery, five other GATA proteins have been identified in vertebrates [43–46], and orthologs exist in invertebrates as well [47–49]. The sequences of these related proteins are conserved only in the two zinc finger domains as well as the consecutive basic domain following them; outside of this region they bear little resemblance to each other in amino acid sequence [50]. They function as transcription factors in a broad range of settings, which also include non-hematopoietic cells, and have been demonstrated to regulate both differentiation and cell-fate determination. GATA-1, -2, and -3 have been identified in various hematopoietic cell types, and can negatively or positively regulate genes specific to the hematopoietic lineages in which they are expressed [51–53]. Similarly, GATA-4, -5, and -6 are expressed primarily in the heart and gut, and activate genes in tissues derived from the gut endoderm [54]. The GATA ortholog *serpent* is necessary for formation of the midgut endoderm in *Drosophila* and is expressed in the developing foregut and hindgut known as the fat body [47,49]. In *Drosophila*, this primitive organ is the functional analog of the mammalian immune system, liver, and possibly the site for energy storage. The similarity of the *Drosophila* fat body to mammalian adipose tissue has prompted examination of the role of GATA transcription factors in adipose tissue formation and metabolism using mammalian experimental systems.

3.1. *GATA transcription factors in adipogenesis*

Of the six GATA proteins, GATA-2 and GATA-3 are expressed abundantly in white adipose, while GATA-2 but not -3 is expressed in brown adipose tissue. Interestingly, GATA expression is restricted to early stages of preadipocyte differentiation in clonal cell lines as well as in the stromal–vascular fraction of adipose tissue, which contains preadipocytes and other cell types. This unique expression pattern suggests that transcriptional downregulation of GATA factors may be a feature of adipogenesis. Indeed, in adipogenic cell lines, constitutive GATA expression throughout differentiation down regulates expression of functionally critical genes. In white adipocytes, ectopic GATA expression results in dramatic decreases in transcript levels of PPARγ and C/EBPα as well as late adipocyte markers such as aP2 and adipsin. Along with this altered gene profile is inhibition of lipid accumulation, as the preadipocytes expressing GATA-2 or -3 appear to be locked in the preadipocyte stage [55]. The relevance of GATA-2 and GATA-3 for metabolism is underscored by the expression pattern in adipose tissue of genetically obese mouse models compared to their lean counterparts. GATA-2 and GATA-3 transcripts are strikingly diminished in white adipose tissue of obese animals when compared to age-matched lean controls from three different genetic backgrounds [55]. This suggests that obesity is associated with inappropriately low expression levels of GATA that otherwise exist as a molecular barrier to adipocyte differentiation.

3.2. *Role of GATA factors in cell-fate determination*

The effects of GATA deficiency on adipogenesis have been studied using GATA-3$^{-/-}$ and GATA2$^{-/-}$ embryonic stem cells [55]. *In vitro* differentiation of GATA-3$^{-/-}$ ES cells to white adipocytes was significantly improved compared to wild-type ES cells, as judged by the number of embryoid bodies that supported differentiation and expression of adipogenic genes. Since brown adipocytes only express GATA-2, *in vitro* differentiated GATA-2$^{-/-}$ ES cells were used to investigate the role of GATA factors in brown adipocyte differentiation. There was no significant difference in expression of UCP-1, PGC-1α, or aP2 in GATA-2$^{-/-}$ versus wild-type ES cells [56]. This indicates that although GATA-2 may not be required for adipocyte-lineage determination, it may become relevant at a later developmental stage, such as in the conversion of the committed preadipocyte to a mature phenotype. However, the ES cell system is not suitable to examine brown adipogenesis accurately. Indeed, conditional somatic inactivation of a GATA-2 allele resulted in increased expression of genes associated with the mature brown adipocyte upon differentiation [56].

Loss-of-function studies in whole animals is more technically challenging because GATA-2$^{-/-}$ embryos die from severe anemia [57], while GATA-3$^{-/-}$ embryos die from a panoply of hematopoietic abnormalities, including massive internal hemorrhages, anemia, and neural tube defects [58]. To overcome these setbacks, an alternative experimental system was generated in order to study the role of GATA-2 in brown or white adipose development. Chimeric animals were created using GATA-2$^{-/-}$ ES cells [56]. An analysis of tissues from these animals demonstrated that GATA-2$^{-/-}$ cells were not excluded from brown or white adipose tissue, and moreover, GATA-2$^{-/-}$ and wild type cells contributed to brown adipose tissue formation in a ratio similar to the degree of chimerism. While there are limitations associated with this experimental paradigm, this finding suggests that GATA deficiency at an earlier developmental stage does not interfere with commitment of precursor cells toward brown adipocyte formation during development, and is consistent with the null effect observed with *in vitro* differentiation of GATA-2$^{-/-}$ ES cells.

Clearly, the investigation of GATA deficiency *in vivo* awaits the development of more sophisticated experimental systems. Such tools would aid the comparison of the functional significance of GATA in brown versus white adipogenesis. A potentially interesting role for GATA-3 in totipotent cells as they progress toward the adipocyte

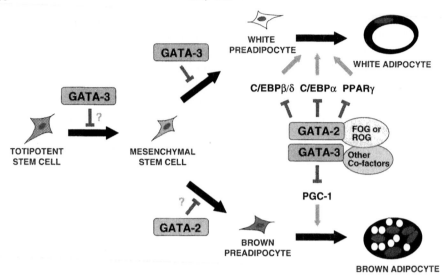

Fig. 1. Precursor cells of mesenchymal origin give rise to adipocytes. While it is not clear whether white and brown adipocytes emerge from a common precursor such as a mesenchymal stem cell, many developmental mechanisms are common to both cell types. In this same context, whether GATA factors contribute to lineage development of white and/or brown adipocytes is currently unknown. On the other hand, it is established that both GATA-2 and GATA-3 control the transition from a preadipocyte to adipocyte. To control this critical transition, GATA factors interfere with the activity of at least two key groups of molecules that govern terminal differentiation, the C/EBP family and PPARγ. In the brown adipogenesis, PGC-1 is also targeted by GATA and several transcriptional co-factors are likely contributors to their actions. See Plate 8 in Colour Plate Section.

lineage is that of a gatekeeper at various stages of adipose tissue formation. It is possible that as the cell makes decisions about its fate, active inhibition of GATA-3 preferentially drives the uncommitted cell to the white lineage, while otherwise endogenous expression of GATA commits the cell to the brown lineage by default (Fig. 1). Alternatively, GATA-3 might silence genes germane to the white adipose lineage until presented with the appropriate cues to derepress transcriptional activation of such genes. Further study of GATA factors in white and brown adipogenesis using gain- and loss-of-function genetic models in cells and whole animals will provide valuable insight into these questions.

3.3. *Possible mechanisms of GATA action during adipogenesis*

The mechanism by which GATA factors function in adipocyte differentiation has not yet been fully resolved, although there are several possibilities that are currently under investigation. Studies on the PPARγ 5′ flanking region have elucidated several potential GATA-binding sites. Further analyses of the 0.6 kb PPARγ promoter demonstrated that either GATA-2 or -3 can suppress basal promoter activity via direct interactions with two of these GATA binding sites. GATA-mediated suppression of PPARγ promoter activity requires both zinc fingers, as only the deletion of both fingers completely abolishes suppression of the PPARγ promoter [55]. Introduction of PPARγ into preadipocytes can rescue the inhibitory effects of GATA factors, but since this rescue is not complete, additional molecular mechanisms are likely to be involved.

The temporal co-expression of GATA with members of the C/EBP protein family during adipocyte differentiation suggests that GATA may also suppress adipogenesis through interactions with C/EBP factors. Co-precipitation studies show that both GATA-2 and GATA-3 can form protein complexes with either C/EBPα or C/EBPβ [59]. The interaction domain between these molecules was mapped to the bZip region of C/EBPα and amino acid residues 381–385 following the carboxyl zinc finger of GATA-2. This interaction is functionally significant, since isolated disruption of C/EBP interaction impairs the ability of GATA to suppress adipocyte differentiation. While the focus of this study was the interaction of GATA with C/EBPα, GATA might interact with other members of the C/EBP family through homologous regions. However, since GATA down regulation partially overlaps with C/EBPα induction, it remains possible that even under normal conditions GATA factors can interact with C/EBPα, perhaps in order to limit its ability to activate the adipogenic program. Considering the strong inhibitory effect of GATA on adipogenesis, and the modest phenotype of C/EBP$\beta^{-/-}$ animals [13], it seems likely that GATA-mediated suppression of differentiation may require multiple lines of regulation. Additionally, the ability of GATA to interact with multiple C/EBP isoforms of various temporal expression patterns suggests that their pro-adipogenic contribution might be counterregulated by GATA in a stage-specific fashion.

Thus, so far there is evidence that GATA can regulate adipogenesis by antagonizing two principal transcription factors of this process, PPARγ and C/EBPα. The dual mechanism by which GATA acts underscores the necessity for tight control of the initiation of adipogenesis in preadipocytes, such that perturbation of either pathway may result in only partial loss of GATA suppression of adipocyte differentiation. By the same token, GATA may exert its effects through its well-recognized property as a DNA-binding transcription factor, but may also do so through interactions with co-factors and proteins involved in other functions. Interaction with such proteins may introduce additional levels of regulation, such as alteration of DNA-binding specificity, or acquisition of transcriptional activity. In other cellular contexts, post-translational modification of GATA has been recognized as an important feature of its regulation of target genes. For example, acetylation of GATA-1 has been reported to increase the stoichiometric ratio of GATA bound to DNA as well as activate transcription of GATA-dependent genes in hematopoiesis [60]. In fact, deletion of preferentially acetylated amino acids on the GATA protein results in reduced megakaryocytic differentiation *in vivo* [38]. It is noteworthy that acetylation is a key modification that is known to regulate transcription by modulating the activity of histones, a class of proteins which associate and dissociate with transcriptionally active chromatin based on its acetylation state. Transcription factors such as GATA that interact directly with DNA to control transcription may be regulated likewise in the context of adipogenesis. Phosphorylation has also been observed on GATA-1 upon exposure to certain stimuli; however, disruption of the phosphorylation site has not been found to significantly interfere with the ability of GATA to bind DNA, or transactivate target genes [61]. Nonetheless, it has not been ruled out that phosphorylation can induce subtle conformational changes which can result in more pronounced consequences such as altering the specificity of GATA for a target gene or protein co-factor. An interesting study recently reported phosphorylation of GATA-2 by Akt at the serine 401 residue [62]. This phosphorylation impairs GATA activity in preadipocytes. Unlike the wild type molecule, a GATA-2 molecule with a mutation at this site can no longer prevent adipocyte differentiation *in vitro* and *in vivo* [62]. As Akt activation is a critical component of insulin action and adipocyte differentiation, this study demonstrated that GATA regulation is also integrated into this signaling system controlling differentiation of fat cells [62]. Furthermore, these results indicate that post-translational suppression of GATA activity through a specific phosphorylation event mediated by Akt is a critical regulatory step in adipogenesis [62].

4. A role for GATA co-factors in adipogenesis?

The recent identification of novel factors that interact with GATA also opens up new possibilities for investigating the mechanism of GATA during adipogenesis. Friend of GATA-1 (FOG-1) is a GATA co-factor identified by a yeast two-hybrid screen of an erythroleukemia cell line (MEL) cDNA library using the N-terminal finger of GATA-1 as bait, since the requirement for the GATA-1 N-finger in erythropoiesis had previously been established [63]. Similarly, repressor of GATA (ROG) was also identified using a yeast two-hybrid screen of a Th-2 cell cDNA library using a GATA-3 zinc finger domain as bait [64]. Friend of GATA-2 (FOG-2) was cloned using 5'- and 3'- RACE technology using degenerate primers against a sequence encoding conserved zinc fingers of FOG-1 [65]. The essential role of FOG proteins has been demonstrated by phenotypes of animals with targeted mutations of these genes. FOG-1$^{-/-}$ mice die at gestational day 10.5–11.5 (e10.5–11.5) due to arrested erythroid maturation, similar to the pathology of GATA-1$^{-/-}$ mice [66]. FOG-2$^{-/-}$ mice die from various cardiac defects [67,68], and knock-in mutations that render FOG-2 incapable of interacting with the cardiac expressed GATA factor GATA-4 result in the same phenotype [69]. These results illustrate the need for intact FOG–GATA interactions in these developmental programs. *In vivo* studies of targeted mutations of ROG have not yet been demonstrated. The role of these co-factors in adipogenesis remains to be examined. FOG co-factors contain multiple zinc fingers that can interact with multiple GATA molecules [70], and may thus function to bring together multiple GATA proteins bound to a number of otherwise distal *cis*-acting regulatory sequences. GATA co-factors could also influence binding specificity to certain target gene-regulatory sequences, or perhaps serve a more general purpose such as the stabilization of protein–DNA interactions during transcription. Alternatively, they may stabilize or even reinforce GATA expression at an early stage of differentiation to silence genes until the cell is cued to enter adipogenesis or even thereafter. In fact, this mechanism has been observed with GATA-2 in erythropoiesis, where expression of a constitutively activated Notch1 receptor prevents down regulation of GATA during erythrocyte differentiation and thus results in acute lymphoblastic leukemia [71].

In addition to assistance by co-factors, GATA proteins are also known to interact with transcriptional co-activators, which contain inherent histone acetyl transferase (HAT) activity, such as CREB-binding protein (CBP/p300). CBP/p300 has been reported to co-precipitate with GATA-1 in nuclear extracts of erythrocytes, and stimulates GATA-1 transcriptional activity in reporter gene assays. CBP/p300 interaction with GATA-1 is mediated by the C-terminal zinc finger on GATA-1 [72], although the N-terminal finger remains a possible mediator as well. CBP/p300 was also reported to transactivate genes dependent on GATA-2, -3, and -4, and co-activate promoters of cardiac and smooth muscle cell genes which are dependent on GATA-4, -5, and -6 [72–75]. On the other hand, GATA can also interact with histone deacetylase (HDAC) proteins. A recent report demonstrated GATA-2 uniquely interacts with HDAC-3 and not other HDAC proteins in hematopoietic cells, and this interaction is abolished when both GATA-2 zinc fingers are deleted. In this study, HDAC-3 was shown to suppress the transactivation potential of GATA-2 on the promoter of β-globin, a GATA-2 dependent gene [76]. It is feasible that GATA factors can either silence transcriptional activation of adipogenic regulators by recruiting proteins with HDAC activity, or trigger their activity by releasing the bound CBP/p300. It remains to be determined whether GATA factors expressed in adipocytes can indeed modulate acetyl transferase activity to remodel chromatin and effect expression of certain genes at appropriate times during differentiation.

5. Future directions

The discovery of a role for GATA transcription factors in adipocyte differentiation is exciting for the insights it provides to the developmental process of adipocyte formation at the cellular level. Of course, there are currently many more questions than there are answers. There is an abundance of mechanistic possibilities by which GATA might regulate adipocyte differentiation. The study of GATA in an *in vivo* experimental system is also necessary to solidify its role as an important transcriptional regulator of adipogenesis, including targeted mutations of regulatory domains, tissue-specific knockout or mutant knock-ins, and finally the excision of GATA during various stages of differentiation. Finally, it remains to be seen whether GATA factors play a role in driving cell-lineage determination of a pluripotent cell or if one exists, a bipotent adipocyte progenitor.

References

[1] B.B. Lowell, B.M. Spiegelman, Towards a molecular understanding of adaptive thermogenesis, Nature 404 (2000) 652–660.
[2] L.J. Bukowiecki, A. Geloen, A.J. Collet, Proliferation and differentiation of brown adipocytes from interstitial cells during cold acclimation, Am. J. Physiol. 250 (1986) C880–C887.

[3] A. Geloen, A.J. Collet, L.J. Bukowiecki, Role of sympathetic innervation in brown adipocyte proliferation, Am. J. Physiol. 263 (1992) R1176–R1181.

[4] M. Klingenberg, S.G. Huang, Structure and function of the uncoupling protein from brown adipose tissue, Biochim. Biophys. Acta 1415 (1999) 271–296.

[5] D.G. Nicholls, R.M. Locke, Thermogenic mechanisms in brown fat, Physiol. Rev. 64 (1984) 1–64.

[6] A.M. Cassard-Doulcier, C. Gelly, F. Bouillaud, D. Ricquier, Tissue-specific and beta-adrenergic regulation of the mitochondrial uncoupling protein gene: control by *cis*-acting elements in the 5'-flanking region, Mol. Endocrinol. 7 (1993) 497–506.

[7] U.C. Kozak, J. Kopecky, J. Teisinger, S. Enerback, B. Boyer, L.P. Kozack, An upstream enhancer regulating brown-fat-specific expression of the mitochondrial uncoupling protein gene, Mol. Cell Biol. 14 (1994) 59–67.

[8] Y.M. Patel, M.D. Lane, Role of calpain in adipocyte differentiation, Proc. Natl. Acad. Sci. USA 96 (1999) 1279–1284.

[9] Q.Q. Tang, T.C. Otto, M.D. Lane, CCAAT/enhancer-binding protein beta is required for mitotic clonal expansion during adipogenesis, Proc. Natl. Acad. Sci. USA 100 (2003) 850–855.

[10] G. Entenmann, H. Hauner, Relationship between replication and differentiation in cultured human adipocyte precursor cells, Am. J. Physiol. 270 (1996) C1011–C1016.

[11] Z. Cao, R.M. Umek, S.L. McKnight, Regulated expression of three C/EBP isoforms during adipose conversion of 3T3-L1 cells, Genes Dev. 5 (1991) 1538–1552.

[12] W.C. Yeh, Z. Cao, M. Classon, S.L. McKnight, Cascade regulation of terminal adipocyte differentiation by three members of the C/EBP family of leucine zipper proteins, Genes Dev. 9 (1995) 168–181.

[13] T. Tanaka, N. Yoshida, T. Kishimoto, S. Akira, Defective adipocyte differentiation in mice lacking the C/EBPbeta and/or C/EBPdelta gene, EMBO J. 16 (1997) 7432–7443.

[14] Z. Wu, E.D. Rosen, R. Brun, S. Hauser, G. Adelmant, A.E. Troy, C. McKeon, G.J. Darlington, B.M. Spiegelman, Cross-regulation of C/EBP alpha and PPAR gamma controls the transcriptional pathway of adipogenesis and insulin sensitivity, Mol. Cell 3 (1999) 151–158.

[15] E.D. Rosen, P. Sarraf, A.E. Troy, G. Bradwin, K. Moore, D.S. Miltone, B.M. Spiegelman, R.M. Mortensen, PPARγ is required for the differentiation of adipose tissue in vivo and in vitro, Mol. Cell 4 (1999) 611–617.

[16] E.D. Rosen, B.M. Spiegelman, Molecular regulation of adipogenesis, Annu. Rev. Cell Dev. Biol. 16 (2000) 145–171.

[17] S.R. Ross, L. Choy, R.A. Graves, N. Fox, V. Solevjeva, S. Klaus, D. Ricquier, B.M. Spiegelman, Hibernoma formation in transgenic mice and isolation of a brown adipocyte cell line expressing the uncoupling protein gene, Proc. Natl. Acad. Sci. USA 89 (1992) 7561–7565.

[18] Y. Irie, A. Asano, X. Canas, H. Nikami, S. Aizawa, M. Saito, Immortal brown adipocytes from p53-knockout mice: differentiation and expression of uncoupling proteins, Biochem. Biophys. Res. Commun. 255 (1999) 221–225.

[19] P. Puigserver, Z. Wu, C.W. Park, R. Graves, M. Wright, B.M. Spiegelman, A cold-inducible coactivator of nuclear receptors linked to adaptive thermogenesis, Cell 92 (1998) 829–839.

[20] B.M. Spiegelman, J.S. Flier, Obesity and the regulation of energy balance, Cell 104 (2001) 531–543.

[21] H. Hauner, K. Rohrig, T. Petruschke, Effects of epidermal growth factor (EGF), platelet-derived growth factor (PDGF) and fibroblast growth factor (FGF) on human adipocyte development and function, Eur. J. Clin. Invest. 25 (1995) 90–96.

[22] L. Choy, J. Skillington, R. Derynck, Roles of autocrine TGF-beta receptor and Smad signaling in adipocyte differentiation, J. Cell Biol. 149 (2000) 667–682.

[23] M. Navre, G.M. Ringold, Differential effects of fibroblast growth factor and tumor promoters on the initiation and maintenance of adipocyte differentiation, J. Cell Biol. 109 (1989) 1857–1863.

[24] G. Serrero, D. Mills, Physiological role of epidermal growth factor on adipose tissue development *in vivo*, Proc. Natl. Acad. Sci. USA 88 (1991) 3912–3916.

[25] J.M. Stephens, M. Butts, R. Stone, P.H. Pekala, D.A. Bernlohr, Regulation of transcription factor mRNA accumulation during 3T3-L1 preadipocyte differentiation by antagonists of adipogenesis, Mol. Cell Biochem. 123 (1993) 63–71.

[26] L. Choy, R. Derynck, TGF-beta inhibits adipocyte differentiation by Smad3 interacting with C/EBP and repressing C/EBP transactivation function, J. Biol. Chem. 278 (2003) 9609–9619.

[27] E. Hu, J.B. Kim, P. Sarraf, B.M. Spiegelman, Inhibition of adipogenesis through MAP kinase-mediated phosphorylation of PPAR gamma, Science 274 (1996) 2100–2103.

[28] J.K. Sethi, G.S. Hotamisligil, The role of TNF alpha in adipocyte metabolism, Semin. Cell Dev. Biol. 10 (1999) 19–29.

[29] H. Xu, J.K. Sethi, G.S. Hotamisligil, Transmembrane tumor necrosis factor (TNF)-alpha inhibits adipocyte differentiation by selectively activating TNF receptor 1, J. Biol. Chem. 274 (1999) 26287–26295.

[30] H. Xu, G.S. Hotamisligil, Signaling pathways utilized by tumor necrosis factor receptor 1 in adipocytes to suppress differentiation, FEBS Lett. 506 (2001) 97–102.

[31] J. Font de Mora, A. Porras, N. Ahn, E. Santos, Mitogen-activated protein kinase activation is not necessary for, but antagonizes, 3T3-L1 adipocytic differentiation, Mol. Cell Biol. 17 (1997) 6068–6075.

[32] J.A. Engelman, A.H. Berg, R.Y. Lewis, M.P. Lisanti, P.E. Scherer, Tumor necrosis factor alpha-mediated insulin resistance, but not dedifferentiation, is abrogated by MEK1/2 inhibitors in 3T3-L1 adipocytes, Mol. Endocrinol. 14 (2000) 1557–1569.

[33] C.M. Smas, H.S. Sul, Pref-1, a protein containing EGF-like repeats, inhibits adipocyte differentiation, Cell 73 (1993) 725–734.

[34] K. Lee, J.A. Villena, Y.S. Moon, K.H. Kim, S. Lee, C. Kang, H.S. Sul, Inhibition of adipogenesis and development of glucose intolerance by soluble preadipocyte factor-1 (Pref-1), J. Clin. Invest. 111 (2003) 453–461.

[35] S.E. Ross, N. Hemati, K.A. Longo, C.N. Bennett, P.C. Lucas, R.L. Erickson, O.A. MacDougald, Inhibition of adipogenesis by Wnt signaling, Science 289 (2000) 950–953.

[36] C.N. Bennett, S.E. Ross, K.A. Longo, L. Bajnok, N. Hemati, K.W. Johnson, S.D. Harrison, O.A. MacDougald, Regulation of Wnt signaling during adipogenesis, J. Biol. Chem. 277 (2002) 30998–31004.

[37] T. Evans, M. Reitman, G. Felsenfeld, An erythrocyte-specific DNA-binding factor recognizes a regulatory sequence common to all chicken globin genes, Proc. Natl. Acad. Sci. USA 85 (1988) 5976–5980.

[38] J.E. Visvader, M. Crossley, J. Hill, S.H. Orkin, J.M. Adams, The C-terminal zinc finger of GATA-1 or GATA-2 is sufficient to induce megakaryocytic differentiation of an early myeloid cell line, Mol. Cell Biol. 15 (1995) 634–641.

[39] D.I. Martin, S.H. Orkin, Transcriptional activation and DNA binding by the erythroid factor GF-1/NF-E1/Eryf 1, Genes Dev. 4 (1990) 1886–1898.

[40] H.Y. Yang, T. Evans, Distinct roles for the two cGATA-1 finger domains, Mol. Cell Biol. 12 (1992) 4562–4570.

[41] S.H. Orkin, GATA-binding transcription factors in hematopoietic cells, Blood 80 (1992) 575–581.

[42] L. Pevny, M.C. Simon, E. Robertson, W.H. Klein, S.F. Tsai, V. D'Agati, S.H. Orkin, F. Costantini, Erythroid differentiation in chimaeric mice blocked by a targeted mutation in the gene for transcription factor GATA-1, Nature 349 (1991) 257–260.

[43] R.J. Arceci, A.A. King, M.C. Simon, S.H. Orkin, D.B. Wilson, Mouse GATA-4: a retinoic acid-inducible GATA-binding transcription factor expressed in endodermally derived tissues and heart, Mol. Cell Biol. 13 (1993) 2235–2246.

[44] E.E. Morrisey, H.S. Ipsdsd, M.M. Lu, M.S. Parmacek, GATA-6: a zinc finger transcription factor that is expressed in multiple cell lineages derived from lateral mesoderm, Dev. Biol. 177 (1996) 309–322.

[45] E.E. Morrisey, H.S. Ip, Z. Tang, M.M. Lu, M.S. Parmacek, GATA-5: a transcriptional activator expressed in a novel temporally and spatially restricted pattern during embryonic development, Dev. Biol. 183 (1997) 21–36.

[46] M. Yamamoto, L.J. Ko, M.W. Leonard, H. Beug, S.H. Orkin, J.D. Engel, Activity and tissue-specific expression of the transcription factor NF-E1 multigene family, Genes Dev. 4 (1990) 1650–1662.

[47] K.P. Rehorn, H. Thelen, A.M. Michelson, R. Reuter, A molecular aspect of hematopoiesis and endoderm development common to vertebrates and Drosophila, Development 122 (1996) 4023–4031.

[48] P. Ramain, P. Heitzler, M. Haenlin, P. Simpson, Pannier, a negative regulator of achaete and scute in Drosophila, encodes a zinc finger protein with homology to the vertebrate transcription factor GATA-1, Development 119 (1993) 1277–1291.

[49] T. Abel, A.M. Michelson, T.A. Maniatis, Drosophila GATA family member that binds to ADH regulatory sequences is expressed in the developing fat body, Development 119 (1993) 623–633.

[50] L.I. Zon, H. Youssoufian, C. Mather, H.F. Lodish, S.H. Orkin, Activation of the erythropoietin receptor promoter by transcription factor GATA-1, Proc. Natl. Acad. Sci. USA 88 (1991) 10638–10641.

[51] A.B. Cantor, S.H. Orkin, Transcriptional regulation of erythropoiesis: an affair involving multiple partners, Oncogene 21 (2002) 3368–3376.

[52] A.C. Mullen, A.S. Hutchins, A.V. Villarino, H.W. Lee, F.A. High, N. Cereb, S.Y. Yang, X. Hua, S.L. Reiner, Cell cycle controlling the silencing and functioning of mammalian activators, Curr. Biol. 11 (2001) 1695–1699.

[53] R.K. Patient, J.D. McGhee, The GATA family (vertebrates and invertebrates), Curr. Opin. Genet. Dev. 12 (2002) 416–422.

[54] J.D. Molkentin, The zinc finger-containing transcription factors GATA-4, -5, and -6. Ubiquitously expressed regulators of tissue-specific gene expression, J. Biol. Chem. 275 (2000) 38949–38952.

[55] Q. Tong, G. Dalgin, H. Xu, C.N. Ting, J.M. Leiden, G.S. Hotamisligil, Function of GATA transcription factors in preadipocyte–adipocyte transition, Science 290 (2000) 134–138.

[56] J. Tsai, Q. Tong, G. Tan, A.N. Chang, S.H. Orkin, G.S. Hotamisligil, The transcription factor GATA-2 regulates differentiation of brown adipocytes, EMBO Rep. 6 (2005) 879–884.

[57] F.Y. Tsai, G. Keller, F.C. Kuo, M. Weiss, J. Chen, M. Rosenblatt, F.W. Alt, S.H. Orkin, An early haematopoietic defect in mice lacking the transcription factor GATA-2, Nature 371 (1994) 221–226.

[58] P.P. Pandolfi, M.E. Roth, A. Karis, M.W. Leonard, E. Dzierzak, F.G. Grosveld, J.D. Engel, M.H. Lindenbaum, Targeted disruption of the GATA-3 gene causes severe abnormalities in the nervous system and in fetal liver haematopoiesis, Nat. Genet. 11 (1995) 40–44.

[59] Q. Tong, J. Tsai, G. Tan, G. Dalgin, G.S. Hotamisligil, Interaction between GATA and the C/EBP family of transcription factors is critical in GATA-mediated suppression of adipocyte differentiation, Mol. Cell Biol. 25 (2005) 706–715.

[60] J. Boyes, P. Byfield, Y. Nakatani, V. Ogryzko, Regulation of activity of the transcription factor GATA-1 by acetylation, Nature 396 (1998) 594–598.

[61] M. Crossley, S.H. Orkin, Phosphorylation of the erythroid transcription factor GATA-1, J. Biol. Chem. 269 (1994) 16589–16596.

[62] R. Menghini, V. Marchetti, M. Cardellini, M.L. Hribal, A. Mauriello, D. Lauro, P. Sbraccia, R. Lauro, M. Federici, Phosphorylation of GATA-2 by Akt increases adipose tissue differentiation and reduces adipose tissue-related inflammation: a novel pathway linking obesity to atherosclerosis, Circulation 111 (2005) 1946–1953.

[63] A.P. Tsang, J.E. Visvader, C.A. Turner, Y. Fujiwara, C. Yu, M.J. Weiss, M. Crossley, S.H. Orkin, FOG, a multitype zinc finger protein, acts as a cofactor for transcription factor GATA-1 in erythroid and megakaryocytic differentiation, Cell 90 (1997) 109–119.

[64] S.C. Miaw, A. Choi, E. Yu, H. Kishikawa, I.C. Ho, ROG, repressor of GATA, regulates the expression of cytokine genes, Immunity 12 (2000) 323–333.

[65] M. Holmes, J. Turner, A. Fox, O. Chisholm, M. Crossley, B. Chong, hFOG-2, a novel zinc finger protein, binds the co-repressor mCtBP2 and modulates GATA-mediated activation, J. Biol. Chem. 274 (1999) 23491–23498.

[66] A.P. Tsang, Y. Fujiwara, D.B. Hom, S.H. Orkin, Failure of megakaryopoiesis and arrested erythropoiesis in mice lacking the GATA-1 transcriptional cofactor FOG, Genes Dev. 12 (1998) 1176–1188.

[67] S.G. Tevosian, A.E. Deconinck, M. Tanaka, M. Schinke, S.H. Litovsky, S. Izumo, Y. Fujiwara, S.H. Orkin, FOG-2, a cofactor for GATA transcription factors, is essential for heart morphogenesis and development of coronary vessels from epicardium, Cell 101 (2000) 729–739.

[68] E.C. Svensson, G.S. Huggins, H. Lin, C. Clendenin, F. Jiang, R. Tufts, F.B. Dardik, J.M. Leiden, A syndrome of tricuspid atresia in mice with a targeted mutation of the gene encoding Fog-2, Nat. Genet. 25 (2000) 353–356.

[69] J.D. Crispino, M.B. Lodish, B.L. Thurberg, S.H. Litovsky, T. Collins, J.D. Molkentin, S.H. Orkin, Proper coronary vascular development and heart morphogenesis depend on interaction of GATA-4 with FOG cofactors, Genes Dev. 15 (2001) 839–844.

[70] A.H. Fox, C. Liew, M. Holmes, K. Kowalski, J. MacKay, M. Crossley, Transcriptional cofactors of the FOG family interact with GATA proteins by means of multiple zinc fingers, EMBO J. 18 (1999) 2812–2822.

[71] K. Kumano, S. Chiba, K. Shimizu, T. Yamagata, N. Hosoya, T. Saito, T. Takahashi, Y. Hamada, H. Hirai, Notch1 inhibits differentiation of hematopoietic cells by sustaining GATA-2 expression, Blood 98 (2001) 3283–3289.

[72] G.A. Blobel, T. Nakajima, R. Eckner, M. Montminy, S.H. Orkin, CREB-binding protein cooperates with transcription factor GATA-1 and is required for erythroid differentiation, Proc. Natl. Acad. Sci. USA 95 (1998) 2061–2066.

[73] Y.S. Dai, B.E. Markham, p300 Functions as a coactivator of transcription factor GATA-4, J. Biol. Chem. 276 (2001) 37178–37185.

[74] T. Kakita, K. Hasegawa, T. Morimoto, S. Kaburagi, H. Wada, S. Sasayama, p300 protein as a coactivator of GATA-5 in the transcription of cardiac-restricted atrial natriuretic factor gene, J. Biol. Chem. 274 (1999) 34096–34102.

[75] H. Wada, K. Hasegawa, T. Morimoto, T. Kakita, T. Yanazume, S. Sasayama, A p300 protein as a coactivator of GATA-6 in the transcription of the smooth muscle-myosin heavy chain gene, J. Biol. Chem. 275 (2000) 25330–25335.

[76] Y. Ozawa, M. Towatari, S. Tsuzuki, F. Hayakawa, T. Maeda, Y. Miyata, M. Tanimoto, H. Saito, Histone deacetylase 3 associates with and represses the transcription factor GATA-2, Blood 98 (2001) 2116–2123.

Chapter 10

Forkhead proteins and the regulation of hepatic gene expression

Andreas Barthel[1], Stephan Herzig[2], Dieter Schmoll[3]

[1]*Department of Medicine I, kliniken Bergmannsheil, Ruhr-University Bochum, Bochum, Germany;*
[2]*Department of Molecular Metabolic Control, German Cancer Research Center, Heidelberg, Germany,*
[3]*DG Metabolic Diseases, Aventis pharma Deutschland, Industriepark Höchst, Frankfurt, Germany*

Abstract

The FoxO proteins belong to a subfamily of forkhead transcription factors, which all have the so-called 'winged-helix' like DNA-binding structure in common. The FoxO-proteins in mammals are homologues of Daf-16 in *Caenorrhabditis elegans*. Based on genetic studies, Daf-16 was initially identified as a factor that is involved in the regulation of the life span of the organism and that is regulated by an insulin-like signaling cascade in *C. elegans*. In mammals, three major insulin-regulated Daf-16 homologues FoxO-family transcription factors have been identified so far: FoxO1 (FKHR), FoxO3a (FKHRL1), and FoxO4 (AFX). In addition to the N-terminal 'winged-helix-domain', these three FoxO-proteins share several structural and functional characteristics. All of them have a C-terminal transactivation domain, a nuclear localization signal (NLS), a nuclear exclusion sequence (NES), and three RxRxxS/T consensus sites for phosphorylation by protein kinase B (PKB), a serine-/threonine kinase, which is activated after stimulation of cells with insulin and other growth factors. Phosphorylation of FoxO-proteins by PKB results in transcriptional inactivation and nuclear exclusion. Initially, the FoxO-transcription factors were thought to bind to the so-called insulin-responsive structures (IRS; (C/G)(A/T)AAA (C/A)A) that are typically present in the promoters of several insulin-regulated genes playing an important role in fuel metabolism, e.g. the phosphoenolpyruvate carboxykinase (PEPCK) and the glucose-6-phosphatase catalytic subunit (G6 Pase). However, FoxO-proteins have pleiotropic biological functions serving as a crossroad to a variety of signaling pathways. Here, we will summarize the role of FoxO-proteins in hepatic gene expression and metabolism.

1. Hepatic fuel metabolism

The quick adaptation to changing environmental conditions represents one of the major achievements in the evolution of higher mammals. In particular, the discontinuous

ADVANCES IN MOLECULAR AND CELLULAR ENDOCRINOLOGY
VOLUME 5 ISSN 1569-2566/DOI 10.1016/S1569-2566(06)05010-1

availability and access to food imposes a major challenge for the survival of the organism. In response, mammals have evolved efficient metabolic systems that allow the critical adaptation to extended periods of starvation and food deprivation [1].

Given its central location within the systemic circulation, the liver serves as the body's critical organ compartment for the conversion, storage, and re-distribution of nutrients and food components. Consequently, as the predominant metabolic checkpoint, the liver plays an essential role in the adaptive response to alterations in food availability such as fasting, caloric restriction, or exercise, and is largely responsible for the maintenance of systemic energy homeostasis [2–4].

1.1. *Regulation of hepatic metabolism by hormones*

Hepatic glucose and lipid metabolism is controlled by the action of counter-regulatory hormones like insulin on the one hand and glucagon, glucocorticoids, and catecholamines on the other [1]. In liver, high-circulating insulin levels favor the synthesis of glycogen and promote the esterification of free fatty acids (FFA) to triglycerides and their packaging into very-low-density lipoprotein (VLDL) particles that are exported to other tissues [5–7]. Simultaneously, apart from its stimulatory effect on glycogen formation and lipogenesis, insulin effectively blocks hepatic glucose production [8,9].

Low concentrations of plasma glucose during fasting, stress, and exercise trigger a series of hormonal cues that promote a switch in whole body energy usage toward catabolic processes. Along with a drop in insulin levels, fasting results in an increased secretion of glucagon from pancreatic α cells, whereas exercise and stress stimulate catecholamine and glucocorticoid release from the adrenal medulla and cortex, respectively [10–13]. These hormones activate triglyceride breakdown via the induction of hormone-sensitive lipase in white adipose tissue and contribute to glycogen degradation in the liver, thereby leading to the release of previously stored glucose depots [14]. The high availability of circulating, adipose tissue-derived lipids determines the enhanced mitochondrial oxidation of FFA in the liver. The entry of long-chain fatty acids into the mitochondria is controlled through the carnitine palmitoyltransferase (CPT) enzyme family in which CPTI is considered to be rate limiting [15]. CPTI transcription is enhanced upon glucagon administration and inhibited by insulin [16,17]. The oxidation end product, acetyl-CoA, serves as substrate for the synthesis of ketone bodies that are used as primary energy source by skeletal muscle or brain after prolonged starvation periods. Apart from providing acetyl-CoA, FFA β-oxidation represents a critical energy provider for hepatic *de novo* glucose synthesis, a process called gluconeogenesis. The gluconeogenic pathway that mainly occurs in parenchymal hepatocytes of the periportal zone represents a prominent feature of liver metabolism. Gluconeogenesis acts as the primary defence mechanism against hypoglycemic conditions through the provision of glucose for extra-hepatic tissues such as erythrocytes, renal medulla, and brain. In the gluconeogenic mode, the human liver can synthesize at least 240 g of glucose per day, representing about twice the amount required by the nervous tissue and erythrocytes in 1 day of food restriction [18–24].

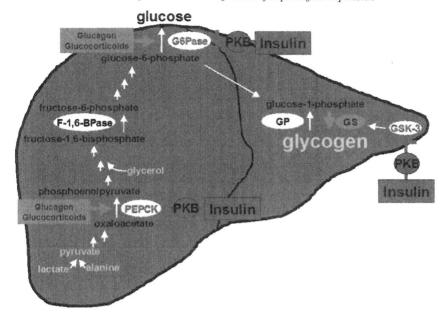

Fig. 1. Regulation of hepatic glucose production. *Note*: Glucagon and glucocorticoids increase hepatic gluconeogenesis by inducing the expression of PEPCK and G6 Pase, two key gluconeogenic enzymes (left). In contrast, insulin inhibits hepatic glucose production by inhibiting gluconeogenesis on the level of G6 Pase and PEPCK gene expression and by stimulating glycogen storage via inhibition of GSK-3 (right). Activation of PKB is a central mechanism in the mediation of the metabolic effects of insulin and parts of the effects of PKB on gene expression are mediated by FoxO-transcription factors. See Plate 9 in Colour Plate Section.

During fasting, lipid- or protein-derived precursors from extra-hepatic tissues, such as lactate (erythrocytes, skeletal muscle) and alanine (muscle), are channelled into the gluconeogenic pathway in which consecutive biochemical steps convert pyruvate to glucose. Main regulatory enzymes comprise pyruvate carboxylase (PC) converting pyruvate into oxaloacetate, PEPCK promoting the decarboxylation of oxaloacetate to phosphoenolpyruvate (see below), and G6 Pase, hydrolysing glucose-6-phosphate into inorganic phosphate and free glucose, which is then delivered into the blood stream [14,19–21,25]. The hormonal regulation of hepatic glucose production is summarized in Fig. 1.

1.2. *Molecular control of hepatic metabolism*

Metabolic control over gluconeogenesis is effectively exerted not only by substrate availability, but in particular through transcriptional regulation of gluconeogenic key enzymes [19,21]. In this regard, PEPCK is considered to be one of the rate-limiting steps in the gluconeogenic pathway. During fasting, expression of the cytosolic form of PEPCK is induced synergistically by glucagon and glucocorticoids, whereas a carbohydrate-rich meal and the concomitant increase in plasma insulin levels acutely inhibit its synthesis rate. The hormonal counter-regulation of PEPCK gene transcription by glucagon, acting through the intracellular second messenger cAMP, and glucocorticoids on the one hand and insulin on the other has been established as the major regulatory axis for PEPCK activity in response to the fasting to feeding transition [21,26–33].

Extensive work over the past years has identified critical hormone-responsive DNA elements within the PEPCK promoter region and their corresponding binding factors. In this regard, several *cis*-acting elements of the PEPCK promoter have been shown to mediate cAMP responsiveness, in particular the so-called cAMP-responsive element (CRE), which is a direct target sequence for the cAMP-responsive element-binding transcription factor (CREB) [34–36] and is located at around −100 bp relative to the PEPCK transcription start site [21,37–39]. Upon binding to this site, CREB mediates cAMP-dependent as well as basal promoter activity [39–43]. Importantly, a functional CRE site is also required for the full glucocorticoid response of the PEPCK promoter, which is conferred by a glucocorticoid-response unit (GRU) located between base pairs −467 and −349 within the PEPCK proximal promoter region. The GRU represents a binding site for multiple transcriptional activators including the glucocorticoid receptor and hepatocyte nuclear factor 4 (HNF-4) [19,43–46].

The molecular basis for the synergism between glucagon and glucocorticoids (e.g. CREB and GRU-binding factors) in the stimulation of PEPCK gene transcription [19,21,42,44,47] has been examined in mouse models harboring a chronic or acute defect in hepatocellular cAMP/CREB signaling. Both transgenic as well as adenovirus-infected mice, expressing a dominant-negative CREB protein [48,49] specifically in liver are profoundly hypoglycemic, and the hepatic RNA levels for the gluconeogenic enzymes PEPCK and G6 Pase are reduced in these animals compared to control littermates [50]. The fact that the G6 Pase promoter lacks a discernable CRE [51] and that the PC gene contains only a weak CRE half-site [52] suggested an indirect role for CREB in the regulation of these gluconeogenic genes and led to the identification of one of the major cAMP/CREB target genes in liver, the nuclear receptor co-activator PGC-1.

Following the early fasting period, in which transcriptional activation of CREB in response to catecholamine and glucagon stimulation induces certain gluconeogenic enzymes (PEPCK) via a direct effect, CREB further potentiates gluconeogenic genes (PEPCK, PC, and G6 Pase) during extended fasting by inducing expression of PGC-1 in liver.

PGC-1 was initially cloned as a co-activator for the nuclear receptor PPARγ in brown adipocytes, responsible for the tissue-specific induction of thermogenesis in response to cold-exposure and β-adrenergic signaling. Subsequent studies identified PGC-1 as a co-activator for multiple nuclear receptors, including the glucocorticoid receptor [53,54] in various cell types [55–58].

In liver, PGC-1 mRNA expression is barely detectable under ad libitum fed conditions. During fasting and in diabetes, however, PGC-1 expression is dramatically upregulated. Studies in isolated hepatocytes demonstrated the ability of PGC-1 to stimulate gluconeogenic enzymes upon overexpression [59]. Importantly, PGC-1 mRNA expression is blocked in the absence of functional cAMP/CREB activity, and the PGC-1 gene promoter was shown to represent a direct CREB target *in vivo*. Consistently, in cultured hepatocytes, PGC-1 promoter activity is efficiently induced by elevated cAMP levels, the effect of which is blocked by dominant-negative CREB, and co-infection with a PGC-1 adenovirus restores fasting glucose levels to near normal and rescues gluconeogenic gene expression in mice lacking functional cAMP-signaling in liver [50].

PGC-1 mediates activation of the PEPCK gene and the entire gluconeogenic program in response to glucocorticoid signals via its interaction with GRU-binding transcription factors, glucocorticoid receptor, and HNF-4 [50,59–61]. This mechanism is likely to explain the long-known observation that the GRU in the PEPCK gene is abnormally activated in type-2 diabetes, and that treatment with glucocorticoid antagonist reduces blood glucose levels in db/db diabetic mice [62]. The induction of PGC-1 by CREB, therefore, serves as a prototypic example of metabolic pathway control through a signal-dependent transcriptional co-activator and provides a molecular rationale for the synergism between glucagon and glucocorticoid signaling in the induction of the gluconeogenic pathway in liver during fasting.

In addition to glucose metabolism, PGC-1 also impacts hepatic lipid metabolism. Toward this end, a direct regulatory function of PGC-1 in the control of CPTI gene expression has been demonstrated, the effect of which is dependent on the interaction with HNF-4 [63]. Also, PGC-1 serves as a potent activator of nuclear receptors PPARα and FXR, thereby promoting FFA combustion in response to fasting signals via the transcriptional induction of mitochondrial β-oxidation enzyme genes [64,65].

1.3. *Pathophysiology of the liver in diabetes*

The most common form of diabetes, the so-called type-2 diabetes, is characterized by the progressive resistance of peripheral tissues to insulin action and the concomitant chronic activation of counter-regulatory hormonal pathways [66].

Molecular analysis has shown that defects in hepatic insulin signaling importantly contribute to the development of systemic peripheral insulin resistance and the concomitant metabolic abnormalities such as hyperglycemia and hyperlipidemia [67]. Transgenic mice with a targeted disruption of the insulin receptor gene in liver (LIRKO mice) display hyperglycemia, hyperinsulinemia, and impaired glucose tolerance, along with aberrant expression of metabolic key enzymes [68].

In the liver, metabolism in diabetes is characterized by an excessive glucose output due to uncontrolled gluconeogenesis, which significantly contributes to diabetic hyperglycemia [14]. In this setting, high-systemic FFA availability attenuates the ability of insulin to suppress glucose production and – via enhanced FFA oxidation – provides acetyl-CoA as a critical substrate for gluconeogenic key enzymes. At the same time, by interfering with pyruvate dehydrogenase activity, acetyl-CoA inhibits glucose utilization, thereby, further promoting cellular insulin resistance and hepatic glucose output [69].

It is commonly accepted that major phenotypic features of diabetic liver metabolism can be attributed to the aberrant expression of corresponding key enzyme genes in the insulin-resistant state [70]. In this regard, elevated expression of PEPCK has been demonstrated in diabetic patients, and overexpression of the PEPCK gene in mice is sufficient to induce hyperglycemia [62,71,72].

As mediators of the counter-regulatory hormonal system, the CREB-PGC-1 pathway is an integral part of the transcriptional machinery controlling PEPCK gene expression. Coincident with elevated blood glucose levels in db/db diabetic mice, PGC-1 and PEPCK mRNA levels are significantly higher in fasted db/db mice relative to wild-type animals. Ablation of CREB activity leads to normoglycemia in db/db mice under fasting conditions and PGC-1 as well as PEPCK RNA levels return to normal. In parallel with the reduction in blood glucose levels, insulin sensitivity is improved in db/db mice deficient in hepatic CREB activity. The improvements in glycemia and insulin resistance due to hepatic inactivation of CREB are likely explained by the inhibition of PGC-1 gene expression and the consequent block of counter-regulatory hormone signaling via glucagon and glucocorticoids. Indeed, liver-specific ablation of PGC-1 mediated by adenoviral-RNA interference strongly improves glucose and insulin tolerance in db/db diabetic animals and reduces gluconeogenic gene expression [73].

In a combinatory fashion, chronically elevated insulin and FFA levels in type-2 diabetes also promote the hepatic overproduction and secretion of VLDLs, thereby significantly contributing to diabetic dyslipidemia [74]. This process seems to be transcriptionally mediated by sterol-regulatory element-binding factor-1c (SREBP-1c; also known as adipocyte differentiation and determination factor ADD-1 [75]). SREBP-1c represents a key factor in the control of insulin-dependent lipogenesis in liver and is overexpressed in mouse models of type-2 diabetes in this tissue [76–80]. Taken together, in the diabetic state the liver shows a mixed pattern of insulin resistance (elevated gluconeogenesis) and insulin sensitivity (increased lipid production). These metabolic properties significantly aggravate systemic insulin resistance and diabetic symptoms and strongly depend on the aberrant activity of distinct transcriptional regulators in liver.

2. Foxo proteins: molecular targets of hormonal regulation

Under normal conditions, the execution of gluconeogenesis and FFA oxidation during fasting and the consequent provision of energy substrates are supported by the concomitant inhibition of insulin-dependent anabolic pathways. In this regard, under the influence of glucagon and glucocorticoids mitochondrial FFA utilization is promoted by the simultaneous repression of insulin-dependent hepatic lipid storage and synthesis (lipogenesis), and end products of FFA oxidation, acetyl-CoA and NADH, serve as allosteric inhibitors of insulin-dependent glycolytic enzymes, isocitrate dehydrogenase, and pyruvate dehydrogenase [14,69,81–84]. On the other hand, insulin efficiently and actively blocks counter-regulatory gluconeogenic and β-oxidation pathways to ensure appropriate energy storage in the fed state [85,86].

The molecular mechanisms controlling the physiological switch from the fed to the fasted state (and vice versa) in response to antagonizing hormonal signals, thus, represent critical checkpoints for the overall metabolic adaptation of liver metabolism to dietary and environmental challenges. The aberrant activity of these control switches is, therefore, importantly involved in the manifestation of insulin resistance and metabolic complications in type-2 diabetes.

All of the actions of insulin are mediated through its membrane-bound receptor, a member of the tyrosine kinase receptor family [87]. Upon insulin binding, the intrinsic tyrosine kinase activity of the insulin receptor at the cell surface becomes activated and leads to the subsequent tyrosine phosphorylation of multiple-signaling components, thereby transducing the insulin signal to downstream cytoplasmic and nuclear effectors [87–92]. Similar to glucagon or glucocorticoids, insulin signal transduction then exerts control over biochemical pathways through either covalent modifications, e.g. phosphorylation/dephosphorylation, of metabolic key enzymes, or through the stimulation or inhibition of the transcriptional activity of its metabolic targets [14,20,25,70,87,93,94].

The FoxO family of transcriptional regulators has been established as one of the key mediators of hormone action on metabolic target gene regulation in the liver.

2.1. *Structure of FoxO-proteins*

Based on common structural similarities of the DNA-binding domain, the FoxO-proteins belong to the family of forkhead transcription factors. FoxO-proteins are highly mobile proteins shuttling between the nucleus and the cytosol within the cell. Multiple structural elements involved in the dynamic regulation of nuclear/cytoplasmic distribution of FoxO-proteins have been identified. So far, two nuclear localization elements (L1 and L2) have been mapped in close proximity to the DNA-binding domain, whereas the three elements identified so far promoting cytoplasmic localization (E1–E3) have been localized in both N-terminal (E1 and E2) and C-terminal (E3) of the DNA-binding domain [95]. FoxO-proteins are highly phosphorylated proteins and phosphorylation is one important mechanism to regulate FoxO-transcriptional activity, DNA binding, and subcellular localization. In *C. elegans*, DAF-16 contains multiple consensus motifs (RXRXXS/T) for phosphorylation by Akt1/2, the homologue to protein kinase B in this worm. The fact that three of these consensus motifs are conserved in the mammalian homologues of DAF-16, FoxO1, FoxO3, and FoxO4, respectively led to the recognition that the PKB-dependent effects of insulin on gene transcription are at least in some cases mediated via PKB-dependent regulation of this group of transcription factors. In addition to phosphorylation by PKB, these FoxO-proteins are substrates of several other kinases including the serum and glucocorticoid-regulated kinase (SGK), casein kinase 1 (CK1), DYRK1, and IkappaB kinase (IKK).

The arrangement and relationship of these regulatory structures (summarized in Fig. 2) is of central importance for the regulation of FoxO-function.

2.2. *Regulation of FoxO-function*

The transcriptional activity of FoxO-proteins is regulated at multiple levels. Covalent modifications of FoxO-proteins include phosphorylation and acetylation events. Other mechanisms of controlling FoxO-activity include modulation of the cellular

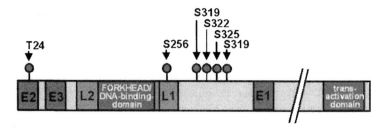

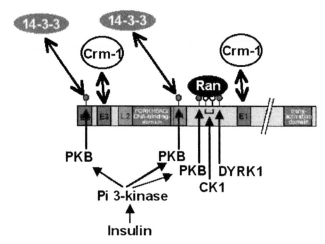

Fig. 2. The structure and regulation of FoxO-proteins. *Note*: Upper panel: phosphorylation sites and structural elements involved in the nuclear/cytoplasmic distribution of FoxO1. Lower panel: phosphorylation of FoxO-proteins by PKB, CK1, and DYRK1 results in inactivation and cytoplasmic localization by facilitating the interaction of FoxO-proteins with proteins of the nuclear export machinery like Crm1, 14-3-3, and Ran. See Plate 10 in Colour Plate Section.

FoxO-protein level by affecting FoxO-protein stability or FoxO-gene expression and also regulation of FoxO-activity by protein–protein interactions.

2.2.1. *Phosphorylation and acetylation of FoxO-proteins*
The phosphorylation of FoxO-proteins in response to insulin reduces the transcriptional activity of the transcription factor by a combination of multiple processes: a decrease of DNA-binding affinity, the nuclear exclusion of the transcription factor, and the prevention of interaction with other proteins of the transcriptional machinery.

First, in the case of FoxO1 the phosphorylation of serine 256 by PKB has been reported to decrease the DNA-binding ability of FoxO1 [96]. *In-vitro* studies have shown that mutation of the serine residue 256 into the amino acid aspartate strongly reduces the binding affinity of FoxO1 proteins to double-stranded oligonucleotides in gel-shift assays. This could be explained by the electrostatic repulsion of the introduced negatively charged aspartate residue, since serine 256 is located within a basic region that plays a role in DNA binding. It is thought that introduction of negative charges into this region by phosphorylation of the serine residue acts in a similar way.

Second, an additional level of regulation of FoxO-activity is the nuclear exclusion of the transcription factor in response to insulin. This shift of the equilibrium from the nuclear toward the cytosolic fraction of the protein might be due to several mechanisms. For example, it is possible that a reduced retention of the phosphorylated protein in the nucleus arises simply by the decreased DNA-binding ability after phosphorylation of serine 256, although other, more complicated mechanisms may exist. In contrast, the phosphorylated FoxO proteins could also be retained in the cytoplasm. This could be due to masking of the NLS within the FoxO-protein, thereby preventing access of the nuclear import machinery to the transcription factor. It is possible that this masking process is mediated by the phosphorylation of threonine 24 or serine 256 itself resulting in conformational changes of the transcription factor or by the interaction of FoxO-proteins with 14-3-3 proteins, since these proteins have been found to bind to the phosphorylated FoxO-proteins [95,97–99]. Hyperphosphorylation of FoxO-proteins could also promote the nuclear export. The phosphorylation of serine 256 in FoxO1 is regarded as gatekeeper for the subsequent phosphorylation of threonine 24 and serine 319 [100]. The phosphorylation of threonine 24 and serine 319 by PKB, serine 329 by DYRK1 as well as phosphorylation of serine 322 and 325 by casein kinase 1 have all been described as critical for the subcellular localization of FoxO [96,101,102]. Even more complex, there is a tight functional interdependence between phosphorylation of the serine residues 319, 322, and 325, since phosphorylation of serine 319 has been described to be a prerequisite for phosphorylation of the latter serine residues [102]. The precise molecular mechanisms of the nuclear export of hyperphosphorylated FoxO-proteins are not fully characterized. The fact that the nuclear exclusion of FoxO-proteins is sensitive to leptomycin B indicates a participation of Crm1, a nuclear export receptor that binds to the small GTPase Ran [98,102]. In addition, phosphorylation of the residues serine 322 and 325 in FoxO1 has been demonstrated to enhance the association with a complex containing the GTPase Ran and might thereby stimulate the export [102].

Recently, two different groups proposed the regulation of FoxO-activity by covalent modification with acetyl residues [103,104]. In this scenario, FoxO-proteins become acetylated by the acetyltransferase activity of CBP/p300. This process is reversed by the enzymatic activity of Sirtuins, a family of deacetylases, adding FoxOs to the list of Sirtuin targets. However, the functional implications of acetylation/deacetylation of FoxO-proteins are currently unclear.

The regulation of FoxO-proteins by posttranslational covalent mechanisms is summarized in Table 1.

2.2.2. *FoxO-stability and FoxO-gene expression*

FoxO-activity is not only regulated by posttranslational mechanisms, but also by regulation of FoxO-gene expression. For example, starvation has been described to

Table 1
Summary of posttranslational modifications of FoxO-proteins

Modifying enzyme	Type of modification	Site	Effect on FoxO	Reference
PKB/SGK	Phosphorylation	Thr-24 (FoxO1), Thr-32 (FoxO3A), Thr-29 (FoxO4)	14-3-3 binding, nuclear exlusion, blocking of DNA binding	95,97,136,137
PKB	Phosphorylation	Ser-256 (FoxO1), Ser-253 (FoxO3A), Ser-193 (FoxO4)	14-3-3 binding, nuclear exclusion, reduction of DNA binding, inhibition of transactivation	95–97,99
PKB/SGK	Phosphorylation	Ser-319 (FoxO1), Ser-315 (FoxO3a), Ser-258 (FoxO4)	Nuclear exclusion	95,102,136
CKI	Phosphorylation	Ser-322/Ser-325 (FoxO1)	Nuclear exclusion	102
DYRK	Phosphorylation	Ser-329 (FoxO1), Ser-269 (FoxO4)	Nuclear exclusion	101
IKK	Phosphorylation	Ser-644 (FoxO3A)	Ubiquitination and degradation	138
? (Ras/Ral-regulated kinase)	Phosphorylation	Thr-447/Thr-451 (FoxO4)	Transactivation activity, potentiation of PKB regulation	139
CBP/p300	Acetylation	Lys-242/Lys-245/Lys-262 (FoxO1)	Gene-specific modulation of transactivation activity	103,104,140,141
SIR2	Deacetylation	Lys-242/Lys-245/Lys-262 (FoxO1)	Gene-specific modulation of transactivation activity	103,104,140,141
	Ubiquitination		Proteosomal degradation	138

result in an increase of FoxO1, 3, and 4 expression in liver and of FoxO1 and 3 in muscle [105,106]. The levels of FoxO-proteins are also elevated in db/db and streptozotocin-induced diabetic mice [105–107]. The molecular background of the regulation of FoxO-gene transcription is not yet clear.

Another major mechanism of regulating FoxO-activity is based on specific degradation of FoxO-proteins. It has been reported recently that activaton of PI 3-kinase/PKB-signaling results in ubiquitination of FoxO1a and FoxO3 with consecutive proteasomal degradation [108,109]. Interestingly, targeting of the FoxO-proteins to the proteasome depends on the same phosphorylation events that result in nuclear export of the forkhead proteins into the cytosol [108]. This combination of multiple regulatory mechanisms makes sense from the mechanistic point of view, because proteasomal degradation takes place in the cytoplasm. Ubiquitination and proteasomal degradation of FoxO1a is also a potential mechanism that may occur after activation of AMP-kinase, a kinase that may mimick some insulin-like biological effects, e.g. inhibition of gluconeogenesis in hepatic cells [110]. Other, less well-characterized mechanisms of proteolytic regulation of FoxO-proteins include the caspase-3-dependent degradation of FoxO3a during apoptosis in T lymphocytes [111].

2.2.3. *FoxO-interacting proteins*

Besides by covalent modification and changes of gene expression, FoxO-protein activity is also controlled by direct protein–protein interactions (Table 2). This mechanism can modulate DNA-binding affinity or subcellular localization of FoxO-proteins, as exemplified by the interaction with 14-3-3 proteins [112,113]. The docking of 14-3-3 to FoxO is special among those proteins listed in Table 1, as it requires FoxO to be phosphorylated at the P1 (threonine 24) and P2 (serine 256) sites, whereas the other interaction partners bind to the unphosphorylated form. Furthermore, protein–protein interactions also allow the recruitment of co-activators, such as CBP, p300, SRC-1, and peroxisome proliferator-activated receptor-γ co-activator 1α (PGC-1α) to gene promoters with a FoxO-binding site [56,114,115]. These co-activators mediate the contact to the transcriptional machinery. CBP, p300, and SRC-1 also re-model the structure of the chromatin by their histone acetyl-transferase activity (HAT), which modulates the access of transcription factors to a gene promoter. The acetyltransferase activity of the co-activator proteins could also control the transcriptional activity by the direct acetylation of FoxO proteins (see above). Nasrin et al. [114] describe differences among the members of the FoxO family in the ability to bind to co-activator proteins. FoxO1 and FoxO3A bind to CBP, p300, and SRC-1, but FoxO4 only to CBP and p300. The data suggest that the C-terminus of all FoxO-proteins may interact with the KIX domain of CBP and p300. In addition, FoxO1 and FoxO3A bind via an additional site to the C/H3 domain of CBP and to SRC. This site could be located within the N-terminus of the FoxO proteins, as the first 52 amino acids at the N-terminus of FoxO3A are able to interact with p300 [115]. Differential recruitment of co-activators through FoxO proteins could explain why, in contrast to FoxO1 and FoxO3A, overexpressed FoxO4 stimulated only basal expression, and not glucocorticoid induction of the IGFBP-1 gene [114]. PGC-1α binds to the C-terminus of FoxO1 and is an additional co-activator of FoxO-dependent gene transcription in liver [56]. PGC-1α lacks HAT activity and induces gene expression probably by the recruitment of additional co-activators, such as CBP, p300, and SRC-1. The prevention of the interaction between FoxO1 and PGC-1α by insulin-induced phosphorylation of FoxO1 mediates in part the suppression of G6 Pase and PEPCK expression by this hormone [56].

G6 Pase promoter activity is also stimulated by the interaction between FoxO1 and DYRK1, while the DYRK2 isoform has no effect [116]. This stimulation was

Table 2
Overview on FoxO-interacting proteins in hepatic cells

Interacting protein	Proposed physiological function	Reference
14-3-3	Decrease of FoxO-dependent gene expression by suppression of DNA binding and promotion of nuclear export as well as cytosolic sequestration of phosphorylated FoxO	112,113
CBP, p300	Regulation of cell cycle and apoptosis in erythroid progenitor cells in the absence of erythropoietin	115
CBP/p300/ SRC	Basal and glucocorticoid-induced expression of FoxO-regulated genes such as IGFBP-1	114
PGC-1α	Induction of FoxO-regulated genes such as G6 Pase and PEPCK	56
ER	Estrogen–mediated regulation of ER-dependent gene expression: repression of ER-dependent gene expression (HepG2), stimulation of ER-dependent gene expression (MCF7 cells), repression of FoxO-dependent gene expression, regulation of cell proliferation	124,125
SHP	Repression of gluconeogenic key enzymes, such as G6 Pase, in response to bile acids	117
CAR, PXR	Co-activation of CAR- and PXR-mediated transcription of drug-metabolizing enzymes. Inhibition of FoxO1-mediated induction of gluconeogenic genes	118
DYRK	Stimulation of the expression of FoxO-regulated genes, such as G6 Pase	116
STAT3	Stimulation of IL6-regulated genes, such as α2-macroglobulin	142
HNF-4	Inhibition of HNF-4-dependent gene expression, regulation of glycolysis/gluconeogenesis (?)	123

also observed with a kinase-deficient DYRK1. The mechanism for the co-activation of promoter activity by DYRK1 is not known.

FoxO1 binds with its C-terminus to the N-terminus of the atypical orphan nuclear receptor small heterodimer partner (SHP) [117]. This prevents the docking of co-activator proteins, such as CBP. As bile acids induce SHP expression in liver, a competition between co-activators and SHP for FoxO1 could explain the mechanism by which bile acids reduce the expression of key gluconeogenic enzymes, such as G6 Pase.

Apart from co-activator proteins, FoxO proteins can also form complexes with other transcription factors on gene promoters. In liver, FoxO1 has been shown to act as a co-activator for CAR and PXR in the stimulation of drug-metabolizing enzymes, such as cytochrom P450. On the other hand, following the activation of PXR and CAR by phentobarbital, the transcription factors block the induction of genes by FoxO1-encoding gluconeogenic enzymes [118]. Additional transcription factors interacting with FoxO proteins are SMAD3, SMAD4, and C/EBPβ [119,120]. In the latter case, FoxO1 and C/EBPβ bind to adjacent sites within the decidual prolactin

domain, led to a reduction of both fed and fasted blood glucose levels by approximately 25% within 4 days [107]. Similar results were obtained by using diabetic db/db mice. Furthermore, the hepatic expression of the key gluconeogenic enzymes G6 Pase and PEPCK was significantly decreased. These data are supported by the phenotype of mice that overexpress a constitutively active FoxO1 mutant (FoxO1-S253A) in the liver. These animals become glucose intolerant with a fasting hyperglycemia and hyper-insulinemia, and increased expression of G6 Pase. These animal models suggest a role of FoxO1 in the control of hepatic glucose metabolism by the regulation of genes such as G6 Pase. The potential role of FoxO1 in promoting hepatic glucose production is supported by the observation that FoxO1 protein levels are increased during starvation. The plasma concentration of the gluconeogenic substrate lactate and the hepatic gly-cogen content was not significantly changed in these models [107,129]. Therefore, in order to assess whether gluconeogenesis is the main target of FoxO1 *in vivo*, a detailed analysis of the metabolic fluxes in the respective animals models is required. Further-more, additional studies are necessary to exploit an *in-vivo* function of FoxO proteins in the regulation of ketogenesis, drug metabolism, and the expression of acute phase proteins, which has been suggested by *in-vitro* data.

One particular animal model has directly linked FoxO1 with insulin action in liver: the partial knockout of the FoxO1 gene almost completely reverses insulin resistance in an animal model with haploinsufficiency of the *insulin receptor* gene and protects it against the development of diabetes [129]. This could be due to improved hepatic insulin sensitivity, because G6 Pase gene expression as well as plasma insulin levels was decreased. Interestingly, in the diabetic db/db mouse model, the levels of FoxO1 expression were increased and, in contrast to the heterozygous mice, FoxO1 was localized mainly in the nucleus. This may reflect the impaired insulin signaling [107].

However, FoxO-proteins do not only control metabolism and the effects of insulin on the liver, but also in pancreatic β cells, adipocytes, and skeletal muscle. For example, overexpression of a constitutively active FoxO1 mutant in β cells promotes the onset of diabetes by β-cell dysfunction, whereas haploinsufficiency of FoxO1 protects against β-cell failure in IRS2 null mice [130]. This points to an important role of FoxO1 in β-cell differentiation, perhaps by its ability to repress the expression of the key regulator of β-cell development PDX-1 in a Foxa2-dependent way [130]. Furthermore, a constitutively active FoxO1 mutant prevents the differentiation of adipocytes *in vitro* and FoxO1 (+/−) mice are protected against diet-induced diabetes [132]. Although these animals become obese, they do not show fat cell hypertrophy. In addition, they have reduced levels of the adipokines TNFα and resistin, which have been associated with the development of insulin resistance. These observations have been explained by the ability of FoxO1 to upregulate the cell cycle inhibitor p21 in preadipocytes. This prevents their clonal expansion and subsequent differentiation [132]. An additional mechanism for the control of adipogenesis by FoxO proteins could be due to their ability to suppress the function of PPARγ by a direct protein–protein interaction [122] as discussed above. Furthermore, in skeletal muscle the oxidative phosphorylation of glucose is decreased, whereas the utilization of lipids is increased during starvation and exercise as well as in an animal model of type-1 diabetes. This is associated with an increased expression of pyruvate dehydrogenase kinase 4 (PDK4) and lipoprotein lipase (LPL) in muscle, which decreases flux through pyruvate dehydrogenase and enhances uptake of fatty acids, respectively. Interestingly, under these conditions FoxO1 and FoxO3A protein levels are increased in muscle and these proteins have been shown to stimulate the expression of PDK4 and LPL in muscle cells *in vitro* [106,133,134]. These data suggest that FoxO proteins also possess an important regulatory function for muscle metabolism.

FoxO-proteins and FoxO1 in particular may be regarded as opponents of insulin action. Furthermore, their inactivation seems to be an important part of intracellular insulin signaling *in vivo* and a central mechanism for the control of metabolism by this hormone. In addition, increased FoxO-activity can contribute to the diabetic phenotype in several animal models by the induction of hepatic insulin resistance and an impaired β-cell development and adipocyte differentiation. However, there may be exceptions from the assumption that FoxO-proteins are generally insulin antagonists with pro-diabetic function. For example, FoxO1 has been recently shown to be involved in the induction of the gene encoding the adiponectin receptor adipoR1/2 during starvation [135]. As adiponectin is regarded as a mediator of insulin sensitivity, an upregulation of adipoR1/2 can be postulated as a mechanism for the treatment of diabetes.

4. Conclusions

Based on several experimental approaches, forkhead proteins of the FoxO family of transcription factors have been recognized as central master switches and integrators of hepatic fuel metabolism. We have now accumulated compelling evidence that FoxO-proteins are critical elements in the mediation of a variety of metabolic responses of the organism to insulin and in particular in the regulation of hepatic glucose production. Furthermore, an impairment of FoxO-functions results in characteristic pathophysiological changes in metabolism culminating in a diabetic phenotype. Thus, FoxO-proteins and their function can be regarded as rational drug targets for the treatment of diabetes. Accordingly, the recognition that FoxO proteins are of central importance in the regulation of hepatic gene expression and metabolism and the detailed understanding of FoxO-functions forms a promising basis for the translational approach toward more effective strategies to treat this disease.

References

[1] G. van den Berghe, The role of the liver in metabolic homeostasis: implications for inborn errors of metabolism, J. Inherit Metab. Dis. 14 (1991) 407–420.
[2] K. Casteels, C. Mathieu, Diabetic ketoacidosis, Rev. Endoc. Metab. Disord. 4 (2003) 159–166.
[3] V.A. Zammit, A.M. Moir, Monitoring the partitioning of hepatic fatty acids *in vivo*: keeping track of control, Trends Biochem. Sci. 19 (1994) 313–317.
[4] V.A. Zammit, Role of insulin in hepatic fatty acid partitioning: emerging concepts, Biochem. J. 314 (1996) 1–14.
[5] B. Desvergne, W. Wahli, Peroxisome proliferator-activated receptors: nuclear control of metabolism, Endocr. Rev. 20 (1999) 649–688.

[6] J.M. Duerden, S.M. Bartlett, G.F. Gibbons, Regulation of very-low-density-lipoprotein lipid secretion in hepatocyte cultures derived from diabetic animals, Biochem. J. 262 (1989) 313–319.

[7] J.M. Argiles, S. Busquets, F.J. Lopez-Soriano, Metabolic interrelationships between liver and skeletal muscle in pathological states, Life Sci. 69 (2001) 1345–1361.

[8] Y.T. Kruszynska, J.M. Olefsky, Cellular and molecular mechanisms of non-insulin dependent diabetes mellitus, J. Investig. Med. 44 (1996) 413–428.

[9] R.M. O'Brien, D.K. Granner, Regulation of gene expression by insulin, Biochem. J. 278 (1991) 609–619.

[10] R.C. Andrews, B.R. Walker, Glucocorticoids and insulin resistance: old hormones, new targets, Clin. Sci. (Lond.) 96 (1999) 513–523.

[11] R. Rosmond, P. Bjorntorp, The hypothalamic-pituitary-adrenal axis activity as a predictor of cardiovascular disease, type 2 diabetes and stroke, J. Intern. Med. 247 (2000) 188–197.

[12] R.H. Unger, L. Orc, Glucagon and the A cell: physiology and pathophysiology (second of two parts), N. Engl. J. Med. 304 (1981) 1575–1580.

[13] R.H. Unger, L. Orc, Glucagon and the A cell: physiology and pathophysiology (first two parts), N. Engl. J. Med. 304 (1981) 1518–1524.

[14] A.R. Saltiel, New perspectives into the molecular pathogenesis and treatment of type 2 diabetes, Cell 104 (2001) 517–529.

[15] J.D. McGarry, N.F. Brown, The mitochondrial carnitine palmitoyltransferase system. From concept to molecular analysis, Eur. J. Biochem. 244 (1997) 1–14.

[16] F. Chatelain, C. Kohl, V. Esser, J.D. McGarry, J. Girard, J.P. Pegorier, Cyclic AMP and fatty acids increase carnitine palmitoyltransferase I gene transcription in cultured fetal rat hepatocytes, Eur. J. Biochem. 235 (1996) 789–798.

[17] J.F. Louet, C. Le May, J.P. Pegorier, J.F. Decaux, J. Girard, Regulation of liver carnitine palmitoyltransferase I gene expression by hormones and fatty acids, Biochem. Soc. Trans. 29 (2001) 310–316.

[18] A. Consoli, Role of liver in pathophysiology of NIDDM, Diabetes Care 15 (1992) 430–441.

[19] F.P. Lemaigre, G.G. Rousseau, Transcriptional control of genes that regulate glycolysis and gluconeogenesis in adult liver, Biochem. J. 303 (1994) 1–14.

[20] R.C. Nordlie, J.D. Foster, A.J. Lange, Regulation of glucose production by the liver, Annu. Rev. Nutr. 19 (1999) 379–406.

[21] R.W. Hanson, L. Reshef, Regulation of phosphoenolpyruvate carboxykinase (GTP) gene expression, Annu. Rev. Biochem. 66 (1997) 581–611.

[22] K. Jungermann, Metabolic zonation of liver parenchyma, Semin. Liver Dis. 8 (1988) 329–341.

[23] K. Jungermann, N. Katz, Functional specialization of different hepatocyte populations, Physiol. Rev. 69 (1989) 708–764.

[24] K. Jungermann, T. Kietzmann, Zonation of parenchymal and nonparenchymal metabolism in liver, Annu. Rev. Nutr. 16 (1996) 179–203.

[25] S.J. Pilkis, D.K. Granner, Molecular physiology of the regulation of hepatic gluconeogenesis and glycolysis, Annu. Rev. Physiol. 54 (1992) 885–909.

[26] J.M. Gunn, R.W. Hanson, O. Meyuhas, L. Reshef, F.J. Ballard, Glucocorticoids and the regulation of phosphoenolpyruvate carboxykinase (guanosine triphosphate) in the rat, Biochem. J. 150 (1975) 195–203.

[27] D. Kioussis, J. Reshef, H. Cohen, S.M. Tilghman, P.B. Iynedjian, F.J. Ballard, R.W. Hanson, Alterations in translatable messenger RNA coding for phosphoenolpyruvate carboxykinase (GTP) in rat liver cytosol during deinduction, J. Biol. Chem. 253 (1978) 4327–4332.

[28] S.M. Tilghman, J.M. Gunn, L.M. Fisher, R.W. Hanson, Deinduction of phosphoenolpyruvate carboxykinase (guanosine triphosphate) synthesis in Reuber H-35 cells, J. Biol. Chem. 250 (1975) 3322–3329.

[29] S.M. Tilghman, R.W. Hanson, L. Reshef, M.F. Hopgood, F.J. Ballard, Rapid loss of translatable messenger RNA of phosphoenolpyruvate carboxykinase during glucose repression in liver, Proc. Natl. Acad. Sci. USA 71 (1974) 1304–1308.

[30] P.B. Iynedjian, F.J. Ballard, R.W. Hanson, The regulation of phosphoenolpyruvate carboxykinase (GTP) synthesis in rat kidney cortex. The role of acid–base balance and glucocorticoids, J. Biol. Chem. 250 (1975) 5596–5603.

[31] P.B. Iynedjian, R.W. Hanson, Messenger RNA for renal phosphoenolpyruvate carboxykinase (GTP). Its translation in a heterologous cell-free system and its regulation by glucocorticoids and by changes in acid–base balance, J. Biol. Chem. 252 (1977) 8398–8403.

[32] P.B. Iynedjian, R.W. Hanson, Increase in level of functional messenger RNA coding for phosphoenolpyruvate carboxykinase (GTP) during induction by cyclic adenosine 3':5'-monophosphate, J. Biol. Chem. 252 (1977) 655–662.

[33] D.S. Loose, D.K. Cameron, H.P. Short, R.W. Hanson, Thyroid hormone regulates transcription of the gene for cytosolic phosphoenolpyruvate carboxykinase (GTP) in rat liver, Biochemistry 24 (1985) 4509–4512.

[34] M.R. Montminy, G.A. Gonzalez, K.K. Yamamoto, Regulation of cAMP-inducible genes by CREB, Trends Neurosci. 13 (1990) 184–188.

[35] M.R. Montminy, K.A. Sevarino, J.A. Wagner, G. Mandel, R.H. Goodman, Identification of a cyclic-AMP-responsive element within the rat somatostatin gene, Proc. Natl. Acad. Sci. USA 83 (1986) 6682–6686.

[36] M. Montminy, Transcriptional regulation by cyclic AMP, Annu. Rev. Biochem. 66 (1997) 807–822.

[37] W.J. Roesler, G.R. Vandenbark, R.W. Hanson, Identification of multiple protein binding domains in the promoter-regulatory region of the phosphoenolpyruvate carboxykinase (GTP) gene, J. Biol. Chem. 264 (1989) 9657–9664.

[38] J.M. Short, A. Wynshaw-Boris, H.P. Short, R.W. Hanson, Characterization of the phosphoenolpyruvate carboxykinase (GTP) promoter-regulatory region. II. Identification of cAMP and glucocorticoid regulatory domains, J. Biol. Chem. 261 (1986) 9721–9726.

[39] E.A. Park, A.L. Gurney, S.E. Nizielski, P. Hakimi, Z. Cao, A. Moorman, R.W. Hanson, Relative roles of CCAAT/enhancer-binding protein beta and cAMP regulatory element-binding protein in controlling transcription of the gene for phosphoenolpyruvate carboxykinase (GTP), J. Biol. Chem. 268 (1993) 613–619.

[40] J.S. Liu, E.A. Park, A.L. Gurney, W.J. Roesler, R.W. Hanson, Cyclic AMP induction of phosphoenolpyruvate carboxykinase (GTP) gene transcription is mediated by multiple promoter elements, J. Biol. Chem. 266 (1991) 19095–19102.

[41] P.G. Quinn, D.K. Granner, Cyclic AMP-dependent protein kinase regulates transcription of the phosphoenolpyruvate carboxykinase gene but not binding of nuclear factors to the cyclic AMP regulatory element, Mol. Cell Biol. 10 (1990) 3357–3364.

[42] E. Imai, J.N. Miner, J.A. Mitchell, K.R. Yamamoto, D.K. Granner, Glucocorticoid receptor-cAMP response element-binding protein interaction and the response of the phosphoenolpyruvate carboxykinase gene to glucocorticoids, J. Biol. Chem. 268 (1993) 5353–5356.

[43] L. Xing, P.G. Quinn, Involvement of 3',5'-cyclic adenosine monophosphate regulatory element binding protein (CREB) in both basal and hormone-mediated expression of the phosphoenolpyruvate carboxykinase (PEPCK) gene, Mol. Endocrinol. 7 (1993) 1484–1494.

[44] E. Imai, P.E. Stromstedt, P.G. Quinn, J. Carlstedt-Duke, J.A. Gustafsson, D.K. Granner, Characterization of a complex glucocorticoid response unit in the phosphoenolpyruvate carboxykinase gene, Mol. Cell Biol. 10 (1990) 4712–4719.

[45] R.K. Hall, D.K. Scott, E.L. Noisin, P.C. Lucas, D.K. Granner, Activation of the phosphoenolpyruvate carboxykinase gene retinoic acid response element is dependent on a retinoic acid receptor/coregulator complex, Mol. Cell Biol. 12 (1992) 5527–5535.

[46] H. Meisner, D.S. Loose, R.W. Hanson, Effect of hormones on transcription of the gene for cytosolic phosphoenolpyruvate carboxykinase (GTP) in rat kidney, Biochemistry 24 (1985) 421–425.

[47] P.O. Angrand, C. Coffinier, M.C. Weiss, Response of the phosphoenolpyruvate carboxykinase gene to glucocorticoids depends on the integrity of the cAMP pathway, Cell Growth Differ. 5 (1994) 957–966.

[48] F. Long, E. Schipani, H. Asahara, H. Kronenberg, M. Montminy, The CREB family of activators is required for endochondral bone development, Development 128 (2001) 541–550.

[49] S. Ahn, M. Olive, S. Aggarwal, D. Krylov, D.D. Ginty, C. Vinson, Dominant-negative inhibitor of CREB reveals that it is a general mediator of stimulus-dependent transcription of c-fos, Mol. Cell Biol. 18 (1998) 967–977.

[50] S. Herzig, F. Long, U.S. Jhala, S. Hedrick, R. Quinn, A. Bauer, D. Rudolph, G. Schutz, C. Yoon, P. Puigserver, B. Spiegelman, M. Montminy, CREB regulates hepatic gluconeogenesis through the coactivator PGC-1, Nature 413 (2001) 179–183.

[51] D. Schmoll, C. Wasner, C.J. Hinds, B.B. Allan, R. Walther, A. Burchell, Identification of a cAMP response element within the glucose-6-phosphatase hydrolytic subunit gene promoter which is involved in the transcriptional regulation by cAMP and glucocorticoids in H4IIE hepatoma cells, Biochem. J. 338 (1999) 457–463.

[52] S. Jitrapakdee, G.W. Booker, A.I. Cassady, J.C. Wallace, The rat pyruvate carboxylase gene structure. Alternate promoters generate multiple transcripts with the 5′-end heterogeneity,, J. Biol. Chem. 272 (1997) 20522–20530.

[53] D. Knutti, A. Kaul, A. Kralli, A tissue-specific coactivator of steroid receptors, identified in a functional genetic screen, Mol. Cell Biol. 20 (2000) 2411–2422.

[54] D. Knutti, A. Kralli, PGC-1, a versatile coactivator, Trends Endocrinol. Metab. 12 (2001) 360–365.

[55] P. Puigserver, Z. Wu, C.W. Park, R. Graves, M. Wright, B.M. Spiegelman, A cold-inducible coactivator of nuclear receptors linked to adaptive thermogenesis, Cell 92 (1998) 829–839.

[56] P. Puigserver, J. Rhee, J. Donovan, C.J. Walkey, J.C. Yoon, F. Oriente, Y. Kitamura, J. Altomonte, H. Dong, D. Accili, B.M. Spiegelman, Insulin-regulated hepatic gluconeogenesis through FOXO1-PGC-1alpha interaction, Nature 423 (2003) 550–555.

[57] P. Puigserver, B.M. Spiegelman, Peroxisome proliferator-activated receptor-gamma coactivator 1 alpha (PGC-1 alpha): transcriptional coactivator and metabolic regulator, Endocr. Rev. 24 (2003) 78–90.

[58] P. Puigserver, G. Adelmant, Z. Wu, M. Fan, J. Xu, B. O'Malley, B.M. Spiegelman, Activation of PPARgamma coactivator-1 through transcription factor docking, Science 286 (1999) 1368–1371.

[59] J.C. Yoon, P. Puigserver, G. Chen, J. Donovan, Z. Wu, J. Rhee, G. Adelmant, J. Stafford, C.R. Kahn, D.K. Granner, C.B. Newgard, B.M. Spiegelman, Control of hepatic gluconeogenesis through the transcriptional coactivator PGC-1, Nature 413 (2001) 131–138.

[60] J. Rhee, Y. Inoue, J.C. Yoon, P. Puigserver, M. Fan, F.J. Gonzalez, B.M. Spiegelman, Regulation of hepatic fasting response by PPARgamma coactivator-1alpha (PGC-1): requirement for hepatocyte nuclear factor 4alpha in gluconeogenesis, Proc. Natl. Acad. Sci. USA 100 (2003) 4012–4017.

[61] J.N. Boustead, B.T. Stadelmaier, A.M. Eeds, P.O. Wiebe, C.A. Svitek, J.K. Oeser, R.M. O'Brien, Hepatocyte nuclear factor-4 alpha mediates the stimulatory effect of peroxisome proliferator-activated receptor gamma co-activator-1 alpha (PGC-1 alpha) on glucose-6-phosphatase catalytic subunit gene transcription in H4IIE cells, Biochem. J. 369 (2003) 17–22.

[62] J.E. Friedman, Y. Sun, T. Ishizuka, C.J. Farrell, S.E. McCormack, L.M. Herron, P. Hakimi, P. Lechner, J.S. Yun, Phosphoenolpyruvate carboxykinase (GTP) gene transcription and hyperglycemia are regulated by glucocorticoids in genetically obese db/db transgenic mice, J. Biol. Chem. 272 (1997) 31475–31481.

[63] J.F. Louet, G. Hayhurst, F.J. Gonzalez, J. Girard, J.F. Decaux, The coactivator PGC-1 is involved in the regulation of the liver carnitine palmitoyltransferase I gene expression by cAMP in combination with HNF4 alpha and cAMP-response element-binding protein (CREB), J. Biol. Chem. 277 (2002) 37991–38000.

[64] Y. Zhang, L.W. Castellani, C.J. Sinal, F.J. Gonzalez, P. Edwards, Peroxisome proliferator-activated receptor-gamma coactivator 1alpha (PGC-1alpha) regulates triglyceride metabolism by activation of the nuclear receptor FXR, Genes Dev. 18 (2004) 157–169.

[65] R.B. Vega, J.M. Huss, D.P. Kelly, The coactivator PGC-1 cooperates with peroxisome proliferator-activated receptor alpha in transcriptional control of nuclear genes encoding mitochondrial fatty acid oxidation enzymes, Mol. Cell Biol. 20 (2000) 1868–1876.

[66] J.E. Pessin, A.R. Saltiel, Signaling pathways in insulin action: molecular targets of insulin resistance, J. Clin. Invest. 106 (2000) 165–169.

[67] J.K. Kim, O. Gavrilova, Y. Chen, M.L. Reitman, G.I. Shulman, Mechanism of insulin resistance in A-ZIP/F-1 fatless mice, J. Biol. Chem. 275 (2000) 8456–8460.

[68] M.D. Michael, R.N. Kulkarni, C. Postic, S.F. Previs, G.I. Shulman, M.A. Magnuson, C.R. Kahn, Loss of insulin signaling in hepatocytes leads to severe insulin resistance and progressive hepatic dysfunction, Mol. Cell 6 (2000) 87–97.

[69] G.I. Shulman, Cellular mechanisms of insulin resistance, J. Clin. Invest. 106 (2000) 171–176.

[70] A.R. Saltiel, C.R. Kahn, Insulin signalling and the regulation of glucose and lipid metabolism, Nature 414 (2001) 799–806.

[71] J.E. Friedman, J.S. Yun, Y.M. Patel, M.M. McGrane, R.W. Hanson, Glucocorticoids regulate the induction of phosphoenolpyruvate carboxykinase (GTP) gene transcription during diabetes, J. Biol. Chem. 268 (1993) 12952–12957.

[72] A. Valera, A. Pujol, M. Pelegrin, F. Bosch, Transgenic mice overexpressing phosphoenolpyruvate carboxykinase develop non-insulin-dependent diabetes mellitus, Proc. Natl. Acad. Sci. USA 91 (1994) 9151–9154.

[73] S.H. Koo, H. Satoh, S. Herzig, C.H. Lee, S. Hedrick, R. Kulkarni, R.M. Evans, J. Olefsky, M. Montminy, PGC-1 promotes insulin resistance in liver through PPAR-alpha-dependent induction of TRB-3, Nat. Med. 10 (2004) 530–534.

[74] K.E. Watson, B.N. Horowitz, G. Matson, Lipid abnormalities in insulin resistant states, Rev. Cardiovasc. Med. 4 (2003) 228–236.

[75] J.B. Kim, B.M. Spiegelman, ADD1/SREBP1 promotes adipocyte differentiation and gene expression linked to fatty acid metabolism, Genes Dev. 10 (1996) 1096–1107.

[76] I. Shimomura, H. Shimano, B.S. Korn, Y. Bashmakov, J.D. Horton, Nuclear sterol regulatory element-binding proteins activate genes responsible for the entire program of unsaturated fatty acid biosynthesis in transgenic mouse liver, J. Biol. Chem. 273 (1998) 35299–35306.

[77] I. Shimomura, R.E. Hammer, J.A. Richardson, S. Ikemoto, Y. Bashmakov, J.L. Goldstein, M.S. Brown, Insulin resistance and diabetes mellitus in transgenic mice expressing nuclear SREBP-1c in adipose tissue: model for congenital generalized lipodystrophy,, Genes Dev. 12 (1998) 3182–3194.

[78] I. Shimomura, M. Matsuda, R.E. Hammer, Y. Bashmakov, M.S. Brown, J.L. Goldstein, Insulin selectively increases SREBP-1c mRNA in the livers of rats with streptozotocin-induced diabetes, Proc. Natl. Acad. Sci. USA 96 (1999) 13656–13661.

[79] I. Shimomura, Y. Bashmakov, J.D. Horton, Increased levels of nuclear SREBP-1c associated with fatty livers in two mouse models of diabetes mellitus, J. Biol. Chem. 274 (1999) 30028–30032.

[80] I. Shimomura, M. Matsuda, R.E. Hammer, Y. Bashmakov, M.S. Brown, J.L. Goldstein, Decreased IRS-2 and increased SREBP-1c lead to mixed insulin resistance and sensitivity in livers of lipo-dystrophic and ob/ob mice, Mol. Cell 6 (2000) 77–86.

[81] T.K. Lam, Mechanisms of the free fatty acid-induced increase in hepatic glucose production, Am. J. Physiol. Endocrinol. Metab. 284 (2003) E863–E873.

[82] P.J. Randle, P.B. Garland, C.N. Hales, E.A. Newsholme, The glucose fatty-acid cycle. Its role in insulin sensitivity and the metabolic disturbances of diabetes mellitus,, Lancet 1 (1963) 785–789.

[83] P.J. Randle, E.A. Newsholme, P.B. Garland, Regulation of glucose uptake by muscle. 8. Effects of fatty acids, ketone bodies and pyruvate, and of alloxan-diabetes and starvation, on the uptake and metabolic fate of glucose in rat heart and diaphragm muscles, Biochem. J. 93 (1964) 652–665.

[84] P.J. Randle, P.B. Garland, E.A. Newsholme, C.N. Hales, The glucose fatty acid cycle in obesity and maturity onset diabetes mellitus, Ann. N.Y. Acad. Sci. 131 (1965) 324–333.

[85] G.F. Gibbons, K. Islam, R.J. Pease, Mobilisation of triacylglycerol stores, Biochim. Biophys. Acta. 1483 (2000) 37–57.

[86] E. Duplus, M. Glorian, C. Forest, Fatty acid regulation of gene transcription, J. Biol. Chem. 275 (2000) 30749–30752.

[87] A.R. Saltiel, J.E. Pessin, Insulin signaling pathways in time and space, Trends Cell Biol. 12 (2002) 65–71.

[88] E. Araki, M.A. Lipes, M.E. Patti, J.C. Brunning, B. Haag 3rd, R.S. Johnson, C.R. Kahn, Alternative pathway of insulin signalling in mice with targeted disruption of the IRS-1 gene, Nature 372 (1994) 186–190.

[89] A. Kharitonenkov, Z. Chen, I. Sures, H. Wang, J. Schilling, A. Ullrich, A family of proteins that inhibit signalling through tyrosine kinase receptors, Nature 386 (1997) 181–186.

[90] M.F. White, The IRS-signalling system: a network of docking proteins that mediate insulin action, Mol. Cell Biochem. 182 (1998) 3–11.

[91] G. Sesti, M. Federici, M.L. Hribal, D. Lauro, P. Sbraccia, R. Lauro, Defects of the insulin receptor substrate (IRS) system in human metabolic disorders, Faseb J. 15 (2001) 2099–2111.

[92] V. Ribon, A.R. Saltiel, Insulin stimulates tyrosine phosphorylation of the proto-oncogene product of c-Cbl in 3T3-L1 adipocytes, Biochem. J. 324 (1997) 839–845.

[93] R.M. O'Brien, R.S. Streeper, J.E. Ayala, B.T. Stadelmaier, L.A. Hornbuckle Insulin-regulated gene expression,, Biochem. Soc. Trans. 29 (2001) 552–558.

[94] A. Barthel, D. Schmoll, Novel concepts in insulin regulation of hepatic gluconeogenesis, Am. J. Physiol. Endocrinol. Metab. 285 (2003) E685–E692.

[95] X. Zhao, L. Gan, H. Pan, D. Kan, M. Majeski, S.A. Adam, T.G. Unterman, Multiple elements regulate nuclear/cytoplasmic shuttling of FOXO1: characterization of phosphorylation- and 14-3-3- dependent and –independent mechanisms, Biochem. J. 378 (2004) 839–849.

[96] X. Zhang, L. Gan, H. Pan, S. Guo, X. He, S.T. Olson, A. Mesecar, S. Adam, T.G. Unterman, Phosphorylation of serine 256 suppresses transactivation by FKHR (FOXO1) by multiple mechanisms. Direct and indirect effects on nuclear/cytoplasmic shuttling and DNA binding, J. Biol. Chem. 277 (2002) 45276–45284.

[97] A. Bonni, M.J. Zigmond, M.Z. Lin, P. Juo, L.S. Hu, M.J. Anderson, K.C. Arden, J. Blenis, M.E. Greenberg, Akt promotes cell survival by phosphorylating and inhibiting a forkhead transcription factor, Cell 96 (1999) 857–868.

[98] A.M. Brownawell, G.J. Kops, I.G. Macara, B.M. Burgering, Inhibition of nuclear import by protein kinase B (Akt) regulates the subcellular distribution and activity of the forkhead transcription factor AFX, Mol. Cell Biol. 21 (2001) 3534–3546.

[99] G. Rena, A.R. Prescott, S. Guo, P. Cohen, T.G. Unterman, Roles of forkhead in rhabdomyosarcoma (FKHR) phosphorylation sites in regulating 14-3-binding, transactivation and nuclear targeting, Biochem. J. 354 (2001) 605–612.

[100] J. Nakae, B.C. Park, D. Accili, Insulin stimulates phosphorylation of the forkhead transcription factor FKHR on serine 253 through a Wortmannin-sensitive pathway, J. Biol. Chem. 274 (1999) 15982–15985.

[101] Y.L. Woods, The kinase DYRK1A phosphorylates the transcription factor FKHR at Ser329 *in vitro*, a novel *in vivo* phosphorylation site, Biochem. J. 355 (2001) 597–607.

[102] G. Rena, Y.L. Woods, A.R. Prescott, M. Peggie, T.G. Unterman, M.R. Williams, P. Cohen, Two novel phosphorylation sites on FKHR that are critical for its nuclear exclusion, EMBO J. 21 (2002) 2263–2271.

[103] M.C. Motta, N. Divecha, M. Lemieux, C. Kamel, D. Chen, W. Gu, Y. Bultsma, M. McBurney, L. Guarente, Mammalian SIRT1 represses forkhead transcription factors, Cell 116 (2004) 551–563.

[104] A. Brunet, L.B. Sweeney, J.F. Sturgill, K.F. Chua, P.L. Greer, Y. Lin, H. Tran, S.E. Ross, R. Mostoslavsky, H.Y. Cohen, L.S. Hu, H.L. Cheng, M.P. Jedrychowski, S.P. Gygi, D.A. Sinclair, F.W. Alt, M.E. Greenberg, Stress-dependent regulation of FOXO transcription factors by the SIRT1 deacetylase, Science 303 (2004) 2011–2015.

[105] M. Imae, Z. Fu, A. Yoshida, T. Noguchi, H. Kato, Nutritional and hormonal factors control the gene expression of FoxOs, the mammalian homologues of DAF-16, J. Mol. Endocrinol. 30 (2003) 253–262.

[106] Y. Kamei, J. Mizukami, S. Miura, M. Suzuki, N. Takahashi, T. Kawada, T. Taniguchi, O. Ezaki, A forkhead transcription factor FKHR up-regulates lipoprotein lipase expression in skeletal muscle, FEBS Lett. 536 (2003) 232–236.

[107] J. Altomonte, A. Richter, S. Harbaran, J. Suriawinata, J. Nakae, S.N. Thung, M. Meseck, D. Accili, H. Dong, Inhibition of Foxo1 function is associated with improved fasting glycemia in diabetic mice, Am. J. Physiol. Endocrinol. Metab. 285 (2003) E718–E728.

[108] H. Matsuzaki, H. Daitoku, M. Hatta, K. Tanaka, A. Fukamizu, Insulin-induced phosphorylation of FKHR (Foxo1) targets to proteasomal degradation, Proc. Natl. Acad. Sci. USA 100 (2003) 11285–11290.

[109] D.R. Plas, C.B. Thompson, Akt activation promotes degradation of tuberin and FOXO3a via the proteasome, J. Biol. Chem. 278 (2003) 12361–12366.

[110] A. Barthel, D. Schmoll, K.D. Kruger, R.A. Roth, H.G. Joost, Regulation of the forkhead transcription factor FKHR (FOXO1a) by glucose starvation and AICAR, an activator of AMP-activated protein kinase, Endocrinology 143 (2002) 3183–3186.

[111] C. Charvet, I. Alberti, F. Luciano, A. Jacquel, A. Bernard, P. Auberger, M. Deckert, Proteolytic regulation of forkhead transcription factor FOXO3a by caspase-3-like proteases, Oncogene 22 (2003) 4557–4568.

[112] A. Brunet, F. Kanai, J. Stehn, J. Xu, D. Sarbassova, J.V. Frangioni, S.N. Dalal, J.A. DeCaprio, M.E. Greenberg, M.B. Yaffe, 14-3-3 transits to the nucleus and participates in dynamic nucleo-cytoplasmic transport, J. Cell. Biol. 156 (2002) 817–828.

[113] T. Obsil, R. Ghirlando, D.E. Anderson, A.B. Hickman, F. Dyda, Two 14-3-3 binding motifs are required for stable association of forkhead transcription factor FOXO4 with 14-3-3 proteins and inhibition of DNA binding, Biochemistry 42 (2003) 15264–15272.

[114] N. Nasrin, S. Ogg, C.M. Cahill, W. Biggs, S. Nui, J. Dore, D. Calvo, Y. Shi, G. Ruvkun, M.C. Alexander-Bridges, DAF-16 recruits the CREB-binding protein coactivator complex to the insulin-like growth factor binding protein 1 promoter in HepG2 cells, Proc. Natl. Acad. Sci. USA 97 (2000) 10412–10417.

[115] D.L. Mahmud, M. G-Amlak, D.K. Deb, L.C. Platanias, S. Uddin, A. Wickrema, Phosphorylation of forkhead transcription factors by erythropoietin and stem cell factor prevents acetylation and their interaction with coactivator p300 in erythroid progenitor cells, Oncogene 21 (2002) 1556–1562.

[116] F. von Groote-Bidlingmaier, D. Schmoll, H.M. Orth, H. Joost, W. Becker, A. Barthel, DYRK1 is a co-activator of FKHR (FOXO1a)-dependent glucose-6-phosphatase gene expression, Biochem. Biophys. Res. Commun. 300 (2003) 764–769.

[117] K. Yamagata, H. Daitoku, Y. Shimamoto, H. Matsuzaki, K. Hirota, J. Ishida, A. Fukamizu, Bile acids regulate gluconeogenic gene expression via small heterodimer partner-mediated repression of hepatocyte nuclear factor 4 and Foxo1, J. Biol. Chem. 279 (2004) 23158–23165.

[118] S. Kodama, C. Koike, M. Negishi, Y. Yamamoto, Nuclear receptors CAR and PXR cross talk with FOXO1 to regulate genes that encode drug-metabolizing and gluconeogenic enzymes, Mol. Cell. Biol. 24 (2004) 7931–7940.

[119] J. Seoane, H.V. Le, L. Shen, S.A. Anderson, J. Massague, Integration of Smad and forkhead pathways in the control of neuroepithelial and glioblastoma cell proliferation, Cell 117 (2004) 211–223.

[120] M. Christian, X. Zhang, T. Schneider-Merck, T.G. Unterman, B. Gellersen, J.O. White, J.J. Brosens, Cyclic AMP-induced forkhead transcription factor, FKHR, cooperates with CCAAT/enhancer-binding protein beta in differentiating human endometrial stromal cells, J. Biol. Chem. 277 (2002) 20825–20832.

[121] C.M. Croniger, C. Millward, J. Yang, Y. Kawai, I.J. Arinze, S. Liu, M. Harada-Shiba, K. Chakravarty, J.E. Friedman, V. Poli, R.W. Hanson, Mice with a deletion in the gene for CCAAT/enhancer-binding protein beta have an attenuated response to cAMP and impaired carbohydrate metabolism, J. Biol. Chem. 276 (2001) 629–638.

[122] P. Dowell, T.C. Otto, S. Adi, M.D. Lane, Convergence of peroxisome proliferator-activated receptor gamma and Foxo1 signaling pathways, J. Biol. Chem. 278 (2003) 45485–45491.

[123] K. Hirota, H. Daitoku, H. Matsuzaki, N. Araya, K. Yamagata, S. Asada, T. Sugaya, A. Fukamizu, Hepatocyte nuclear factor-4 is a novel downstream target of insulin via FKHR as a signal-regulated transcriptional inhibitor, J. Biol. Chem. 278 (2003) 13056–13060.

[124] H.H. Zhao, R.E. Herrera, E. Coronado-Heinsohn, M.C. Yang, J.H. Ludes-Meyers, K.J. Seybold-Tilson, Z. Nawaz, D. Yee, F.G. Barr, S.G. Diab, P.H. Brown, S.A. Fuqua, C.K. Osborne, Forkhead homologue in rhabdomyosarcoma functions as a bifunctional nuclear receptor-interacting protein with both coactivator and corepressor functions, J. Biol. Chem. 276 (2001) 27907–27912.

[125] E.R. Schuur, A.V. Loktev, M. Sharma, Z. Sun, R.A. Roth, R.J. Weigel, Ligand-dependent inter-action of estrogen receptor-alpha with members of the forkhead transcription factor family, J. Biol. Chem. 276 (2001) 33554–33560.

] P. Li, H. Lee, S. Guo, T.G. Unterman, G. Jenster, W. Bai, AKT-independent protection of prostate cancer cells from apoptosis mediated through complex formation between the androgen receptor and FKHR, Mol. Cell Biol. 23 (2003) 104–118.

] T.G. Unterman, A. Fareeduddin, M.A. Harris, R.G. Goswami, A. Porcella, R.H. Costa, R.G. Lacson, Hepatocyte nuclear factor-3 (HNF-3) binds to the insulin response sequence in the IGF binding protein-1 (IGFBP-1) promoter and enhances promoter function, Biochem. Biophys. Res. Commun. 203 (1994) 1835–1841.

] R.S. Streeper, C.A. Svitek, S. Chapman, L.E. Greenbaum, R. Taub, R.M. O'Brien, A multicomponent insulin response sequence mediates a strong repression of mouse glucose-6-phosphatase gene transcription by insulin, J. Biol. Chem. 272 (1997) 11698–11701.

] J. Nakae, W.H. Biggs 3rd, T. Kitamura, W.K. Cavenee, C.V. Wright, K.C. Arden, D. Accili, Regulation of insulin action and pancreatic beta-cell function by mutated alleles of the gene encoding forkhead transcription factor Foxo1, Nat. Genet. 32 (2002) 245–253.

] T. Kitamura, J. Nakae, Y. Kitamura, Y. Kido, W.H. Biggs 3rd, C.V. Wright, M.F. White, K.C. Arden, D. Accili, The forkhead transcription factor Foxo1 links insulin signaling to Pdx1 regulation of pancreatic beta cell growth, J. Clin. Invest. 110 (2002) 1839–1847.

] T. Hosaka, W.H. Biggs 3rd, D. Tieu, A.D. Boyer, N.M. Varki, W.K. Cavenee, K.C. Arden, Disruption of forkhead transcription factor (FOXO) family members in mice reveals their functional diversification, Proc. Natl. Acad. Sci. USA 101 (2004) 2975–2980.

] J. Nakae, T. Kitamura, Y. Kitamura, W.H. Biggs 3rd, K.C. Arden, D. Accili, The forkhead transcription factor Foxo1 regulates adipocyte differentiation, Dev. Cell 4 (2003) 119–129.

] G. Kwon, B. Huang, T.G. Unterman, R.A. Harris, Protein kinase B-alpha inhibits human pyruvate dehydrogenase kinase-4 gene induction by dexamethasone through inactivation of FOXO transcription factors, Diabetes 53 (2004) 899–910.

] T. Furuyama, K. Kitayama, H. Yamashita, N. Mori, Forkhead transcription factor FOXO1 (FKHR)-dependent induction of PDK4 gene expression in skeletal muscle during energy deprivation, Biochem. J. 375 (2003) 365–371.

] A. Tsuchida, T. Yamauchi, Y. Ito, Y. Hada, T. Maki, S. Takekawa, J. Kamon, M. Kobayashi, R. Suzuki, K. Hara, N. Kubota, Y. Terauchi, P. Froguel, J. Nakae, M. Kasuga, D. Accili, K. Tobe, K. Ueki, R. Nagai, T. Kadowaki, Insulin/Foxo1 pathway regulates expression levels of adiponectin receptors and adiponectin sensitivity, J. Biol. Chem. 279 (2004) 30817–30822.

A. Brunet, J. Park, H. Tran, L.S. Hu, B.A. Hemmings, M.E. Greenberg, Protein kinase SGK mediates survival signals by phosphorylating the forkhead transcription factor FKHRL1 (FOXO3a), Mol. Cell. Biol. 21 (2001) 952–965.

C.M. Cahill, G. Tzivion, N. Nasrin, S. Ogg, J. Dore, G. Ruvkun, M. Alexander-Bridges, Phosphatidylinositol 3-kinase signaling inhibits DAF-16 DNA binding and function via 14-3-3-dependent and 14-3-3-independent pathways, J. Biol. Chem. 276 (2001) 13402–13410.

M.C. Hu, D.F. Lee, W. Xia, L.S. Golfman, F. Ou-Yang, J.Y. Yang, Y. Zou, S. Bao, N. Hanada, H. Saso, R. Kobayashi, M.C. Hung, IkappaB kinase promotes tumorigenesis through inhibition of forkhead FOXO3a, Cell 117 (2004) 225–237.

N.D. De Ruiter, B.M. Burgering, J.L. Bos, Regulation of the forkhead transcription factor AFX by Ral-dependent phosphorylation of threonines 447 and 451, Mol. Cell Biol. 21 (2001) 8225–8235.

A. van der Horst, L.G. Tertoolen, L.M. de Vries-Smits, R.A. Frye, R.H. Medema, B.M. Burgering, FOXO4 is acetylated upon peroxide stress and deacetylated by the longevity protein hSir2(SIRT1), J. Biol. Chem. 279 (2004) 28873–28879.

H. Daitoku, M. Hatta, H. Matsuzaki, S. Aratani, T. Ohshima, M. Miyagishi, T. Nakajima, A. Fukamizu, Silent information regulator 2 potentiates Foxo1-mediated transcription through its deacetylase activity, Proc. Natl. Acad. Sci. USA 101 (2004) 10042–10047.

M. Kortylewski, F. Feld, K.D. Kruger, G. Bahrenberg, R.A. Roth, H.G. Joost, P.C. Heinrich, I. Behrmann, A. Barthel, Akt modulates STAT3-mediated gene expression through a FKHR (FOXO1a)-dependent mechanism, J. Biol. Chem. 278 (2003) 5242–5249.

D. Schmoll, K.S. Walker, D.R. Alessi, R. Grempler, A. Burchell, S. Guo, R. Walther, T.G. Unterman, Regulation of glucose-6-phosphatase gene expression by protein kinase B alpha and the forkhead transcription factor FKHR. Evidence for insulin response unit-dependent and -independent effects of insulin on promoter activity, J. Biol. Chem. 275 (2000) 36324–36333.

[144] J. Nakae, T. Kitamura, D.L. Silver, D. Accili, The forkhead transcription factor Foxo1 (Fkhr) confers insulin sensitivity onto glucose-6-phosphatase expression, J. Clin. Invest. 108 (2001) 1359–1367.

[145] A. Kallwellis-Opara, X. Zaho, U. Zimmermann, T.G. Unterman, R. Walther, D. Schmoll, Characterization of cis-elements mediating the stimulation of glucose-6-phosphate transporter promoter activity by glucocorticoids, Gene. 320 (2003) 59–66.

[146] R.K. Hall, T. Yamasaki, T. Kucera, M. Waltner-Law, R. O'Brien, D.K. Granner, Regulation of phosphoenolpyruvate carboxykinase and insulin-like growth factor-binding protein-1 gene expression by insulin. The role of winged helix/forkhead proteins, J. Biol. Chem. 275 (2000) 30169–30175.

[147] S. Guo, G. Rena, S. Cichy, X. He, P. Cohen, T. Unterman, Phosphorylation of serine 256 by protein kinase B disrupts transactivation by FKHR and mediates effects of insulin on insulin-like growth factor-binding protein-1 promoter activity through a conserved insulin response sequence, J. Biol. Chem. 274 (1999) 17184–17192.

[148] H. Daitoku, K. Yamagata, H. Matsuzaki, M. Hatta, A. Fukamizu, Regulation of PGC-1 promoter activity by protein kinase B and the forkhead transcription factor FKHR, Diabetes 52 (2003) 642–649.

[149] A. Nadal, P.F. Marrero, D. Haro, Down-regulation of the mitochondrial 3-hydroxy-3-methyl-glutaryl-CoA synthase gene by insulin: the role of the forkhead transcription factor FKHRL1, Biochem. J. 366 (2002) 289–297.

Chapter 11

Disruption of CREB regulated of gene expression in diabetes

Jane E.B. Reusch[1], Peter A. Watson[2], Subbiah Pugazhenthi[3]

[1]University of Colorado, Staff Endocrinologist, Denver VA Medical Center, Denver, CO, USA;
[2]University of Colorado, Senior Research Associate, Denver VA Medical Center, Denver, CO, USA,
[3]University of Colorado, Denver, CO, USA

Abstract

Cardiovascular disease it is the leading cause of death in diabetes. In light of this, diabetes has recently been named and a cardiovascular disease equivalent. The molecular mechanisms that place persons with diabetes at excess vascular risk are numerous, including dyslipidemia, hypertension, hyperglycemia chronic inflammation and oxidative stress. These different factors place the diabetic vasculature in a state of chronic metabolic stress and this stress leads to vascular dysfunction. Our laboratory has focused on gaining a better understanding of the impact of diabetes and insulin resistance (IR) upon vascular smooth muscle cell gene regulation. Specifically, we have observed that the transcription factor CREB (cAMP response element binding protein) is critical for the maintenance of healthy quiescent (contractile and non-proliferative) vascular smooth muscle cell (SMC) function. In rodent models of diabetes and IR there is decreased expression of CREB protein in the vasculature. Loss of vascular CREB expression is associated with simultaneous increased expression of pro-atherogenic transcriptional regulators, such as NF-kB and C/EBP delta (CCAAT enhancer binding protein). This imbalance promotes SMC activation (proliferation, migration, matrix production and apoptosis) and may be important for excess vascular disease in diabetes. The evidence for CREB regulation of SMC function and its disruption in models of diabetes and atherosclerosis will be discussed in this chapter.

In addition to macrovascular disease, many other target organs are injured by the metabolic stress of diabetes including pancreatic beta cells (which contribute to disease progression) and cardiac and neuronal cells (which contribute to complications). We have identified a pattern of changes in gene regulation, loss of CREB function and augmentation of stress induced gene expression, that may contribute to the multi-organ dysfunction observed in diabetes.

ADVANCES IN MOLECULAR AND CELLULAR ENDOCRINOLOGY
VOLUME 5 ISSN 1569-2566/DOI 10.1016/S1569-2566(06)05011-3

1. Introduction

Under normal circumstances, the vascular smooth muscle cell or medial component of the blood vessel wall is quiescent. Quiescent vascular smooth muscle cells are contractile, have low proliferative capacity and low migratory activities. In response to acute injury, vascular smooth muscle cells (SMC) change phenotype to a synthetic or active phenotype. This process is called phenotypic modulation and it is important for normal response to injury. Phenotypic modulation in excess is the hallmark of atherosclerosis. The activated SMC is migratory and has increased proliferative capacity. Activated SMC are able to synthesize matrix proteins, growth factors and cytokines. The ability for vascular SMC to change phenotype in response to injury or acute stress is necessary for the maintenance of vascular integrity. In disease states of the vasculature, such as atherosclerosis, pulmonary hypertension or hypertension, SMC phenotypic modulation becomes exaggerated leading to medial hypertrophy or in the case of atherosclerosis, intimal proliferation, stiffening of blood vessels and vascular disease. Many inciting paradigms for induction of SMC activation have been reported including chronic hypertension, chronic hypoxia (pulmonary hypertension), high low-density lipoprotein (LDL) -cholesterol, chronic inflammation or diabetes. Characterization of the molecular response to local factors, such as angiotensin and endothelin-1 in hypertension, cytokines and platelet derived growth factor (PDGF) in pulmonary hypertension and oxidized LDL and chronic inflammation in atherosclerosis has been an exciting area of work in the past few years. There are numerous reports of pathological gene regulatory responses and interventions to prevent these negative events. Our group has focused upon the transcription factor CREB (cAMP Response Element Binding Protein) that plays a pivotal role in acute SMC responses to trophic and toxic stimuli and appears to be essential normal SMC function.

Our laboratory is interested in the impact of the transcription factor CREB on SMC function. The group of the late Russell Ross beautifully characterized the impact of cyclic AMP as a mitogenic gate for inhibiting SMC activation in healthy blood vessels [1-3]. CREB was initially defined as a target for the cyclic AMP dependent protein kinase, protein kinase A (PKA). Our early studies were designed to assess whether CREB was the nuclear target for cyclic AMP in serving as the mitogenic gate and keeping SMC in the quiescent or highly differentiated state. The background for this question was based on observations in our lab and by other groups indicating that CREB was important for differentiation of a number of cell types including neurons, adipocytes and cardiac myocytes. We made the observation, as will be outlined in this chapter, that CREB is associated with highly differentiated SMC contractile phenotype and that overexpression of CREB restrains SMC proliferation and migration in response to growth factor stimulation or oxidant SMC injury. We believe this observation to be important because we have observed loss of medial CREB protein content in a number of rodent and porcine models of vascular disease. These models include streptozotocin (STZ) induced diabetes, genetically induced insulin resistance (IR) diabetes in mice, pigs and rats, autoimmune diabetes in the non-obese diabetic (NOD) mouse, high-fat feeding in the LDL receptor knockout mouse and in aging rodents. CREB, in collaboration with the transcriptional activator CCAAT enhancer binding protein beta (C/EBP), C/EBP β, seems to counter balance the pro-atherogenic transcriptional regulators C/EBP δ, egr-1 and NF kappa B *in vivo* and *in vitro*. In this chapter, we will review the data that supports the theory that CREB is associated with SMC differentiation and that it has in an inverse relationship with pro-inflammatory transcription factors. The result of this yin-yang transcriptional balance dictates SMC phenotype. We will also briefly highlight the occurrence of similar changes in gene expression and their relevance for development of diabetes and its attendant complications.

2. CREB and C/EBP involvement in cellular differentiation

Others and we have shown that CREB plays an important role in differentiation of numerous tissues including adipocytes, neurons, cardiac myocytes and SMC.

2.1. *Adipose tissue differentiation*

A considerable body of work has defined a critical role for timed expression and function of members of the C/EBP transcription factor family in the process of adipogenesis. This work will not be reviewed here, but readers are referred to review this work in the literature [4,5]. Work from our laboratory, in collaboration with Dr Dwight Klemm, has shown that the transcription factor CREB is a target for extracellular agents and intracellular signaling systems that induce adipogenesis [6,7]. This suggested that CREB could be mechanistically important for SMC differentiation. Ectopic expression of a constitutively active, chimeric VP16-CREB protein was sufficient to induce adipogenesis, whereas expression of a dominant negative form of CREB, KCREB, blocked the adipogenic program. CREB functions in concert with C/EBP proteins to achieve this impact on adipocyte differentiation.

In more recent studies [8], our group has detailed how CREB impacts adipocyte number through regulation of adipocyte apoptosis. When KCREB is expressed in mature adipocytes, a loss of triacylglycerol vesicles and cells with typical adipocyte morphology over a 4–8-day period is observed. This loss could be due to lipolysis or to dedifferentiation of fat cells or to adipocyte apoptosis. Results indicate that ectopic expression of KCREB leads to apoptosis of mature adipocytes, which are replaced by undifferentiated pre-adipocytes in culture. Apoptosis was concomitant with an increase in several pro-apoptotic genes and down-regulation of the anti-apoptotic PKB/Akt. It was also observed that ectopic expression of constitutively active forms of CREB block adipocyte apoptosis in response to exposure to tumor necrosis factor (TNF)-α. These results indicate that CREB acts as a survival factor in mature adipocytes and may play a role in regulating adipose tissue mass and controlling insulin sensitivity.

2.2. *Neuronal cell differentiation*

Similar roles to those described above for CREB in adipose tissue have been observed in neuronal cells where it participates in differentiation and neurite outgrowth

[9–11]. In contrast to adipocytes, CREB activation alone is not sufficient to support neuronal differentiation. Other factors stimulated by nerve growth factor (NGF) are required. CREB also serves as a potent survival factor in neurons preventing apoptosis due to neurotrophin withdrawal [12–14]. Aspects of neuronal maturation have also been linked to CREB expression and activity. C/EBP β is widely expressed in the central nervous system of adult mice, including cells of the hippocampus and dentate gyrus and cerebellar Purkinje and granule cells [15]. Studies in PC12 cells, which can undergo differentiation to neuron-like cells in response to NGF, demonstrate that C/EBP β protein and gene are direct downstream targets of the NGF receptor, and suggest that C/EBP β may play a role in neurotrophin signaling in the brain [15]. The relationship between CREB and C/EBPb in neuronal tissues has not been examined.

2.3. *Cardiac and skeletal muscle cell differentiation and growth*

Work from other laboratories indicates that CREB may play a role in normal differentiation and development of the heart. Three critical, published observations involving heart-specific transgenic mouse models, in which CREB function has been modified, indicate that CREB function is important for normal physiological cardiac function. Transgenic ablation in the heart of the activity of the transcription factor CREB, the Cyclic-nucleotide Regulatory Element Binding Protein, is sufficient to induce dilated cardiomyopathy [16] accompanied by reduced left ventricular contractility and decreased cardiac reserve [17]. The absence of CREB function in this transgenic, dominant negative CREB animal also prevents improvement of survival and cardiac pathology in response to exercise [18]. Increased expression of the negative regulator of CREB transactivation, inducible cAMP early repressor (ICER), occurs during pathological hypertrophy induced by β-adrenergic stimulation, and results in diminished expression of bcl-2 and increased cardiac myocyte apoptosis *in vivo* [19]. Overexpression of either ICER or dominant-negative CREB (Ser133 to Ala 133 mutation) mimics the response to β-adrenergic stimulation, inducing apoptosis in cultured cardiac myocytes [19]. In addition, studies into the mechanisms underlying hypertrophy in response to ischemia/hypoxia indicate that activation of CREB occurs concurrent with reoxygenation and subsequent hypertrophy, and expression of dominant negative CREB abrogates hypertrophy in response to hypoxia/reoxygenation [20].

2.4. *Studies in isolated cardiac myocytes demonstrate that chronic stimulation of the cAMP-signaling pathway (which lead to congestive failure of the heart) leads to chronic CREB phosphorylation and subsequent loss of CREB protein content [21]*

The loss of CREB protein is accompanied by significant loss of CRE-mediated transcription, which may contribute to congestive heart failure. Recent work from our laboratory (in review) further support a role for CREB in cardiac remodeling and restoration of normal compensated cardiac function following cardiac hypertrophy. Three significant conclusions derive from these results. (1) Loss of CREB activity is a common feature of the early stages of cardiac hypertrophy, compensated and decompensated. (2) Restoration of CREB function occurs concurrent with the establishment of a compensated hypertrophic state, but not with decompensated cardiac failure. (3) Expression of the anti-apoptotic, CREB-dependent protein bcl-2, decreases in parallel with the loss of CREB function in response to pathological stimuli, along with increase in active caspase 9 and 3. This loss of bcl-2 protein and activation of caspases is reversed by exercise, concurrent with restoration of CREB function.

Our results demonstrate dynamic regulation of CREB function during hypertrophic remodeling, and restoration of CREB function only with compensation of exercise-induced hypertrophy. Our results also suggest that the transient loss of CREB function during hypertrophic remodeling may be permissive for cardiac remodeling. Quantitative changes in ventricular mass accompany early responses to both physiological and pathological stimuli for growth of the heart. The results presented in this data set indicate that while CREB activity may not be crucial for these quantitative changes in heart mass, CREB function may be crucial for the qualitative phenotypic that define physiological hypertrophy. Exercise, even of moderate intensity, increased CREB Ser133 phosphorylation and increased survival of SHHF rats with hypertension and cardiac failure. We speculate that this improvement in CREB activity and accompanying improvement in apoptotic status in the heart are responsible for the improved survival of these animals. The necessity for restoration of CREB function for compensation is supported by work; the aforementioned work in transgenic mice expressing dominant-negative CREB, which develop dilated cardiomyopathy [16] but fail to manifest improved morbidity and mortality in response to exercise training [18].

Retinoblastoma (RB) gene transcription, induced by MyoD, is a key event in skeletal muscle cell differentiation. MyoD regulation of RB gene transcription occurs independently of MyoD binding to the RB gene promoter. Studies demonstrate that CREB protein content and CREB Ser133 phosphorylation rapidly increase at the onset of muscle differentiation and both remain elevated during the myogenic process [22]. These studies demonstrate that MyoD associates with CREB, and these two proteins are targeted to a CRE element in the RB gene promoter along with the transcriptional co-factor CREB-Binding Protein (CBP)/p300, which stimulates RB gene transcription [22]. Studies by Polesskaya, et al. [23] indicate that CBP/p300 histone acetylase (HAT) activity is critical for specific events in muscle cell differentiation; cell fusion and muscle specific gene expression. Expression of a negative transdominant mutant of CBP/p300, or chemical inhibition of HAT activity of these proteins prevents muscle cell terminal differentiation [23]. This indicates that CREB accumulation and activation is necessary for skeletal muscle myogenesis.

3. CREB and C/EBP proteins in the vasculature

Work from our laboratory and the laboratories of many others have defined CREB and members of the C/EBP family of transcription factors as contributing factors to phenotypic modulation in vascular SMC during health and disease. In this section, we will review the published work regarding the contribution of SMC phenotype to vascular disease, and the impact of CREB and C/EBP transcription factors on these processes.

3.1. Smooth muscle cell phenotype and phenotypic modulation

Recent advances have greatly improved our understanding of vascular biology and the physiology of atherosclerosis and restenosis [24–28]. As mentioned in the introduction, diabetic vascular disease is characterized by changes in SMC phenotype. The transition of arterial SMC from a contractile to a synthetic, proliferative state appears to be an early event in the pathogenesis of atherosclerosis [24–28]. The vascular SMC in mature animals is a highly specialized cell whose principal function is contraction. The fully differentiated or mature vascular SMC proliferates at an extremely low rate. Mature SMCs express specific proteins and signaling elements that function to serve this contractile state. Investigation of phenotypic modulation is made difficult by the fact that merely placing vascular SMC into culture leads to a switch in phenotype. Rapid and reversible changes in SMC phenotype occur in response to local environmental cues for normal blood vessel maintenance. Numerous studies using SMCs from diabetic animals and humans have demonstrated an increased migratory and proliferative phenotype [29–32]. Additionally, a recent study has demonstrated that the phenotypic modulation in primary SMC cultures from STZ rats occurs more rapidly and more dramatically [33–35].

3.2. Cyclic AMP-cyclic GMP and "gating" of SMC proliferation

Much attention has been paid to abnormal function of the vasculature. Before discussing pathophysiology, it is essential to understand the factors that are important for mature normal SMC function. Cyclic nucleotides (cAMP and cGMP) promote SMC quiescence in vitro and in vivo. Beta-adrenergic stimulation of cAMP signaling is important for SMC quiescence and contractile function under normal conditions. Activation of PKA is capable of supporting the maintenance of a contractile, proliferation resistant phenotype in SMC. Accumulation of cyclic AMP and cGMP appears to be important for inhibition of MAP kinases, p70 S6 kinases and cdk4, which effectively block the entry into G1 from the G0 phase of the cell cycle [36–40]. Cells are released into cell cycle under circumstances that induce phenotypic modulation. Studies from our laboratory and others demonstrate alterations in SMC cytoskeletal markers, migration and proliferation with inhibitors of PKA (unpublished, Watson, 2000). Alternatively, treatment of SMC with dibutyrl cAMP significantly attenuated cellular migration in response to 100 pM PDGF. The response to cAMP accumulation may depend upon cellular context [41]. In injury models, agents such as endothelin, thrombin and angiotensin (all stimulate cAMP and CREB phosphorylation) lead to SMC proliferation. In these settings, CREB is activated simultaneously with pro-inflammatory transcriptional regulators, such as egr-1 and NF-kB. As such, the balance of transcriptional regulators and their nuclear targets ultimately determines the phenotypic response. It would be overly simplistic to think of CREB, or any transcriptional regulator, as 'good' or 'bad'. In the next section of this chapter, we will outline studies emerging from our lab that suggest CREB as a key molecular switch in vascular response to injury.

4. CREB regulation of smooth muscle cell phenotype

Cyclic nucleotides have been recognized for some time as important for the maintenance of mature SMC phenotype. The importance of CREB as a downstream target of cAMP (and in some reports cGMP) has only recently been elucidated. CREB is an important nuclear target of cyclic nucleotide signaling and is a widely expressed DNA binding protein. Classically, CREB functional state is regulated by phosphorylation on serine 133, which permits binding to the co-activator protein CREB binding protein (CBP) and leads to gene regulation [42]. We hypothesized that CREB was an important nuclear target of cyclic nucleotides, their impact on SMC quiescence. Vascular expression of CREB is high in the highly differentiated medial SMC compartment of the large blood vessel (Fig. 1). These studies were followed with a set of experiments in fetal calves exposed to chronic hypoxia. This model of pulmonary hypertension develops of pulmonary vascular SMC proliferation and permits evaluation of SMC proliferation *in vivo*. As such this is an excellent model for *in vivo* SMC proliferation. CREB content correlated inversely with SMC proliferation as detected by Ki67. These two experiments suggested that CREB was a marker of SMC differentiation. To define whether CREB was mechanistically important for SMC differentiation, functional CREB content was manipulated using either inducible expression vectors or by infection with adenovirus encoding constitutively active or dominant negative CREB. Expression of active CREB blunted serum and PDGF mediated SMC proliferation (Fig. 2) [2]. PDGF stimulated migration was blunted by active CREB and augmented with dominant negative CREB [2,3]. These

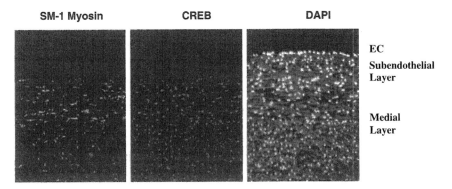

Fig. 1. Correlation between CREB content and SMC differentiation markers *in vivo*: fluorescent immunostaining of bovine aorta for cellularity (blue- DAPI), SMC (green-SM Myosin 1) and CREB (red). CREB staining co-localized with medial SMC. For experimental detail, see ref. [1]. *Source:* Adapted figure reproduced with permission ref. [1]. See Plate 11 in Colour Plate Section.

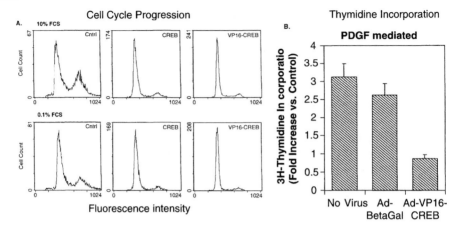

Fig. 2. CREB regulation of SMC Proliferation. (A) Stably transfected adult bovine SMC with ponas-
terone inducible expression of wild-type CREB or constitutively active CREB (VP-16 CREB) were treated
cultured in either 10% FBS (upper) or 0.1% FBS, as indicated. Expression of CREB or VP-16 CREB was
induced with 1 μM muristerone for 24 hours. Cells were fixed, stained with propidium iodide and subjected
to flow cytometric analysis. Cells expressing CREB or CA CREB showed decreased entry into cell cycle.
(B) SMC were infected with adenovirus (1 × 10 m.o.i. per 400,000 cells) encoding control (β-galactosidase),
or constitutively active CREB (VP-16 CREB). SMC were then exposed to PDG for 24 hours and [3 H]
thymidine for the final 3 hours. Thymidine incorporation was quantified and normalized for protein. For
additional experimental detail, see ref. [1]. *Source:* Adapted figure reproduced with permission ref. [1].

studies illustrated that CREB functional CREB activity is important for maintenance
of the differentiated SMC phenotype (quiescent, non-proliferative, non-migratory).

4.1. *CREB regulates a panel of genes consistent with quiescence*

To better understand the mechanism whereby CREB decreased mitogen-stimulated
SMC proliferation we performed a cDNA array to identify CREB target genes [2].
Active CREB decreased the expression of a number of cell cycle and mitogenic genes,
providing a potential mechanism for the impact of CREB on SMC behavior (Fig. 3)
[2]. Our group has carefully analyzed the impact of CREB on the PDGF receptor
alpha promoter (PRGFRα). CREB decreases expression of PRGFRα and its
ligand PDGF–AA [1] (unpublished results). PRGFRα is defined to be a marker of
SMC dedifferentiation and acquisition of the proliferative phenotype [43]. We have
employed PDGFRα as a marker of CREB activity in the vasculature.

4.2. *Vascular CREB expression decreases in diabetes, IR and other disease states*

Diabetes (DM) and IR are associated with increased vascular disease and in many
reports SMC isolated from rodents with DM and IR are activated, as mentioned
above [24–27,44]. Examination of aortic lystates from genetic and overfeeding models
of IR demonstrates decreased expression of CREB protein in aortic lysates (Fig. 4) [1].
Interestingly CREB content is also decreased in aortic lysates from 12 week STZ rats

CREB regulated gene expression

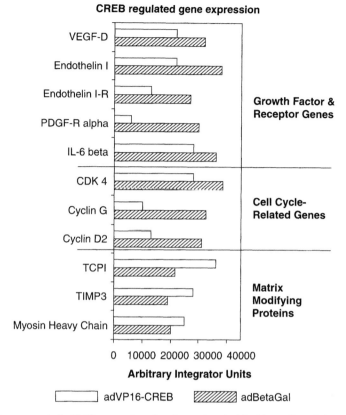

Fig. 3. cDNA array analysis: SMC were cultured and transduced with either adBetaGal or adVP16CREB as described above. Cells were extracted for total RNA using Trizol Reagent (GIBCO/BRL). Single-strand cDNA probes were generated from total RNA using ^{32}P-dATP and reagents and protocols provided by Clontech. These probes were used for hybridization to separate rat cDNA array membranes using protocols and reagents provided by the manufacturer (Clontech). Arrays were subjected to autoradiography at $-80°C$ using Kodak Lightning Plus Screens. Scanned Arrays were analyzed using Atlas Image Software, comparing relative intensities of specific cDNA "spots," which were corrected for differences in housekeeping genes between membranes prior to analysis. Three separate array analyses were performed with probes generated from RNA resulting from 2 different experiments. Results for cDNAs depicted below are the mean of these 3 separate determinations. Data is presented as mRNA content in adVP16CREB treated cells relative to mRNA content in adBetaGal treated cells. *Source:* Reproduced with permission from ref. [1].

(Fig. 4) [1]. Loss of vascular CREB protein appears to be functionally important because it correlates with increased expression of vascular PDGFR, a gene repressed by CREB [1]. One common feature of vascular injury in IR diabetes and STZ or insulin deficient diabetes is oxidative stress. Oxidative stress has been proposed as the "common soil" for vascular injury and atherosclerosis [45]. In unpublished studies, we have examined other models that develop vascular oxidant stress to determine if decreased CREB expression was observed. In the high-fat fed LDL receptor null mouse and in mouse and rat aging models CREB protein content is low (unpublished Reusch,

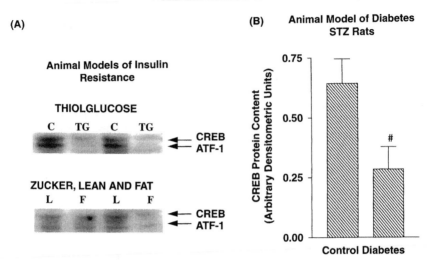

Fig. 4. Aorta CREB protein content from animal models of IR and diabetes. Aortic lysates were analyzed for CREB protein expression by Western analysis as previously described [2]. CREB protein content in the vasculature of animal with feeding induced (thioglucose) or genetically determined (Zucker) IR was significantly decreased. In 12-week STZ animals, there was also significantly decreased CREB protein content. For experimental details, see ref. [2]. *Source:* Adapted figure reproduced with permission from ref. [2].

O'Brien, 2003 and Reusch, Levi, 2003). This observation of decreased vascular CREB expression across numerous models of vascular disease suggested a common mechanism of down-regulation. Two possibilities likely present themselves, oxidative stress and chronic inflammation. We have explored oxidative stress in detail.

4.3. *CREB expression is diminished by oxidative stress and other inflammatory insults*

Glucose, advanced glycation end-products (AGE), lipids and cytokines all increase intracellular oxidant load. To mimic this situation *in vitro*, we exposed SMC and endothelial cells to oxidants. We have previously reported that CREB content decreased in SMC exposed to oxidants (Fig. 5) (unpublished). To extend that observation, we examined CREB content in SMC and endothelial cells exposed to oxidative stress and observed that CREB content is decreased in both vascular cell types by oxidants (Fig. 5) [3] (Watson, unpublished results). The functional relevance of loss of CREB protein expression in endothelial cells is not known at this time. In pancreatic beta cells cytokines decrease CREB expression (Pugazhenthi and Reusch, unpublished observations). We observe a similar response to cytokines in SMC (unpublished, Reusch and Jobin, 2003).

4.4. *Summary of the CREB effects in the vasculature*

CREB plays an important role is the maintenance of SMC differentiation by limiting SMC proliferation and migration. It decreases the expression of a number of growth

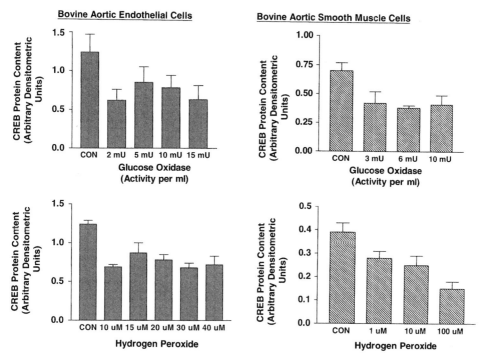

Fig. 5. CREB protein content in bovine aortic SMCs and endothelial cells. SMC and EC were cultured to 90% confluence and exposed to either glucose oxidase or hydrogen peroxide in the doses noted. Cells were treated for 48 hours and harvested in LSB. Lysates were analyzed for protein and 20 ug of protein was run on a 12% SDS/PAGE gel. CREB protein was analyzed by Western analysis and quantified using the Kodak image station. The above results are a summary of four experiments run in duplicate.

factor and cell cycle regulatory proteins. In rodent models of vascular injury and atherosclerosis, CREB protein content is decreased and there is increased expression of the CREB dependent gene PDFGRα. Loss of CREB is likely a consequence of chronic low-grade oxidative stress, cytokine stress or both. It remains to be examined how the depletion of vascular CREB and disruption of signaling to CREB in chronic metabolic disease affects acute stress responses.

4.5. Caveat

In contrast to the chronic metabolic stress models presented above, it is critical to mention that CREB is an immediate early gene. As such, it is activated acutely by numerous signals both trophic and toxic. For example, treatment of cells with oxidants, interleukin −1b (IL-1b), hypoxia, thrombin and numerous other toxic insults results in acute CREB phosphorylation. This leads to expression of a panel of genes that are regulated in concert with other immediate early genes, such as ets, erg-1 and NF-kB. In a recent paper examining induction of gene expression in response to oxidized phospholipids, CREB-mediated regulation of heme-oxygenase-1 was

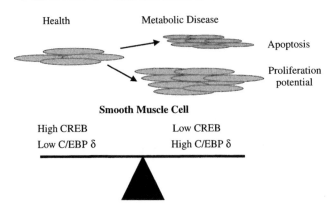

Fig. 6. Working model: Vascular gene regulatory response to metabolic and cytokine stress.

defined. Heme oxygenase-1 (HO-1) catalyzes the rate-limiting step in heme degradation, protects against oxidative stress and shows potent anti-inflammatory effects. These authors concluded that "CREB may represent a feedback mechanism to limit inflammation and associated tissue damage" [46]. This assertion is consistent with our *in vitro* observations and supported by the loss of CREB in animals models prone to atherosclerosis. Since CREB is critical for cellular differentiation and survival in a number of cell types, we suspect that decreased CREB content and function will interfere will normal cellular responses to acute stress, In the instance of vascular disease we are led to the following working model (Fig. 6).

5. Impact of C/EBP isoforms on SMC activation

A considerable body of work supports a role for members of the C/EBP family of transcription factors as targets of activating stimuli, and as agents of activation in SMC. Recent work from our laboratory indicates that members of the C/EBP protein family can contribute to both activation and quiescence in SMC, and this transcriptional family is regulated by CREB activity. Below we review the evidence supporting the contribution of C/EBP proteins to SMC phenotype.

5.1. *Inflammatory cytokines stimulate C/EBPδ and SMC activation*

SMC activation in response to injury is accompanied by a localized or generalized inflammatory response, involving the release of cytokines by infiltrating blood cells. Members of the C/EBP family are frequently a target for cytokine-mediated signaling pathways and have been shown to be involved in acute regulation of injury-response genes in SMC. Induction of genes, such as cyclooxygenase II (COX II) [47,48], interleukin-18 (IL-18) and interleukin -6 (IL-6) involve the actions of C/EBP family members [49]. Other factors present in the lumen in response to injury, such as thrombin [50,51] and angiotensin II [52] may also lead to modulation of C/EBP family members through their impact on CREB activation.

The actions of growth factors and cytokines released by infiltrating macrophages, including PDGFs and IL-1β, have been implicated in the etiology of atherosclerosis [25,53,54]. IL-1β increases expression of C/EBPβ in SMC. This effect is described in a series of papers from Hiwada's group, focusing on the regulation of transcription of the gene encoding the platelet-derived growth factor receptor-α (PDGFRα [55–57]. This group generated a transgenic mouse in which overexpression of C/EBPδ was targeted to vascular SMC [58]. The SMC from this animal demonstrated, in addition to an increased expression of PDGFRα a significant increase in growth and proliferation as compared to SMC isolated from vessels in their non-transgenic littermates. As such, this result indicates that increased C/EBPδ expression is capable of driving SMC proliferation *in vivo*. Indeed, recent studies in hypercholesterolemic rabbits demonstrate the efficacy of C/EBP decoy oligonucleotide in suppressing development of macrophage-rich vascular lesion formation [59]. It is interesting to note that the vascular inflammatory response through activation of C/EBPδ is negatively autoregulated through the ability of C/EBPδ to transactivate Peroxisome Proliferator-Activated Receptor-γ (PPARγ) gene expression [60]. We have observed that CREB activity in SMC is augmented by treatment with PPARγ agonists (thiazolidinediones or TZDs), and that CREB activity suppresses C/EBPδ expression, at least in part through suppression of transcription (unpublished, Reusch and Watson, 2003). As such, augmented CREB content may act coordinately with upregulation of PPARγ to suppress inflammatory responses in SMC by reducing C/EBPδ expression.

Expression of PDGFRα appears to be a strong marker of SMC activation and dysfunction. Changes in the content and function of PDGFRα have been associated with vascular pathology. These pathologies include genetic hypertension in Spontaneously Hypertensive Rats (SHR), atherogenesis and inflammatory responses in the vasculature, particularly in response to inflammatory cytokines such as IL-1 β. Induction of PDGFRα expression in an angioplasty model of vascular injury was recently reported [61]. Recent studies indicate that C/EBPδ may be involved in upregulation of PDGFRα gene expression and protein content in response to IL-1β [55–58]. Treatment of SMC with the PPARγ-agonist troglitazone inhibits IL-1β stimulation of PDGFRα gene expression [57]. Increased expression of PPARγ has been observed in the vasculature in response to vascular insults. Treatment of atherosclerosis-prone animals with PPARγ ligands decreases plaque burden [62]. Thus, increase PPARγ expression is thought to limit excessive vascular remodeling in atherosclerosis [63–67].

One of the actions of IL-1β is to increase the expression of PDGFRα and enhance the release of PDGF-AA from SMC [68–71]. Thus, cytokines augment PDGF action in the vasculature by increasing both PDGFRα ligand and receptor. PDGFRα was recently reported to play a critical role in susceptibility of vascular SMC to proliferation [56,58]. PDGFRα is upregulated by C/EBP δ and downregulated by the CREB and PPARγ ligand troglitazone [55–57].

Evidence also exists supporting a role for C/EBPδ (and its modulation of PDGFRα) in vascular pathology in the microvaculature in certain disease states. One such piece of *in vivo* evidence comes from studies in models of diabetic microvascular disease, such as proliferative retinopathy. In this study, PDGFRα expression is increased and treatment with agents that interfere with PDGFRα action block proliferative retinopathy [72]. It is likely that this increase in PDGFRα expression is linked to diabetes-induced loss of CREB content and subsequent upregulation of stimulatory C/EBPδ.

5.2. *Evidence supporting C/EBPβ as an intermediate of CREB-induced suppression of SMC activation*

As described above, studies in animal models of insulin-resistance and diabetes demonstrate significant loss of CREB protein associated with vascular dysfunction and increased expression of PDGFRα. Studies in cultured SMC demonstrate loss of CREB protein in the presence of diabetogenic toxins. For example, we observed a decrease in CREB content in the vasculature of rodents with IR and STZ diabetes, which was accompanied by a loss of C/EBPβ protein and accumulation of PDGFRα [73]. Also, we observed a restoration of CREB content, along with C/EBPβ, in the vascular stroma of Ob/Ob mice treated with the PPARγ ligand rosiglitazone [73]. Rosiglitazone simultaneously downregulates PDGFRα content. In all cases tested, loss of CREB protein content is mirrored by the loss of C/EBPβ protein and increased content of C/EBPδ and PDGFRαproteins. Further studies, performed in cultured SMC indicate that this relationship may be more than coincidental.

Recent work from our laboratory indicates that CREB's ability to suppress PDGFRα gene transcription [1] is mimicked by overexpression of another member of the CCAAT enhancer-binding protein family, C/EBPβ. CREB activity was shown stimulate accumulation of C/EBPβ in SMC, and to suppress C/EBPδ expression. Overexpression of C/EBPβ in cotransfection experiments in cultured SMC was shown to attenuate basal PDGFRα promoter activity, as well as inhibiting activation by overexpressed C/EBP δ These results suggest a role for C/EBPβ in supporting the normal, quiescent phenotype in vascular SMC.

6. CREB-C/EBP responses in SMC; life and death decisions

Data from our laboratory and others demonstrate a role for CREB in maintaining vascular health through its ability to support quiescent, healthy phenotypes in both vascular SMC and endothelial cells. We have observed that with acute exposure of the cells to vascular toxins, such as oxidant stress, high glucose, cytokines or C-reactive protein, CREB phosphorylation (and thus CREB function) is enhanced. We have interpreted this response as a "protective" response to these vascular insults. Indeed, *in vivo* studies of STZ-induced diabetes (DM) in rats indicate an initial increase in CREB phosphorylation early in the development of diabetes (unpublished, Reusch Watson, 2001). However, prolonged exposure of vascular cells to these toxins (either in cell culture or *in vivo*) results in a loss of CREB protein content, which is accompanied by vascular SMC activation and vascular dysfunction.

7. CREB function beyond the cardiovascular system

7.1. *CREB as a mediator of cell survival*

The nuclear transcription factor, CREB plays an important role in diverse cellular functions including cell survival [74]. This 43 kD protein binds to CRE in the promoter regions of several genes needed for cell growth and survival [75]. Neurotrophin-mediated survival pathways proceed through CREB [76,77]. Tissue specific expression of dominant negative CREB in transgenic mice leads to decreased survival of several cell types [78,79]. The bcl-2 family of proteins is known to regulate the intracellular mitochondrial pathway of apoptosis [80]. They consist of both pro-apoptotic (Bax, tBid, Bad, Bik, etc.) and anti-apoptotic (Bcl-2, Bcl-xL, Brag-1, etc.) proteins. The expression of bcl-2 has been shown to be a key determinant of cell survival [81,82]. It has been shown by our lab and others that CREB plays a positive role in inducing the anti-apoptotic gene bcl-2 [83–85]. The inhibitors of apoptosis (IAP) are another novel conserved family of proteins that inhibit the activity of caspases and play a role in cell survival [86] The enhancer region of the cellular inhibitor of apoptosis (c-IAP2), a member of the IAP family, contains 2 CRE sites and is induced by cAMP [87,88]. Furthermore, CREB gene itself is positively regulated by a CRE site in its promoter [89].

7.2. *CREB in β-cells*

Although CREB-mediated gene expression has been characterized in neurons, limited information is available regarding its role in β-cell function. The 5′ flanking region of rat insulin gene contains a CRE site, which seems to respond to ATF-2 or related CREB family members [90,91]. Membrane depolarization and calcium influx in β-cells have been shown to activate CREB [92]. Glucose-induced upregulation of c-fos expression proceeds through activation of CREB [93]. The role of CREB in improving the survival and the growth factor mediated signaling pathways leading to CREB activation have not been well characterized in β-cells previously. Cytokine-induced β cell apoptosis involves downregulation of bcl-2 [94–96]. Human islets have been shown to be protected from cytokines by the transfer of bcl-2 gene [97]. We have shown that cytokine-induced downregulation of bcl-2 expression in β cells involves impairment of CREB function [98]. Two other recent studies reported that β cell-specific overexpression of CREB antagonists in transgenic mice leads to induction of diabetes [99,100].

8. Summary

The current working hypothesis supported by the observations outlined in this chapter is that CREB is a central component of the intercellular cytoprotective homeostatic response to physiological metabolic stress. We postulate that chronic metabolic and inflammatory stress leads to inappropriate regulation of CREB resulting in dedifferentiation or death of many cell types and dysfunction of target organs. We propose as model, wherein CREB is a key element in what might be termed the Starling Curve of the cellular homeostasis where mild intermittent stress enhances CREB function and cellular defenses and chronic stress leads to CREB dysfunction and cellular dysfunction. CREB dysfunction in this context may contribute to beta cell failure and the development of diabetes. It may also contribute to the development of diabetic complications in the nervous system and vasculature.

Acknowledgments

This work is supported by funding via VA Merit Review and REAP; NIH HL56481, DK57516, DK64741, American Heart Association, Juvenile Diabetes Research Foundation International and American Diabetes Association.

Reference

[1] P.A. Watson, C. Vinson, A. Nesterova, J.E.-B. Reusch, Content and activity of cAMP response element-binding protein regulate platelet-derived growth factor receptor-alpha content in vascualr smooth muscles, Endocrinology 143 (2002) 2922–2929.

[2] D.J. Klemm, P.A. Watson, M.G. Frid, E.C. Dempsey, J. Schaack, L.A. Colton, A. Nesterova, K.R. Stenmark, J.E. Reusch, Cyclic AMP response element-binding protein content is a molecular determinant of smooth muscle cell phenotype, J. Biol. Chem. 276 (2001) 46132–46141.

[3] P.A. Watson, A. Nesterova, C.F. Burant, D.J. Klemm, J.E-B. Reusch, Diabetes-related changes in cAMP response element-binding protein content enhance smooth muscle cell proliferation and migration, J. Biol. Chem. 276 (2001) 46142–46150.

[4] S.M. Rangwala, M.A. Lazar, Transcriptional control of adipogenesis, Annu. Rev. Nutr. 20 (2000) 535–559.

[5] O.A. MacDougald, M.D. Lane, Transcriptional regulation of gene expression during adipocyte differentiation, Annu. Rev. Biochem. 64 (1995) 345–373.

[6] J.E. Reusch, L.A. Colton, D.J. Klemm, CREB activation induces adipogenesis in 3T3-L1 cells, *Mol. Cell. Biol.* 20 (0 AD/2/1) 1008–1020.

[7] D. Klemm, J.W. Leitner, P. Watson, A. Nesterova, J.E. Reusch, M. Goalstone, B. Draznin, Insulin-induced adipocyte differentiation, J. Biol. Chem. 276 (2001) 28430–28435.

[8] J.E.B. Reusch, D.J. Klemm, Inhibition of cAMP-response element-binding protein activity decreases protein kinase B/Akt expression in 3T3-L1 adipocytes and induces apoptosis, J. Biol. Chem. 277 (2002) 1426.

[9] A. Shimomura, Y. Okamoto, Y. Hirata, M. Kobayashi, K. Kawakami, K. Kiuchi, T. Wakabayashi, M. Hagiwara, Dominant negative ATF1 blocks cyclic AMP-induced neurite outgrowth in PC12D cells, J. Neurochem. 70 (1998) 1029–1034.

[10] L.E. Heasley, S. Benedit, J. Gleavy, G.L. Johnson, Requirement of the adenovirus E1A transformation domain 1 for inhibition of PC12 cell neuronal differentiation, Cell Regul. 2 (1991) 479–489.

[11] J.Y. Sung, S.W. Shin, Y.S. Ahn, K.C. Chung, Basic fibroblast growth factor-induced activation of Novel CREB kinase during the differentiation of immortalized hippocampal cells, J. Biol. Chem. 276 (2001) 13858.

[12] A. Riccio, S. Ahn, C.M. Davenport, J.A. Blendy, D.D. Ginty, Mediation by a CREB family transcription factor of NGF-dependent survival of sympathetic neurons, Science 286 (1999) 2358–2361.

[13] S. Pugazhenthi, E. Miller, C. Sable, P. Young, K.A. Heidenreich, L.M. Boxer, J.E.B. Reusch, Insulin-like growth factor-I induces bcl-2 promoter through the transcription factor cAMP-response element-binding protein, J. Biol. Chem. 274 (1999) 27529.

[14] S. Pugazhenthi, A. Nesterova, C. Sable, K.A. Heidenreich, L.M. Boxer, L.E. Heasley, J.E.B. Reusch, Akt/protein kinase B up-regulates Bcl-2 expression through cAMP-response element-binding protein, J. Biol. Chem. 275 (2000) 10761.

[15] S. Esta, F.J. Peter, CCAAT/enhancer binding protein is a neuronal transcriptional regulator activated by nerve growth factor receptor signaling, J. Neurochem. 70 (1998) 2424–2433.

[16] R.C. Fentzke, C.E. Korcarz, R.M. Lang, H. Lin, J.M. Leiden, Dilated cardiomyopathy in transgenic mice expressing a dominant-negative CREB transcription factor in the heart, J. Clin. Inves. 101 (1998) 2415–2426.

[17] R. Fentzke, C. Korcarz, S. Shroff, H. Lin, J. Leiden, R. Lang, The left ventricular stress-velocity relation in transgenic mice expressing a dominant negative CREB transgene in the heart, J. Am. Soc. Echocardiogr. 14 (2001) 209–218.

[18] K.T. Spencer, K. Collins, C. Korcarz, R. Fentzke, R.M. Lang, J.M. Leiden, Effects of exercise training on LV performance and mortality in a murine model of dilated cardiomyopathy, Am. J. Physiol. Heart. Circ. Physiol. 279 H210–H215.

[19] H. Tomita, M. Nazmy, K. Kajimoto, G. Yehia, C.A. Molina, J. Sadoshima, Inducible cAMP early repressor (ICER) is a negative-feedback regulator of cardiac hypertrophy and an important mediator of cardiac myocyte apoptosis in response to β-adrenergic stimulation, Circ. Res. 93 (2003) 12–22.

[20] A. El Jamali, C. Freund, C. Rechner, C. Scheidereit, R. Dietz, M.W. Bergmann, Reoxygenation after severe hypoxia induces cardiomyocyte hypertrophy *in vitro*: activation of CREB downstream of GSK3β., FASEB J. 18 (2004) 1096–1098.

[21] F.U. Muller, P. Boknik, J. Knapp, B. Linck, H. Luss, J. Neumann, W. Schmitz, Activation and inactivation of cAMP-response element-mediated gene transcription in cardiac myocytes, Cardiovasc. Res. 52 (2001) 95–102.

[22] A. Magenta, C. Cenciarelli, F. De Santa, P. Fuschi, F. Martelli, M. Caruso, A. Felsani, MyoD stimulates RB promoter activity via the CREB/p300 nuclear transduction pathway, Mol. Cellular Biol. 23 (2003) 2893.

[23] A. Polesskaya, I. Naguibneva, L. Fritsch, A. Duquet, S. Ait-Si-Ali, P. Robin, A. Vervisch, L.L. Pritchard, P. Cole, A. Harel-Bellan, CBP/p300 and muscle differentiation: no HAT, no muscle, EMBO J. 20 (2001) 6816.

[24] K.E. Bornfeldt, Intracellular signaling in arterial smooth muscle migration versus proliferation, Trends Cardiovas. Med. 6 (1996) 143–151.

[25] R. Ross, Cell biology of atherosclerosis, Annu. Rev. Physiol. 57 (1995) 791–804.

[26] G.R. Owens, Regulation of differentiation of vascular smooth muscle cells, Physiol. Rev. 75 (1995) 487–517.

[27] G.K. Owens, S.M. Vernon, C.S. Madsen, Molecular regulation of smooth muscle cell differentiation, J. Hypertens. 14 (1996) S55–S64.

[28] G.K. Owens Molecular control of vascular smooth muscle cell differentiation,, Acta Physiol. Scand. 164 (1998) 623–625.

[29] P.M. Absher, D.J. Schneider, L.C. Baldor, J.C. Russell, B.E. Sobel, Increased proliferation of explanted vascular smooth muscle cells: a marker presaging atherogenesis, Atherosclerosis 131 (1997) 187–194.

[30] R. Avena, M. Mitchell, R. Neville, A. Sidawy, The additive effects of glucose and insulin on the proliferation of infragenicular vascular smooth muscle cells, J. Nasc. Surg. 28 (1998) 1038–1039.

[31] I. Kimura, A. Nagamori, R. Honda, S. Kobayashi, Glycated serum stimulation of macrophages in GK-and streptozotocin-rats for the proliferation of primary smooth muscle cells of the aorta, Immunopharmacology 40 (1998) 105–118.

[32] Y. Wang, P. Zhang, A.B. Rice, J.C. Bonner Regulation of interleukin-1beta-induced platelet-derived growth receptor alpha experssion in rat pulmonary myofibroblasts by p38 mitogen-activated protein kinase,, J. Biol. Chem. 275 (2001) 22550–22557.

[33] P. Absher, D. Schneider, L. Baldor, J. Russell, B. Sobel The retardation of vasculopathy induced by attenuation of insulin resistance in the corpulent JCR: LA-cp rat is reflected by decreased vascular smooth muscle cell differentiation *in vivo*, Atherosclerosis 143 (1999) 245–251.

[34] B. Mompeo, F. Ortega, L. Sarmiento, I. Castano, Ultrastructural analogies between intimal alterations in veins from diabetic patients and animals with STZ-induced diabetes, Ann. Basc. Surg. 13 (1999) 294–301.

[35] P. Etienne, N. Pares-Herbute, L. Mani-Ponset, J. Gabrion, H. Rabesandratana, S. Herbute, L. Monnier, Phenotype modulation in primary cultures of aortic smooth muscle cells from streptozotocin-diabetic rats, Differentiation 63 (1998) 225–236.

[36] J. Chiche, S. Schlutsmeyer, D. Bloch, S. Monte, J.R. Jr, G. Filippov, S. Janssens, A. Rosenzweig, K. Bloch, Adenovirus-mediated gene transfer if cGMP-dependent protein kinase increases the sensitivity of cultured vascular smooth muscle cells to the antiproliferative and pro-apoptotic effects of nitric oxide/cGMP, J. Biol. Chem. 273 (1998) 34263–34271.

[37] Y. Tintut, F. Parhami, K. Bostrom, S. Jackson, L. Demer, cAMP stimulates osteoblast-like differentiation of calcifying vascular cells. Potential signaling pathway for vascular calcification, J. Biol. Chem. 273 (1998) 7547–7553.

[38] M. Hoshiya, M. Awazu, Trapidil inhibits platlet-derived growth factor-stimulated mitogen-activated protein kinase cascade, Hypertension 31 (1998) 665–671.

[39] Y. Li, R. Fiscus, J. Wu, L. Yang, X. Wang, The antiproliferative effects of calcitonin gene-related peptide in different passages of cultured vascular smooth muscle cells, Neuropeptides 31 (1997) 503–509.

[40] P. Vadiveloo, E. Filonzi, H. Stanton, J. Hamilton, G1 phase arrest of human smooth muscle cells by heparin, IL-4 and cAMP is linked to repression of cyclin D1 and cdk2, Atherosclerosis 133 (1997) 61–69.

[41] K.E. Bornfeldt, J.S. Campbell, H. Koyama, G.M. Argast, C.C. Leslie, E.W. Raines, E.G. Krebs, R. Ross, The Mitogen-activated protein kinase pathway can mediate growth inhibtion and proliferation in smooth muscle cells, J. Clin. Invest. 100 (1997) 875–885.

[42] J.R. Cardinaux, J.C. Notis, Q. Zhang, N. Vo, J.C. Craig, D.M. Fass, R.G. Brennan, R.H. Goodman, Recruitment of CREB binding protein is sufficient for CREB-mediated gene activation, Mol. Cell. Biol. 20 (0 AD/3/1) 1546–1552.

[43] G.A. Ferns, E.W. Raines, K.H. Sprugel, A.S. Montani, M.A. Reidy, R. Ross, Inhibition of neointimal smooth muscle accumulation after angioplasty by an antibody to PDGF, Science 253 (1991) 1129–1132.

[44] N.D. Group, Diabetes in America, 2n edition, 1995, NIH, NIDDK NIH PUB 95–1468, pp. 1–733.

[45] M.P. Stern, Perspectives in diabetes: diabetes and cardiovascular disease: the "common soil" hypothesis, Diabetes 44 (1995) 369–374.

[46] G. Kronke, V.N. Bochkov, J. Huber, F. Gruber, S. Bluml, A. Furnkranz, A. Kadl, B.R. Binder N. Leitinger, Oxidized phospholipids induce expression of human heme oxygenase-1 involving activation of cAMP-responsive element binding protein (CREB), J. Biol. Chem. Epub ahead of print 278 (51) (2003) 51006–51014.

[47] Y. Zhu, M.A. Saunders, H. Yeh, W.-G. Deng, K.K. Wu, Dynamic regulation of cyclooxygenase-2 promoter activity by isoforms of CCAAT/enhancer binding proteins, J. Biol. Chem. 277 (2002) 6923–6928.

[48] K. Schroer, Y. Zhu, M.A. Saunders, W.-G. Deng, X.-M. Xu, J. Meyer-Kirchrath, K.K. Wu, Obligatory role of cyclic adenosine monophosphate response element in cyclooxygenase-2 promoter induction and feedback regulation by inflammatory mediators, Circulation 105 (2002) 2760–2765.

[49] E.S. Hungness, G.J. Luo, T.A. Pritts, X. Sun, B.W. Robb, D. Hershko, P.O. Hasselgren, Transcription factors C/EBP-beta and -delta regulate IL-6 production in IL-1beta-stimulated human enterocytes, J. Cell Physiol. 192 (2002) 64–70.

[50] T. Tokunou, T. Ichiki, K. Takeda, Y. Funakoshi, N. Iino, H. Shimokawa, K. Egashira, A. Takeshita, Thrombin induces interleukin-6 expression through the cAMP response element in vascular smooth muscle cells, Arteriosclerosis, Thrombosis, Vasc. Biol. 21 (2001) 1759–1763.

[51] T. Tokunou, T. Ichiki, K. Takeda, Y. Funakoshi, N. Iino, A. Takeshita, cAMP response element-binding protein mediates thrombin-induced proliferation of vascular smooth muscle cells, Arteriosclerosis, Thrombosis,Vasc. Biol. 21 (2001) 1764–1769.

[52] Y. Funakoshi, T. Ichiki, K. Takeda, T. Tokuno, N. Iino, A. Takeshita, Critical role of cAMP-response element-binding protein for angiotensin II-induced hypertrophy of vascular smooth muscle cells, J. Biol. Chem. 277 (2002) 18710–18717.

[53] L. Jonasson, J. Holm, O. Skalli, G. Bondjers, G.K. Hansson, Regional accumulation of T cells, macrophages, and smooth muscle cells in the human atherosclerotic plaque, Arteriosclerosis 6 (1986) 131–138.

[54] I. Joris, T. Zand, J.J. Nunnari, F.J. Krolikowski, G. Majno, Studies on the pathogenesis of atherosclerosis. I. Adhesion and emigration of mononuclear cells in the aorta of hypercholesterolemic rats, Am. J. Pathol. 113 (1983) 341–358.

[55] Y. Kitami, H. Inui, S. Uno, T. Inagami, Molecular structure and transcriptional regulation of the gene for the platelet-derived growth factor alpha receptor in cultured vascular smooth muscle cells, J. Clin. Invest. 96 (1995) 558–567.

[56] T. Fukuoka, Y. Kitami, T. Okura, K. Hiwada, Transcriptional regulation of the platelet-derived growth factor alpha receptor gene via CCAAT/enhancer-binding protein-delta in vascular smooth muscle cells, J. Biol. Chem. 274 (1999) 25576–25582.

[57] Y. Takata, Y. Kitami, T. Okura, K. Hiwada, Peroxisome proliferation-activated receptor-gamma activation inhibits interleukin-1beta-mediated platelet-derived growth factor-alpha receptor gene expression via CCAAT/enhancer-binding protein-delta in vascular smooth muscle cells, J. Biol. Chem. 276 (2001) 12893–12897.

[58] Z.H. Yang, Y. Kitami, Y. Takata, T. Okura, K. Hiwada, Targeted overexpression of CCAAT/enhancer-binding protein-delta evokes enhanced gene transcription of platelet-derived growth factor alpha-receptor in vascular smooth muscle cells, Circ. Res. 89 (2001) 503–508.

[59] U. Kelkenberg, A.H. Wagner, J. Sarhaddar, M. Hecker, H. von der Leyen, CCAAT/enhancer-binding protein decoy oligonucleotide inhibition of macrophage-rich vascular lesion formation in hypercholesterolemic rabbits, Arteriosclerosis, Thrombosis, Vasc. Biol. 22 (2002) 949–954.

[60] Y. Takata, Y. Kitami, Z.-H. Yang, M. Nakamura, T. Okura, K. Hiwada, Vascular inflammation is negatively autoregulated by interaction between CCAAT/enhancer-binding protein-delta and peroxisome proliferator-activated receptor-gamma, Circ. Res. 91 (2002) 427–433.

[61] A. Linqvist, B.O. Nilsson, E. Ekblad, P. Hellstrand, Platelet-derived growth factor receptors expressed in response to injury of differentiated vascular smooth muscle *in vitro*: effects of Ca2 + and growth signals, Acta Physiol. Scand. 173 (2001) 175–184.

[62] W.A. Hsueh, S. Jackson, R.E. Law, Control of vascular cell proliferation and migration by PPAR-gamma: a new approach to the macrovascular complications of diabetes, Diabetes Care 24 (2001) 392–397.

[63] N. Marx, U. Schonbeck, M.A. Lazar, P. Libby, J. Plutzky, Peroxisome proliferator-activated receptor gamma activators inhibit gene expression and migration in human vascular smooth muscle cells, Circ. Res. 83 (1998) 1097–1103.

[64] S. Goetze, X.P. Xi, H. Kawano, T. Gotlibowski, E. Fleck, W.A. Hsueh, R.E. Law, PPAR gamma-ligands inhibit migration mediated by multiple chemoattractants in vascular smooth muscle cells, J. Cardiovasc. Pharmacol. 33 (1999) 798–806.

[65] R.E. Law, W.P. Meehan, X.P. Xi, K. Graf, D.A. Wuthrich, W. Coats, D. Faxon, W.A. Hsueh, Troglitazone inhibits vascular smooth muscle cell growth and intimal hyperplasia, J. Clin. Invest. 98 (1996) 1897–1905.

[66] H. Koshiyama, D. Shimono, N. Kuwamura, J. Minamikawi, Y. Nakamura, Inhibitory effect of pioglitazone on carotid arterial wall thickness in type 2 diabetes, J. Clin. Endocrinol. Metab. 86 (2001) 3452–3456.

[67] J. Minamikawa, S. Tanaka, T. Yamauchi, D. Inoue, H. Koshiyama, Potent inhibitory effects of troglitazone on carotid arterial wall thickness in type 2 diabetes, J. Clin. Endocrinol. Metab. 83 (1998) 1818–1820.

[68] U. Ikeda, M. Ikeda, T. Oohara, S. Kano, T. Yaginuma, Mitogenic action of interleukin-1 on vascular smooth muscle cells mediated by PDGF, Atherosclerosis 84 (1990) 183–188.

[69] E.W. Raines, S.K. Dower, R. Ross, Interleukin-1 mitogenic activity for fibroblasts and smooth muscle cells is due to PDGF-AA, Science 243 (1989) 393–396.

[70] P.D. Bonin, G.J. Fici, J.P. Singh, Interleukin-1 promotes proliferation of vascular smooth muscle cells in coordination with PDGF or a monocyte derived growth factor, Exp. Cell Res. 181 (1989) 475–482.

[71] J.C. Bonner, P.M. Lindroos, A.B. Rice, C.R. Moomaw, D.L. Morgan, Induction of PDGF recep-
      tor-alpha in rat myofibroblasts during pulmonary fibrogenesis *in vivo*, Am. J. Physiol. 274 (1998)
      L72–L80.

[72] Y. Ikuno, A. Kazlasuskas, An *in vivo* gene therapy approach for experimental proliferative
      vitreoretinopathy using the truncated platelet-derived growth factor alpha receptor, Invest.
      Ophthamol. Vis. Sci. 43 (2002) 2406–2411.

[73] P.A. Watson, A. Nesterova, C.F. Burant, D.J. Klemm, J.E. Reusch, Diabetes-related changes in
      CREB content enhance smooth muscle cell proliferation and migration, J. Biol. Chem. 276 (2001)
      46142–46150.

[74] M. Montminy, Transcriptional regulation by cyclic AMP, Annu. Rev. Biochem. 66 (1997) 807–822.

[75] A.J. Shaywitz, M.E. Greenberg, CREB: a stimulus-induced transcription factor activated by a
      diverse array of extracellular signals, Annu. Rev. Biochem. 68 (1999) 821–861.

[76] S. Finkbeiner, CREB couples neurotrophin signals to survival messages, Neuron 25 (2000) 11–14.

[77] S. Finkbeiner, S.F. Tavazoie, A. Maloratsky, K.M. Jacobs, K.M. Harris, M.E. Greenberg, CREB: a
      major mediator of neuronal neurotrophin responses, Neuron 19 (1997) 1031–1047.

[78] R.C. Fentzke, C.E. Korcarz, R.M. Lang, H. Lin, J.M. Leiden, Dilated cardiomyopathy in transgenic
      mice expressing a dominant-negative CREB transcription factor in the heart, J. Clin. Invest. 101
      (1998) 2415–2426.

[79] R.S. Struthers, W.W. Vale, C. Arias, P.E. Sawchenko, M.R. Montminy, Somatotroph hypoplasia
      and darfism in transgenic mice expressing a non-phosphorylatable CREB mutant, Nature 350 (1991)
      622–624.

[80] D.E. Merry, S.J. Korsmeyer, Bcl-2 gene family in the nervous system, Annu. Rev. Neurosci. 20
      (1997) 245–267.

[81] D.V. Novack, S.J. Korsmeyer, Bcl-2 protein expression during murine development, Am. J. Pathol.
      145 (1994) 61–73.

[82] D. Veis, C. Sorenson, J. Shutter, S. Korsmeyer Bcl-2 deficient mice demonstrate fulminant lymphoid
      apoptosis,, polycystic kidneys, and hypopigmented hair, Cell 75 (1993) 229–240.

[83] S. Pugazhenthi, E. Miller, C. Sable, P. Young, K.A. Heidenreich, L.M. Boxer, J.E.-B. Reusch,
      Insulin-like growth factor-I induces bcl-2 promoter through the transcription factor cAMP-response
      element binding protein, J. Biol. Chem. 274 (1999) 27529–27535.

[84] S. Pugazhenthi, A. Nesterova, C. Sable, K. Heidenreich, L. Boxer, L. Heasley, J. Reusch, Akt/
      protein kinase B up-regulates Bcl-2 expression through cAMP-response element-binding protein,
      J. Biol. Chem. 275 (2000) 10761–10766.

[85] B.E. Wilson, E. Mochon, L.M. Boxer, Induction of bcl-2 expression by phosphorylated CREB
      proteins during B-cell activation and rescue from apoptosis, Mol. Cell. Biol. 16 (1996) 5546–5556.

[86] P. Liston, W.G. Fong, R.G. Korneluk, The inhibitors of apoptosis: there is more to life than Bcl2,
      Oncogene 22 (2003) 8568–8580.

[87] H. Nishihara, M. Hwang, S. Kizaka-Kondoh, L. Eckmann, P.A. Insel, Cyclic AMP promotes
      cAMP-responsive element-binding protein-dependent induction of cellular inhibitor of apoptosis
      protein-2 and suppresses apoptosis of colon cancer cells through ERK1/2 and p38 MAPK, J. Biol.
      Chem. 279 (2004) 26176–26183.

[88] H. Nishihara, S. Kizaka-Kondoh, P.A. Insel, L. Eckmann, Inhibition of apoptosis in normal and
      transformed intestinal epithelial cells by cAMP through induction of inhibitor of apoptosis protein
      (IAP)-2, Proc. Natl. Acad. Sci. USA 100 (2003) 8921–8926.

[89] W.H. Walker, L. Fucci, J.F. Habener, Expression of the gene encoding transcription factor cyclic
      adenosine 3′,5′-monophosphate (cAMP) response element-binding protein (CREB): regulation by
      follicle-stimulating hormone-induced cAMP signaling in primary rat Sertoli cells, Endocrinology 136
      (1995) 3534–3545.

[90] A. Eggers, G. Siemann, R. Blume, W. Knepel, Gene-specific transcriptional activity of the insulin
      cAMP-responsive element is conferred by NF-Y in combination with cAMP response element
      binding protein, J. Biol. Chem. 273 (1998) 18499–18508.

[91] N. Ban, Y. Yamada, Y. Someya, Y. Ihara, T. Adachi, A. Kubota, R. Watanabe, A. Kuroe,
      A. Inada, K. Miyawaki, Y. Sunaga, Z.P. Shen, T. Iwakura, K. Tsukiyama, S. Toyokuni, L. Tsuda,

Y. Seino, Activating transcription factor-2 is a positive regulator in CaM kinase IV-induced human insulin gene expression, Diabetes 49 (2000) 1142–1148.

[92] B. Eckert, M. Schwaninger, W. Knepel, Calcium-mobilizing insulin secretagogues stimulate transcription that is directed by the cyclic adenosine 3',5'-monophosphate/calcium response element in a pancreatic islet beta-cell line, Endocrinology 137 (1996) 225–233.

[93] S. Susini, G.V. Haasteren, S. Li, M. Prentki, W. Schlegel, Essentiality of intron control in the induction of c-fos by glucose and glucoincretin peptides in INS-1 beta-cells, FASEB J 14 (2000) 128–136.

[94] M.V.d. Casteele, B.A. Kefas, Z. Ling, H. Heimberg, D.G. Pipeleers, Specific expression of Bax-omega in pancreatic beta-cells is down-regulated by cytokines before the onset of apoptosis, Endocrinology 143 (2002) 320–326.

[95] S. Piro, R. Lupi, F. Dotta, G. Patane, M.A. Rabuazzo, L. Marselli, C. Santangelo, M. Realacci, S. Del Guerra, F. Purrello, P. Marchetti, Bovine islets are less susceptible than human islets to damage by human cytokines, Transplantation 71 (2001) 21–26.

[96] M.L. Trincavelli, L. Marselli, A. Falleni, V. Gremigni, E. Ragge, F. Dotta, C. Santangelo, P. Marchetti, A. Lucacchini, C. Martini, Upregulation of mitochondrial peripheral benzodiazepine receptor expression by cytokine-induced damage of human pancreatic islets, J. Cell Biochem. 84 (2002) 636–644.

[97] A. Rabinovitch, W. Suarez-Pinzon, K. Strynadka, Q. Ju, D. Edelstein, M. Brownlee, G.S. Korbutt, R.V. Rajotte, Transfection of human pancreatic islets with an anti-apoptotic gene (bcl-2) protects beta-cells from cytokine-induced destruction, Diabetes 48 (1999) 1223–1229.

[98] P. Jambal, S. Masterson, A. Nesterova, R. Bouchard, B. Bergman, J.C. Hutton, L.M. Boxer, J.E. Reusch, S. Pugazhenthi, Cytokine-mediated downregulation of the transcription factor CREB in pancreatic beta –cells, J. Biol. Chem. 278 (2003) 23055–23065.

[99] U.S. Jhala, G. Canettieri, R.A. Screaton, R.N. Kulkarni, S. Krajewski, J. Reed, J. Walker, X. Lin, M. White, M. Montminy, cAMP promotes pancreatic beta-cell survival via CREB-mediated induction of IRS2, Genes Dev. 17 (2003) 1575–1580.

[100] A. Inada, Y. Hamamoto, Y. Tsuura, J. Miyazaki, S. Toyokuni, Y. Ihara, K. Nagai, Y. Yamada, S. Bonner-Weir, Y. Seino, Overexpression of inducible cyclic AMP early repressor inhibits transactivation of genes and cell proliferation in pancreatic beta cells, Mol. Cell. Biol. 24 (2004) 2831–2841.

Chapter 12

Regulation of PGC-1 in humans with insulin resistance and type 2 diabetes: Functional implications

Jussi Pihlajamäki, Mary Elizabeth Patti

Research Division, Joslin Diabetes Center, One Joslin Place, Boston, MA 02215 USA

Abstract

The PGC-1 family of coactivator genes has emerged as attractive candidates for type 2 diabetes (T2DM) diabetes for several reasons: (1) they play a central role in regulating expression of genes critical for maintenance of metabolic homeostasis and oxidative metabolism in key target tissues, and (2) expression of PGC-1 and mitochondrial oxidative genes is reduced in skeletal muscle and adipose tissue from humans with diabetes and "prediabetes." In turn, this expression phenotype may be linked to both primary sequence alterations and environmental risk factors for diabetes, including overnutrition, obesity, and inactivity. We postulate that in genetically susceptible individuals, the development of obesity and decreased aerobic capacity due to inactivity may act in concert to reduce PGC-1 expression, contributing to impaired oxidative metabolism and accumulation of lipid in key insulin target tissues, thus increasing diabetes risk. In this chapter, we review the data supporting a potential role for PGC-1 family members as integrators between genetic and environmental risk factors at a molecular level and thus contributors to pathogenesis of T2DM.

1. Introduction

Insulin resistance and type 2 diabetes (T2DM) are major public health problems worldwide. Since inherited factors cannot account for the rapidly increasing prevalence of T2DM over the past few decades, environmental factors are likely to be major contributors to the epidemic of T2DM at both an individual and population level. However, a broader view would suggest that the concomitant increase in obesity, insulin resistance and T2DM reflects the inability of some individuals to cope with a rapidly changing, "Westernized" environment of abundant food and

ADVANCES IN MOLECULAR AND CELLULAR ENDOCRINOLOGY
VOLUME 5 ISSN 1569-2566/DOI 10.1016/S1569-2566(06)05012-5

decreased need for physical activity. Thus, susceptibility to diabetes and obesity may reflect individual differences in gene–environment interactions, which are critical for maintenance of normal metabolic homeostasis.

Interactions between environmental factors and genes are mediated by a network of transcription factors, coactivators, and corepressors. While transcription factors modulate gene expression by binding to DNA, coactivators and corepressors do not bind directly to DNA, but influence transcription by interacting with transcription factors, modifying chromatin, or altering protein–protein interactions within the transcriptional complex. Among the best studied as diabetes candidate genes in this context are the nuclear receptors peroxisome proliferative activated receptors gamma (PPARγ) and alpha (PPARα), and their coactivators, PGC-1α and β (PPARγ co-activators 1 alpha and beta, official gene names PPARGC1A and PPARGC1B). The PGC-1 family of coactivators is particularly attractive as diabetes-related candidate genes given their roles in coactivation of not only PPARγ [1] and PPARα [2], but also nuclear respiratory factors (NRF) regulating mitochondrial biogenesis and respiration [3]. In addition, PGC-1 coactivates other transcription factors critical for metabolic functions, including estrogen-related receptor α (ERRα) [4], hepatic nuclear factor 4α (HNF4α) [5], SREBP1 [6], FOXO1 [7], and others. In this chapter, we review the potential role of PGC-1 family members as integrators of interactions between genetic and environmental risk factors at a molecular level and thus contributors to pathogenesis of T2DM.

2. PGC-1 family members and their interactions with other molecules

The PGC-1 family of coactivators currently encompasses 3 related but distinct gene products. PGC-1α was first identified as a PPARγ-interacting protein in brown fat cells [1]. Subsequent studies implicate a much broader role for PGC-1α in coordinating transcriptional responses to alterations in energy demand in many tissues [8]. PGC-1β shares extensive sequence homology with PGC-1α [9,10]. The third member of the family, PGC-related coactivator (PRC, PPRC) is less homologous [3,11]. Since extensive reviews on the structure and interactions of these transcription factors have been recently published [12,13], only a short introduction will be presented below.

2.1. Structure

PGC-1α and β share a multidomain structure – an N-terminal activation domain, a central regulatory/repression domain with p38 phosphorylation sites, nuclear receptor binding sites, and C-terminal RS (arginine- and serine-rich) and RNA binding domains. While nuclear receptor binding sites and RNA binding domains are typical for a transcriptional coactivator, PGC-1α and β also possess domains that implicate a broader ability to modulate transcription. For example, the N-terminal activation domain can complex with histone acetyltransferase complexes [14,15] and histone deacetylases [16,17] activating transcription via chromatin remodeling and displacement of repressors, and activation of transcription. The C-terminus of all 3 PGC-1-related genes interacts with components of the TRAP/DRIP complex [15] and has an RS domain typical of splicing factors, which may facilitate PGC-1-dependent regulation of splicing [18]. Taken together, the multidomain structure of PGC-1 family members facilitates a versatile, and most likely central, function in coupling extracellular and metabolic signals to the regulation of gene expression.

3. Regulation of PGC-1α and β

Transcriptional activity of PGC-1 can be modulated by alterations in its expression or by post-translational modifications. In the case of PGC-1α, known environmental stimuli regulating expression and activity include cold exposure (in brown adipocytes) [1], fasting (in liver) [19] and exercise (in skeletal muscle) [20] – all states of energy deficiency or energy demand. While the precise tissue-specific pathways mediating expression and/or activation of PGC-1 may vary between tissues, several dominant mechanisms have been identified.

The upregulation of PGC-1α by cold and adrenergic activators, originally observed in rodent brown fat and skeletal muscle, is mediated by CREB-dependent promoter activation [1,21]. This transcriptional mechanism also plays a role in increased PGC-1α expression in the fasting liver [22]. In skeletal muscle, upregulation of PGC-1α expression has also been linked to thyroid hormone [23], calcium-signaling, MEF2, and AMP kinase-linked pathways. Exercise leads to activation of calcineurin A and calcium/calmodulin-dependent protein kinases; transgenic activation of these pathways in mice increases mitochondrial biogenesis [24] and expression of PGC-1α in C2C12 cells [21]. Another important regulator of PGC-1α expression in skeletal muscle is the transcription factor myocyte enhancer factor 2 (MEF2) [25,26]. Interestingly, MEF2 activation is potently initiated by PGC-1α binding to the MEF2 promoter and further enhanced during exercise by calcium – and calcineurin A-dependent signals [21], generating a positive autoregulatory feedback loop. A similar feed-forward loop is created by PGC-1α-dependent upregulation of ERRα expression; subsequent binding of ERRα to the PGC-1α promoter results in further increases in PGC-1 expression [4,27–34]. The AMP kinase pathway, activated in response to low-energy states in muscle, also plays a role in regulation of PGC-1; mice expressing dominant-negative AMP kinase are unable to increase PGC-1 expression following exercise [35]. While the effect of AMP kinase activation on PGC-1 is not mediated by CREB, the downstream effectors remain unknown. Similarly, the components mediating serum-stimulated upregulation of PRC expression are unknown [11] – implying that other transcriptional activators of PGC-1 family members may also exist.

PGC-1 is also under general transcriptional regulation, with increased expression associated with histone acetylation, and decreased expression linked to deacetylation in mouse heart [25]. Furthermore, small heterodimer partner SHP, a general inhibitor of transactivation of nuclear receptors, represses PGC-1α [17].

Post-translational modification can also influence PGC-1 activity. For example, PGC-1α stability and transcriptional activity are increased by p38 MAPK-mediated phosphorylation [23,36–38]; this pathway may contribute to exercise – and fasting-induced increases in PGC-1α [39,40]. Interestingly, PGC-1 interacts with SIRT1 and SIRT3, the human homologs of genes that mediate the effect of caloric restriction on lifespan in yeast [41–43]. Deacetylation of PGC-1α by SIRT1 in an NAD(+)-dependent manner activates the gluconeogenic actions of PGC-1α [41]. Recently, arginine methylation by PRMT1 within the C-terminus of PGC-1α has been proposed to be essential for PGC-1α activation [44]. Taken together, these data indicate that multiple environmental stimuli, acting through cAMP-, calcium-, MEF2-, and p38 MAPK-dependent pathways, among others, can influence PGC-1α expression and activity in response to states of cellular energy deficit or demand.

4. Role of PGC-1α and β in normal physiology

Maintenance of energy supply for vital functions is critical for homeostasis. In higher eukaryotes, energy metabolism must be able to adapt to both short-term (fasting vs. post-meal) and long-term (famine vs. food abundance) nutritional cycles. In this context, regulated changes in PGC-1 expression and/or activity may serve as a key mechanism to ensure energy homeostasis, by linking the ambient nutritional and hormonal environment to appropriate levels of oxidative metabolism and thermogenesis.

As noted above, PGC-1α and β interact with several other nuclear receptors and transcription factors. Thus, PGC1 function, including transcriptional activation [14], repression [16, 45] and mRNA splicing [18], may vary as a result of tissue-specific expression of partner genes. Therefore, when considering the potential role of PGC1 in diabetes risk, it is critical to assess the effects of PGC1 on tissue-specific metabolism and net whole-body physiology.

4.1. *Mitochondrial biogenesis and oxidative phosphorylation*

PGC-1 expression, which is increased in states of cellular energy deficit, stimulates mitochondrial oxidative metabolism in multiple tissues. These effects are mediated to a large extent via increased expression and transcriptional activity of nuclear respiratory factors 1 and 2 (NRF1 and 2), known regulators of mitochondrial biogenesis [11,47] and transcription of nuclear-encoded mitochondrial genes [47,48]. Together, PGC-1 and NRF genes increase expression of mitochondrial transcription factor A (mtTFA) [47] and mitochondrial transcription specificity factors (TFB1 M and TFB2 M) [48], leading to increased transcription of mitochondrial DNA. In addition, PGC-1 coactivation of PPARγ [1], PPARα [2], PPARδ [49], ERRα [30,50], and thyroid hormone receptor β [51] contributes to stimulation of expression of oxidative metabolism genes.

4.2. *Skeletal muscle*

PGC-1α is now recognized to play a key role in multiple metabolic processes in skeletal muscle linked to oxidative function, insulin sensitivity, exercise capacity, and fiber type specification. Overexpression of PGC-1 in cultured myotubes increases oxidative metabolism (e.g. tricarboxylic acid cycle activity, lipid oxidation, and mitochondrial oxidative phosphorylation) and induces mitochondrial biogenesis [47]. In addition, adenoviral expression of PGC-1α increases GLUT4 expression and glucose uptake in both cultured myotubes [52] and rat skeletal muscle [53]. The muscle phenotypes of PGC-1 overexpression share some similarities with transgenic overexpression of NRF1 in skeletal muscle [54]. Moreover, the effects of PGC-1 in cultured myotubes can be blocked by expression of a dominant-negative NRF lacking its transactivation domain [8,46]. Together, these data suggest that the effects of PGC-1 on mitochondrial function and oxidative metabolism in muscle are mediated largely via induction of NRF-mediated transcription.

Exercise potently upregulates PGC-1α expression in humans as early as 2 h after exercise [55,56]; this effect can be sustained for several weeks [57,58]. While these effects have been noted with high-intensity exercise (50% VO2 max), it remains unclear whether lower intensity exercise influences PGC-1 expression. The impact of exercise in humans is particularly prominent in type II fibers, possibly contributing to conversion to oxidative type I fibers [20,57]. Similar fiber-type changes have been observed in transgenic mice or myotubes overexpressing PGC-1α [35,59]. As previously noted, the upregulation of PGC-1α with exercise involves cAMP – and p38-dependent pathways and MEF2-binding elements in the PGC-1α promoter [39,60]. In C2C12 myotubes, fiber type conversion induced by PGC-1 is co-regulated by calcineurin and MEF2 signals [59].

Negative modulation of PGC-1 expression in skeletal muscle may also play an important role in regulation of muscle metabolism in states of inactivity or obesity. For example, downregulation of PGC-1 in skeletal muscle occurs in states of lipid excess, such as high-fat feeding in mice [61–63] and rats [63] or lipid infusion in healthy humans [64]. However, in human myotubes, unsaturated fatty acids *increase* PGC-1α expression, implying that fatty acids may differ in their ability to modify PGC-1 expression [65]. In rat skeletal muscle, the reduction in PGC-1α expression and associated impairments in β-oxidation induced by high-fat feeding can be reversed by exercise [63]. High levels of PGC-1 induced by exercise and/or chronic fitness may permit enhanced oxidation, protecting cells from the negative effects of lipid exposure on oxidative capacity. Nevertheless, links between regulation of PGC-1, physical fitness, and lipid accumulation are complex and incompletely understood, as indicated by the finding that lipid accumulation in highly trained athletes is actually increased [66].

Taken together, these data indicate that PGC-1 plays a key role in skeletal muscle to maintain oxidative capacity, limit lipid toxicity, and facilitate energy supply for contraction. When PGC-1 is limited, as seen in the extreme in mice lacking PGC-1α, mitochondrial biogenesis, oxidative capacity and exercise tolerance are severely impaired [67,68].

4.3. Liver

In the liver, PGC-1α stimulates key metabolic processes involved in maintenance of nutrient homeostasis during fasting, including gluconeogenesis, fat oxidation and ketogenesis. Accordingly, both PGC-1α [19] and β [10,69] are upregulated in the liver with fasting in mice. The regulation of gluconeogenesis by PGC-1α is largely mediated by increased expression of key gluconeogenic enzymes, such as PEPCK, and requires interactions with HNF-4α [5,70], FOXO1 [7], and the glucocorticoid receptor [22]. Appropriate hepatic PGC-1α responses are critical for maintenance of glucose levels during a fast; mice lacking PGC-1α are resistant to hormone-stimulated gluconeogenesis and ketogenesis, and thus develop fasting hypoglycemia [67,71]. By contrast, PGC-1β does not appear to play a major role in gluconeogenesis in the fasting state [69].

Since PGC-1 promotes lipid oxidation, one might expect that PGC-1α deficient mice would have low rates of fat oxidation and thus develop hepatic steatosis. However, results from two independent whole-body PGC-1α knockout mice are discordant. In one model, fasting lipid content was decreased [67], whereas hepatic steatosis was present in the second [68]. The reason for these discrepancies remains unclear at present.

While saturated fatty acids increase expression of both PGC-1α and PGC-1β in the liver [67], PGC-1β has a unique role in lipid metabolism. Increased expression of PGC-1β in mice leads to SREBP1 activation and increased triglyceride and cholesterol synthesis. Accordingly, PGC-1β-deficient mice are resistant to developing dyslipidemia when fed a diet rich in saturated fatty acids [6]. PGC-1α also coactivates LXRα, highlighting a close relationship between PGC-1 and factors regulating lipid metabolism in the liver [72].

4.4. *Adipose tissue*

PGC-1α promotes the conversion of white adipocytes to a more "brown-like" adipocyte. Adenoviral expression of PGC-1 in human adipocytes induces expression of oxidative phosphorylation proteins and UCP1 and increases palmitate oxidation, thus promoting energy dissipation [73]. In brown adipose tissue, PGC-1α promotes thermogenesis [1]; deficiency of PGC-1α leads to cold sensitivity in mice, due at least in part to defective thermogenesis in BAT [67]. While the significance of brown adipose tissue in human physiology is unclear, the activation of PGC-1 in human adipocytes could yield beneficial impacts on thermogenesis and whole-body energy metabolism.

4.5. *Cardiac muscle*

While the heart primarily utilizes fatty acids as its main energy source, metabolic flexibility in nutrient oxidation is maintained by PPARα and PGC-1α-dependent processes [74]. As in skeletal muscle, PGC-1α stimulates mitochondrial biogenesis [75]; not surprisingly, PGC-1α-deficient mice are unable to meet increased demands for ATP and have reduced contractile function [76]. Importantly, either inhibition of PGC-1α by cardiac-specific activation of Cdk9 [77] or inducible *overexpression* of PGC-1α in adult mice leads to cardiomyopathy [78]. Thus, these data demonstrate the critical importance of PGC-1 in maintaining the metabolic flexibility required for normal cardiac homeostasis.

4.6. *Brain*

PGC-1α is widely expressed throughout the brain [79]. While PGC-1α knockout mice exhibit neuronal degeneration [67,68], the potential impact of central nervous system PGC-1 deficiency on whole-body metabolism and regulation of adiposity remains unclear. One strain of PGC-1-deficient mice is hyperactive, lean and resistant to diet-induced obesity [67]; an independent line of PGC-1α deficient mice is not lean, with females even developing diet-induced obesity with aging [68]. Whether these phenotypes reflect integrated peripheral tissue responses, or central nervous system responses to PGC-1 deficiency, will be important to address in future studies.

4.7. *Other tissue effects of PGC-1*

While increased β-oxidation associated with increased PGC-1α expression might be expected to increase generation of reactive oxygen species [80], overexpression of PGC-1α in endothelial cells actually reduces accumulation of reactive oxygen species by increasing expression of genes encoding mitochondrial detoxifying enzymes [81]. PGC-1α is also expressed in pancreatic islets. Limited data from rodent islets demonstrate that saturated fatty acids increase PGC-1 expression [82] and overexpression of PGC-1α may suppress β-cell energy metabolism [83]. PGC-1α also regulates expression of the rate-limiting enzyme in hepatic heme biosynthesis, 5-aminolevulinate synthase – a potential explanation for the effect of fasting to provoke attacks in porphyria [84].

4.8. *What have we learned about the role of PGC-1α and PGC-1β in normal whole-body physiology from these studies?*

We hypothesize that PGC-1α plays an important role to maintain whole-body energy homeostasis, particularly during prolonged fasting and exercise (Fig. 1). In skeletal and cardiac muscle, PGC-1 ensures availability of substrate and ATP for contraction. In the liver, PGC-1α increases expression of genes critical for gluconeogenesis, lipid oxidation, and ketogenesis, thus facilitating energy availability during prolonged fasting (after glycogen stores are depleted). The physiological relevance of PGC-1-induced thermogenesis in BAT in human adults is unclear. However, PGC-1 may regulate whole-body energy balance by promoting oxidative metabolism and/or adipocytokine production in white adipose tissue. Finally, the potential effects of PGC-1 to regulate metabolism via the CNS will likely be a fruitful area of exploration in the near future.

5. Role of PGC-1α and β in pathophysiology of type 2 diabetes

Accumulation of fat within nonadipose tissue, particularly skeletal muscle and liver, is an early marker of T2DM risk [85] (Fig. 2). In fact, intramyocellular lipid accumulation may contribute directly to insulin resistance via downregulation of insulin signalling [85]. Similarly, "ectopic" fat in the liver may lead to insulin

A.   Tissue-Specific Regulation of PGC-1 Expression

	Exercise	Fasting	Fatty Acids (FA)	Obesity / High Fat Diet
Muscle	↑[57]	↔ (24 hr fast, rat) [63] ↑ (5 day fast, obese humans) [98]	↑ in α (unsaturated FAs)[65] ↓ in α, β (saturated FAs)[61,62] ↓ in α (mixed FAs *in vivo*)[64]	↓[61,62]
Liver		↑ in α, β[69]	↑ in α, β (saturated FAs)[6]	↑[6]
Fat				↓[111]

B.   Tissue-Specific Consequences of PGC-1 Expression

MUSCLE	LIVER	FAT	OTHERS
Fat oxidation ↑[47]	Glucose production ↑[5]	Uncoupling ↑[73]	HEART: Fat oxidation ↑[76]
Glucose uptake ↑[53]	Fat oxidation and ketogenesis↑[67]		BRAIN: Altered regulation of energy metabolism?[67]
	Lipid production (PGC-1β) ↑[6]		PANCREAS: Insulin secretion ↓?[83]

Fig. 1. (A) Tissue-specific regulation of PGC-1 expression. (B) Tissue-specific physiological effects in humans and animals. Note that superscripts denote selected references from text.

resistance, unrestrained gluconeogenesis, increased cholesterol and triglyceride synthesis, inflammation, non-alcoholic steatohepatitis, and even liver failure [86]. Lipid accumulation in pancreatic islets may also contribute to the insulin secretory dysfunction associated with obesity and diabetes [87].

Such examples of ectopic lipid accumulation have been proposed to be caused by reduced activity of TCA cycle, β-oxidation, and electron transport pathways [88] and reductions in mitochondrial area [89] and number [90]. In support of this hypothesis, recent studies utilizing ^{31}P NMR spectroscopy in nondiabetic humans with a family history of diabetes have demonstrated reductions in skeletal muscle mitochondrial function and ATP synthesis both in the basal and insulin-stimulated states, in parallel with intramuscular lipid accumulation [91,92]. While ectopic lipid is clearly recognized as a marker of insulin resistance and diabetes risk, it remains unclear whether ectopic lipid (a) is playing a primary pathogenic role in insulin resistance, (b) is linked to an underlying genetic defect in lipid oxidation, or (c) represents "spillover" of excess fat from adipose tissue.

Recent studies utilizing high-density oligonucleotide arrays provide support for the hypothesis that alterations in PGC-1 expression and/or function may contribute to increased lipid accumulation and disruption of oxidative metabolism in human skeletal muscle. In skeletal muscle of patients with type 2 diabetes, expression of PGC-1α and β is reduced, by up to 46% in the fasting state in a Mexican-American population [93] and by approximately 20% during hyperinsulinemia in Swedish Caucasians [94]. In both studies, modest 25–30% reductions in expression of PGC – and NRF-dependent genes were detected using pathway/approaches. Similar changes in OXPHOS gene expression (but not PGC-1) are also a feature of uncontrolled type T2DM in humans [95] and in

GENETICS
- **Sequence Polymorphisms**
- **Haplotype Variation**

DIABETES RISK PHENOTYPES

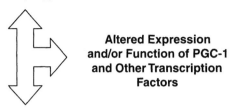

Altered Expression and/or Function of PGC-1 and Other Transcription Factors

SKELETAL MUSCLE
- *Lipid Accumulation*
- *Mitochondrial Dysfunction*
- *↓ Fat Oxidation*
- *Insulin Resistance*

LIVER
- *Steatosis*
- *↑ Gluconeogenesis*
- *↑ Triglyceride Synthesis*

ADIPOSE TISSUE
- *↓ Thermogenesis*
- *Altered Adipocyte Function*

ENVIRONMENT
- **Overnutrition**
- **Suboptimal Diet Composition**
- **Decreased Physical Activity & Fitness**

PANCREAS
- *Insulin Secretory Defect*

Fig. 2. Pathogenesis of type 2 diabetes: potential role of PGC-1 in mediating gene–environment interactions. Possible metabolic defects contributed by dysregulation of PGC-1 are shown in italics.

mice with insulin-deficient diabetes induced by streptozotocin [96]; these changes can be reversed with insulin when insulin receptor signalling is intact [97]. Since these data suggest an important role for hyperglycemia and the diabetes metabolic milieu to modulate changes in PGC-1 and oxidative metabolism gene expression, it is important to note that similar reductions in both PGC-1α and PGC-1β and oxidative gene expression are also observed in insulin resistant, but completely normoglycemic individuals [93] and in obese nondiabetic subjects [98].

Taken together, these data have led to the hypothesis that decreased expression of genes related to mitochondrial oxidative metabolism may contribute to skeletal muscle lipid accumulation in insulin resistance and T2DM. Several findings suggest that decreased PGC-1 expression may be a major, if not primary, contributor to this lipid accumulation and overall diabetes pathophysiology. First, expression of both PGC-1 α and β is significantly reduced in both patients with impaired glucose tolerance [94] and in nondiabetic relatives of T2DM patients [93]. Second, twin studies support the concept that PGC-1 expression in muscle may be influenced by genetic regulation [99]. Finally, polymorphisms in the PGC-1α and β genes have been associated with insulin resistance [100–102], obesity [103] and T2DM [100, 104,105], and may influence lipid oxidation [106] and PGC-1 expression levels [99].

Conversely, we must still consider the possibility that reductions in PGC-1 expression observed in "prediabetic" humans are secondary to insulin resistance and/ or lipid accumulation. As noted previously, obesity, high-fat diet, and lipid infusion are associated with reductions in PGC-1 expression in both mice and humans [61,64]. We believe that it is unlikely that hyperinsulinemia contributes to decreased PGC1 expression, as short-term insulin infusion in humans is associated with variable PGC1 responses [99] and [144], and prolonged insulin treatment of human myotubes is associated with increased PGC1 expression [107]. In fact, normalization of hyperglycemia with insulin in either mice or humans partially reverses decreased

OXPHOS gene expression [95,99]. This effect is blunted in mice with muscle-specific insulin receptor deficiency (MIRKO), suggesting that normal insulin signalling promotes expression of OXPHOS genes. Finally, decreased PGC-1 expression in insulin resistant subjects may be aggravated by inactivity [55–58]. Thus, based on the limited, cross-sectional human data available to date, it is difficult to conclude whether low PGC-1α and β expression in skeletal muscle is a *cause* or a *consequence* of the insulin resistance and diabetes risk. Additional longitudinal studies of individuals with early prediabetes, including assessment of intramuscular lipid accumulation in parallel with gene expression changes, will be required to evaluate the primacy of defects in *PGC-1* expression in skeletal muscle.

The possibility that PGC-1α increases energy dissipation in human fat [108] is intriguing. In adipose tissue from obese humans, expression of PGC-1α is decreased, in parallel with insulin resistance [109–111]. It remains unclear at present whether altered PGC-1 expression and function secondarily reflects excess lipid accumulation in adipose cells, or represents a primary, potentially pathogenic change, which may provide a useful therapeutic target.

Both insulin resistance and insulin secretory dysfunction are critical elements in the development of T2DM. Lipotoxicity has long been proposed to be one explanation for failing insulin secretion in insulin-resistant humans [87], and susceptibility to lipotoxicity may be genetically determined [112]. We speculate that PGC-1α, which is expressed in pancreatic islets, may contribute to that genetic risk. In rat islets, free fatty acids increase PGC-1α expression [82] and may suppress β-cell energy metabolism [83]. In fact, inhibition of PGC-1α using an antisense oligonucleotide ameliorated hyperglycemia in diabetic mice [113]. Thus, data from pancreatic studies, similar to those in liver but in contrast to skeletal muscle, suggest that constantly high PGC-1α expression may not be desirable for optimal pancreatic islet function.

6. Role of genes in the regulation of PGC-1α and β in humans

Because PGC-1α and β can be considered as sensors which mediate metabolic responses to environmental signals, it is plausible that inherited variation in these regulatory genes could contribute to dysregulation of metabolism in insulin resistance and T2DM. This hypothesis may provide an explanation for the well-known clinical observation that there is substantial variability within the population in ability to adapt to a high-energy diet and sedentary lifestyle [114,115].

Genes for PGC-1α and β are mapped to chromosomes 4p15 and 5q33, respectively [10,116]. Interestingly, genome scans have linked the 4p15 region to fasting insulin levels in Pima Indians [117] and to severe obesity in Caucasians [118] and Mexican Americans [119]. Polymorphisms, most often the 482Ser allele in PGC-1α, have been associated with increased prevalence of diabetes in Danish, Japanese, and Korean populations [100,105]. Negative results have been reported for Pima [106] and Caucasian populations [120–122].

Other studies have demonstrated associations between polymorphisms in PGC-1α and phenotypes contributing to diabetes risk, e.g. lipid oxidation [106], insulin

activity in the liver may aggravate fasting hyperglycemia. Second, activation of PGC-1β in the liver increases cholesterol and triglyceride synthesis in mice fed with saturated fatty acids [6]. Third, the activation of PGC-1 in pancreatic islets may suppress β-cell energy metabolism [83], and *inhibition* of PGC-1α in islets can *improve* insulin secretion in diabetic mice [113]. Finally, the effects of whole-body PGC-1α deficiency remain unclear: Two independent mouse models are discordant for obesity – one resistant and the other prone to diet-induced obesity [67,68]. While there are always extensive caveats when considering animal data in light of human disease risk and treatment, these data indicate that PGC-1α activation is not a straightforward treatment for diabetes and/or obesity. Therapeutic modulation of PGC-1α would require a tissue-specific approach – e.g., activation of PGC-1α and β in skeletal muscle and fat, but an inactivation in liver and pancreas (Fig. 2). In addition, the final phenotype in response to PGC-1 modification would likely depend on the amount and distribution of dietary fatty acids.

In conclusion, PGC-1α and β play a central role in adaptive responses to metabolic and environmental cues by modulating expression of genes critical for mitochondrial biogenesis and oxidative function, hepatic gluconeogenesis and lipid metabolism, and thermogenesis. In turn, it is likely that both genetic variation and adverse environmental factors (obesity, fatty acids, inactivity), disrupt appropriate PGC-1 expression and function, leading to deleterious changes in whole-body carbohydrate and lipid metabolism and increased risk for insulin resistance and T2DM. Thus, the PGC-1 family of genes is at the center of interactions between genetics, diet, and exercise – a crucial piece of the puzzle of T2DM pathogenesis and future approaches to tissue-targeted interventions for both therapy and prevention.

Acknowledgments

This work was supported by NIH grants DK062948 and DK060837 (MEP) and the Sigrid Juselius Foundation Fellowship (JP).

References

[1] P. Puigserver, Z. Wu, C.W. Park, R. Graves, M. Wright, B.M. Spiegelman, A cold-inducible co-activator of nuclear receptors linked to adaptive thermogenesis, Cell 92 (6) (1998) 829–839.

[2] R.B. Vega, J.M. Huss, D.P. Kelly, The coactivator PGC-1 cooperates with peroxisome proliferator-activated receptor alpha in transcriptional control of nuclear genes encoding mitochondrial fatty acid oxidation enzymes, Mol. Cell Biol. 20 (5) (2000) 1868–1876.

[3] R.C. Scarpulla, Transcriptional activators and coactivators in the nuclear control of mitochondrial function in mammalian cells, Gene. 286 (1) (2002) 81–89.

[4] I. Tcherepanova, P. Puigserver, J.D. Norris, B.M. Spiegelman, D.P. McDonnell, Modulation of estrogen receptor-alpha transcriptional activity by the coactivator PGC-1, J. Biol. Chem. 275 (21) (2000) 16302–16308.

[5] J. Rhee, Y. Inoue, J.C. Yoon, P. Puigserver, M. Fan, F.J. Gonzalez, et al., Regulation of hepatic fasting response by PPARgamma coactivator-1alpha (PGC-1): requirement for hepatocyte nuclear factor 4alpha in gluconeogenesis, Proc. Natl. Acad. Sci. USA 100 (7) (2003) 4012–4017.

[6] J. Lin, R. Yang, P.T. Tarr, P.H. Wu, C. Handschin, S. Li, et al., Hyperlipidemic effects of dietary saturated fats mediated through PGC-1beta coactivation of SREBP, Cell 120 (2) (2005) 261–273.

[7] P. Puigserver, J. Rhee, J. Donovan, C.J. Walkey, J.C. Yoon, F. Oriente, et al., Insulin-regulated hepatic gluconeogenesis through FOXO1-PGC-1alpha interaction, Nature 423 (6939) (2003) 550–555.

[8] P. Puigserver, B.M. Spiegelman, Peroxisome proliferator-activated receptor-gamma coactivator 1 alpha (PGC-1 alpha): transcriptional coactivator and metabolic regulator, Endocr. Rev. 24 (1) (2003) 78–90.

[9] D. Kressler, S.N. Schreiber, D. Knutti, A. Kralli, The PGC-1-related protein PERC is a selective coactivator of estrogen receptor alpha, J. Biol. Chem. 277 (16) (2002) 13918–13925.

[10] J. Lin, P. Puigserver, J. Donovan, P. Tarr, B.M. Spiegelman, Peroxisome proliferator-activated receptor gamma coactivator 1beta (PGC-1beta), a novel PGC-1-related transcription coactivator associated with host cell factor, J. Biol. Chem. 277 (3) (2002) 1645–1648.

[11] U. Andersson, R.C. Scarpulla, Pgc-1-related coactivator, a novel, serum-inducible coactivator of nuclear respiratory factor 1-dependent transcription in mammalian cells, Mol. Cell Biol. 21 (11) (2001) 3738–3749.

[12] J. Lin, C. Handschin, B.M. Spiegelman, Metabolic control through the PGC-1 family of transcription coactivators, Cell Metab. 1 (6) (2005) 361–370.

[13] P. Puigserver, Tissue-specific regulation of metabolic pathways through the transcriptional coactivator PGC1-alpha, Int. J. Obes. (London) 29 (Suppl 1) (2005) S5–9.

[14] P. Puigserver, G. Adelmant, Z. Wu, M. Fan, J. Xu, B. O'Malley, et al., Activation of PPARgamma coactivator-1 through transcription factor docking, Science 286 (5443) (1999) 1368–1371.

[15] A.E. Wallberg, S. Yamamura, S. Malik, B.M. Spiegelman, R.G. Roeder, Coordination of p300-mediated chromatin remodeling and TRAP/mediator function through coactivator PGC-1alpha, Mol. Cell 12 (5) (2003) 1137–1149.

[16] L.J. Borgius, K.R. Steffensen, J.A. Gustafsson, E. Treuter, Glucocorticoid signaling is perturbed by the atypical orphan receptor and corepressor SHP, J. Biol. Chem. 277 (51) (2002) 49761–49766.

[17] L. Wang, J. Liu, P. Saha, J. Huang, L. Chan, B. Spiegelman, et al. The orphan nuclear receptor SHP regulates PGC-1alpha expression and energy production in brown adipocytes, Cell Metab. 2 (4) (2005) 227–238.

[18] M. Monsalve, Z. Wu, G. Adelmant, P. Puigserver, M. Fan, B.M. Spiegelman, Direct coupling of transcription and mRNA processing through the thermogenic coactivator PGC-1, Mol. Cell 6 (2) (2000) 307–316.

[19] J.C. Yoon, P. Puigserver, G. Chen, J. Donovan, Z. Wu, J. Rhee, et al., Control of hepatic gluconeogenesis through the transcriptional coactivator PGC-1, Nature 413 (6852) (2001) 131–138.

[20] K. Baar, Involvement of PPAR gamma co-activator-1, nuclear respiratory factors 1 and 2, and PPAR alpha in the adaptive response to endurance exercise, Proc. Nutr. Soc. 63 (2) (2004) 269–273.

[21] C. Handschin, J. Rhee, J. Lin, P.T. Tarr, B.M. Spiegelman, An autoregulatory loop controls peroxisome proliferator-activated receptor gamma coactivator 1alpha expression in muscle, Proc. Natl. Acad. Sci. USA 100 (12) (2003) 7111–7116.

[22] S. Herzig, F. Long, U. S. Jhala, S. Hedrick, R. Quinn, Bauer, et al., CREB regulates hepatic gluconeogenesis through the coactivator PGC-1, Nature 413 (6852) (2001) 179–183.

[23] I. Irrcher, P.J. Adhihetty, T. Sheehan, A.M. Joseph, D.A. Hood, PPARgamma coactivator-1alpha expression during thyroid hormone- and contractile activity-induced mitochondrial adaptations, Am. J. Physiol. Cell Physiol. 284 (6) (2003) C1669–1677.

[24] H. Wu, S.B. Kanatous, F.A. Thurmond, T. Gallardo, E. Isotani, E.R. Bassel-Duby, et al., Regulation of mitochondrial biogenesis in skeletal muscle by CaMK, Science 296 (566) (2002) 349–352.

[25] M.P. Czubryt, J. McAnally, G.I. Fishman, E.N. Olson, Regulation of peroxisome proliferator-activated receptor gamma coactivator 1 alpha (PGC-1 alpha) and mitochondrial function by MEF2 and HDAC5, Proc. Natl. Acad. Sci. USA 100 (4) (2003) 1711–1716.

[26] S.L. McGee, M. Hargreaves, Exercise and myocyte enhancer factor 2 regulation in human skeletal muscle, Diabetes 53 (5) (2004) 1208–1214.

[27] M. Ichida, S. Nemoto, T. Finkel, Identification of a specific molecular repressor of the peroxisome proliferator-activated receptor gamma Coactivator-1 alpha (PGC-1alpha), J. Biol. Chem. 277 (52) (2002) 50991–50995.

[28] M. Hentschke, U. Susens, U. Borgmeyer, PGC-1 and PERC, coactivators of the estrogen receptor-related receptor gamma, Biochem. Biophys. Res. Commun. 299 (5) (2002) 872–879.

[29] J. Laganiere, G.B. Tremblay, C.R. Dufour, S. Giroux, F. Rousseau, V. Giguere, A polymorphic autoregulatory hormone response element in the human estrogen-related receptor alpha (ERRalpha) promoter dictates peroxisome proliferator-activated receptor gamma coactivator-1alpha control of ERRalpha expression, J. Biol. Chem. 279 (18) (2004) 18504–18510.

[30] V.K. Mootha, C. Handschin, D. Arlow, X. Xie, J. St Pierre, S. Sihag, et al. Erralpha and Gabpa/b specify PGC-1alpha-dependent oxidative phosphorylation gene expression that is altered in diabetic muscle, Proc. Natl. Acad. Sci. USA 101 (17) (2004) 6570–6755.

[31] J.M. Huss, I.P. Torra, B. Staels, V. Giguere, D.P. Kelly, Estrogen-related receptor alpha directs peroxisome proliferator-activated receptor alpha signaling in the transcriptional control of energy metabolism in cardiac and skeletal muscle, Mol. Cell Biol. 24 (20) (2004) 9079–9091.

[32] J. Kallen, J.M. Schlaeppi, F. Bitsch, I. Filipuzzi, A. Schilb, V. Riou, et al., Evidence for ligand-independent transcriptional activation of the human estrogen-related receptor alpha (ERRalpha): crystal structure of ERRalpha ligand binding domain in complex with peroxisome proliferator-activated receptor coactivator-1alpha, J. Biol. Chem. 279 (47) (2004) 49330–49337.

[33] P.J. Willy, I.R. Murray, J. Qian, B.B. Busch, W.C. Stevens Jr., R. Martin, et al., Regulation of PPARgamma coactivator 1alpha (PGC-1alpha) signaling by an estrogen-related receptor alpha (ERRalpha) ligand, Proc. Natl. Acad. Sci. USA 101 (24) (2004) 8912–8917.

[34] S.N. Schreiber, R. Emter, M.B. Hock, D. Knutti, J. Cardenas, M. Podvinec, et al., The estrogen-related receptor alpha (ERRalpha) functions in PPARgamma coactivator 1alpha (PGC-1alpha)-induced mitochondrial biogenesis, Proc. Natl. Acad. Sci. USA 101 (17) (2004) 6472–6477.

[35] H. Zong, J.M. Ren, L.H. Young, M. Pypaert, J. Mu, M.J. Birnbaum, et al., AMP kinase is required for mitochondrial biogenesis in skeletal muscle in response to chronic energy deprivation, Proc. Natl. Acad. Sci. USA 99 (25) (2002) 15983–15987.

[36] P. Puigserver, J. Rhee, J. Lin, Z. Wu, J.C. Yoon, C.Y. Zhang, et al., Cytokine stimulation of energy expenditure through p38 MAP kinase activation of PPARgamma coactivator-1, Mol. Cell 8 (5) (2001) 971–982.

[37] M. Fan, J. Rhee, J. St-Pierre, C. Handschin, P. Puigserver, J. Lin, et al., Suppression of mitochondrial respiration through recruitment of p160 myb binding protein to PGC-1alpha: modulation by p38 MAPK, Genes Dev. 18 (3) (2004) 278–289.

[38] W. Cao, K.W. Daniel, J. Robidoux, P. Puigserver, A.V. Medvedev, X. Bai, et al., p38 mitogen-activated protein kinase is the central regulator of cyclic AMP-dependent transcription of the brown fat uncoupling protein 1 gene, Mol. Cell Biol. 24 (7) (2004) 3057–3067.

[39] T. Akimoto, S.C. Pohnert, P. Li, M. Zhang, C. Gumbs, P.B. Rosenberg, et al., Exercise stimulates Pgc-1alpha transcription in skeletal muscle through activation of the p38 MAPK pathway, J. Biol. Chem. 280 (20) (2005) 19587–19593.

[40] W. Cao, Q.F. Collins, T.C. Becker, J. Robidoux, E.G. Lupo Jr., Y. Xiong, K.W. Daniel, L. Floering, S. Collins, p38 mitogen-activated protein kinase plays a stimulatory role in hepatic gluconeogenesis, J. Biol. Chem. 280 (52) (2005) 42731–42737.

[41] J.T. Rodgers, C. Lerin, W. Haas, S.P. Gygi, B.M. Spiegelman, P. Puigserver, Nutrient control of glucose homeostasis through a complex of PGC-1alpha and SIRT1, Nature 434 (7029) (2005) 113–118.

[42] T. Shi, F. Wang, E. Stieren, Q. Tong, SIRT3 a mitochondrial sirtuin deacetylase, regulates mitochondrial function and thermogenesis in brown adipocytes, J. Biol. Chem. 280 (14) (2005) 13560–13567.

[43] S. Nemoto, M.M. Fergusson, T. Finkel, SIRT1 functionally interacts with the metabolic regulator and transcriptional coactivator PGC-1{alpha}, J. Biol. Chem. 280 (16) (2005) 16456–16460.

[44] C. Teyssier, H. Ma, R. Emter, A. Kralli, Stallcup MR. Activation of nuclear receptor coactivator PGC-1alpha by arginine methylation, Genes Dev. 19 (12) (2005) 1466–1473.

[45] H.P. Guan, T. Ishizuka, P.C. Chui, M. Lehrke, M.A. Lazar, Corepressors selectively control the transcriptional activity of PPARgamma in adipocytes, Genes Dev. 19 (4) (2005) 453–461.

[46] R.C. Scarpulla, Nuclear activators and coactivators in mammalian mitochondrial biogenesis, Biochim. Biophys. Acta 1576 (1–2) (2002) 1–14.

[47] Z. Wu, P. Puigserver, U. Andersson, C. Zhang, G. Adelmant, V. Mootha, et al., Mechanisms controlling mitochondrial biogenesis and respiration through the thermogenic coactivator PGC-1, Cell 98 (1) (1999) 115–124.

[48] N. Gleyzer, K. Vercauteren, R.C. Scarpulla, Control of mitochondrial transcription specificity factors (TFB1 M and TFB2 M) by nuclear respiratory factors (NRF-1 and NRF-2) and PGC-1 family coactivators, Mol. Cell Biol. 25 (4) (2005) 1354–1366.

[49] Y.X. Wang, C.H. Lee, S. Tiep, R.T. Yu, J. Ham, H. Kang, et al., Peroxisome-proliferator-activated receptor delta activates fat metabolism to prevent obesity, Cell 113 (2) (2003) 159–170.

[50] S.N. Schreiber, D. Knutti, K. Brogli, T. Uhlmann, A. Kralli, The transcriptional coactivator PGC-1 regulates the expression and activity of the orphan nuclear receptor estrogen-related receptor alpha (ERRalpha), J. Biol. Chem. 278 (11) (2003) 9013–9018.

[51] Y. Wu, P. Delerive, W.W. Chin, T.P. Burris, Requirement of helix 1 and the AF-2 domain of the thyroid hormone receptor for coactivation by PGC-1, J. Biol. Chem. 277 (11) (2002) 8898–8905.

[52] L.F. Michael, Z. Wu, R.B. Cheatham, P. Puigserver, G. Adelmant, J.J. Lehman, et al., Restoration of insulin-sensitive glucose transporter (GLUT4) gene expression in muscle cells by the transcriptional coactivator PGC-1, Proc. Natl. Acad. Sci. USA 98 (7) (2001) 3820–3825.

[53] R.L. Oliveira, M. Ueno, C.T. de Souza, M. Pereira-da-Silva, A.L. Gasparetti, R.M. Bezzera, et al., Cold-induced PGC-1alpha expression modulates muscle glucose uptake through an insulin receptor/Akt-independent, AMPK-dependent pathway, Am. J. Physiol. Endocrinol. Metab. 287 (4) (2004) E686–E695.

[54] K. Baar, Z. Song, C.F. Semenkovich, T.E. Jones, D.H. Han, L.A. Nolte, et al., Skeletal muscle overexpression of nuclear respiratory factor 1 increases glucose transport capacity, Faseb J. 17 (12) (2003) 1666–1673.

[55] A.P. Russell, M.K. Hesselink, S.K. Lo, P. Schrauwen, Regulation of metabolic transcriptional coactivators and transcription factors with acute exercise, Faseb J. 19 (8) (2005) 986–988.

[56] R. Cartoni, B. Leger, M.B. Hock, M. Praz, A. Crettenand, S. Pich, et al., Mitofusins 1/2 and ERRalpha expression are increased in human skeletal muscle after physical exercise, J. Physiol. 567 (Pt 1) (2005) 349–358.

[57] A.P. Russell, J. Feilchenfeldt, S. Schreiber, M. Praz, A. Crettenand, C. Gobelet, et al., Endurance training in humans leads to fiber type-specific increases in levels of peroxisome proliferator-activated receptor-gamma coactivator-1 and peroxisome proliferator-activated receptor-alpha in skeletal muscle, Diabetes 52 (12) (2003) 2874–2881.

[58] K.R. Short, J.L. Vittone, M.L. Bigelow, D.N. Proctor, R.A. Rizza, J.M. Coenen-Schimke, et al., Impact of aerobic exercise training on age-related changes in insulin sensitivity and muscle oxidative capacity, Diabetes 52 (8) (2003) 1888–1896.

[59] J. Lin, H. Wu, P.T. Tarr, C.Y. Zhang, Z. Wu, O. Boss, et al., Transcriptional co-activator PGC-1 alpha drives the formation of slow-twitch muscle fibers, Nature 418 (6899) (2002) 797–801.

[60] T. Akimoto, B.S. Sorg, Z. Yan, Real-time imaging of peroxisome proliferator-activated receptor-gamma coactivator-1alpha promoter activity in skeletal muscles of living mice, Am. J. Physiol. Cell Physiol. 287 (3) (2004) C790–C796.

[61] L.M. Sparks, H. Xie, R.A. Koza, R. Mynatt, M.W. Hulver, G.A. Bray, et al., A high-fat diet coordinately downregulates genes required for mitochondrial oxidative phosphorylation in skeletal muscle, Diabetes 54 (7) (2005) 1926–1933.

[62] S. Crunkhorn, H. Gami, K. Barry, R. Faucette, J. Chillaron-Jimenez, M. Patti, Cellular mechanisms regulating PGC1 and NRF-dependent mitochondrial gene expression: potential pathogenic roles in insulin resistance and type 2 DM, Diabetes (53) (2004) A345, abstract.

[63] T.R. Koves, P. Li, J. An, T. Akimoto, D. Slentz, O. Ilkayeva, et al., Peroxisome proliferator-activated receptor-gamma co-activator 1alpha-mediated metabolic remodeling of skeletal myocytes

mimics exercise training and reverses lipid-induced mitochondrial inefficiency, J. Biol. Chem. 280 (39) (2005) 33588–33598.

[64] D.K. Richardson, S. Kashyap, M. Bajaj, K. Cusi, S.J. Mandarino, J. Finlayson, et al., Lipid infusion decreases the expression of nuclear encoded mitochondrial genes and increases the expression of extracellular matrix genes in human skeletal muscle, J. Biol. Chem. 280 (11) (2005) 10290–10297.

[65] H. Staiger, K. Staiger, C. Haas, M. Weisser, F. Machicao, H.U. Haring, Fatty acid-induced differential regulation of the genes encoding peroxisome proliferator-activated receptor-gamma coactivator-1alpha and – 1beta in human skeletal muscle cells that have been differentiated *in vitro*, Diabetologia 48 (10) (2005) 2115–2118.

[66] B.H. Goodpaster, J. He, S. Watkins, D.E. Kelley, Skeletal muscle lipid content and insulin resistance: evidence for a paradox in endurance-trained athletes, J. Clin. Endocrinol. Metab. 86 (12) (2001) 5755–5761.

[67] J. Lin, P.H. Wu, P.T. Tarr, K.S. Lindenberg, J. St-Pierre, C.Y. Zhang, et al., Defects in adaptive energy metabolism with CNS-linked hyperactivity in PGC-1alpha null mice, Cell 119 (1) (2004) 121–135.

[68] T.C. Leone, J.J. Lehman, B.N. Finck, P.J. Schaeffer, A.R. Wende, S. Boudina, et al. PGC-1alpha deficiency causes multi-system energy metabolic derangements: muscle dysfunction, abnormal weight control and hepatic steatosis, PloS Biol. 3 (4) (2005) e101.

[69] J. Lin, P.T. Tarr, R. Yang, J. Rhee, P. Puigserver, C.B. Newgard, et al., PGC-1beta in the regulation of hepatic glucose and energy metabolism, J. Biol. Chem. 278 (33) (2003) 30843–30848.

[70] S. Bhalla, C. Ozalp, S. Fang, L. Xiang, J.K. Kemper, Ligand-activated pregnane X receptor interferes with HNF-4 signaling by targeting a common coactivator PGC-1alpha. Functional implications in hepatic cholesterol and glucose metabolism, J. Biol. Chem. 279 (43) (2004) 45139–45147.

[71] S.H. Koo, H. Satoh, S. Herzig, C.H. Lee, S. Hedrick, R. Kulkarni, et al., PGC-1 promotes insulin resistance in liver through PPAR-alpha-dependent induction of TRB-3, Nat. Med. 10 (5) (2004) 530–534.

[72] H. Oberkofler, E. Schraml, F. Krempler, W. Patsch, Potentiation of liver X receptor transcriptional activity by peroxisome-proliferator-activated receptor gamma co-activator 1 alpha, Biochem. J. 371 (Pt 1) (2003) 89–96.

[73] C. Tiraby, G. Tavernier, C. Lefort, D. Larrouy, F. Bouillaud, D. Ricquier, et al., Acquirement of brown fat cell features by human white adipocytes, J. Biol. Chem. 278 (35) (2003) 33370–33376.

[74] J.M. Huss, R.P. Kopp, D.P. Kelly, Peroxisome proliferator-activated receptor coactivator-1alpha (PGC-1alpha) coactivates the cardiac-enriched nuclear receptors estrogen-related receptor-alpha and -gamma. Identification of novel leucine-rich interaction motif within PGC-1alpha, J. Biol. Chem. 277 (43) (2002) 40265–40274.

[75] J.J. Lehman, P.M. Barger, A. Kovacs, J.E. Saffitz, D.M. Medeiros, D.P. Kelly, Peroxisome proliferator-activated receptor gamma coactivator-1 promotes cardiac mitochondrial biogenesis, J. Clin. Invest. 106 (7) (2000) 847–856.

[76] Z. Arany, H. He, J. Lin, K. Hoyer, C. Handschin, O. Toka, et al., Transcriptional coactivator PGC-1 alpha controls the energy state and contractile function of cardiac muscle, Cell Metab. 1 (4) (2005) 259–271.

[77] M. Sano, S.C. Wang, M. Shirai, F. Scaglia, M. Xie, S. Sakai, et al., Activation of cardiac Cdk9 represses PGC-1 and confers a predisposition to heart failure, EMBO J. 23 (17) (2004) 3559–3569.

[78] L.K. Russell, C.M. Mansfield, J.J. Lehman, A. Kovacs, M. Courtois, J.E. Saffitz, et al., Cardiac-specific induction of the transcriptional coactivator peroxisome proliferator-activated receptor gamma coactivator-1alpha promotes mitochondrial biogenesis and reversible cardiomyopathy in a developmental stage-dependent manner, Circ. Res. 94 (4) (2004) 525–533.

[79] N.A. Tritos, J.W. Mastaitis, E.G. Kokkotou, P. Puigserver, B.M. Spiegelman, E. Maratos-Flier, Characterization of the peroxisome proliferator activated receptor coactivator 1 alpha (PGC 1alpha) expression in the murine brain, Brain Res. 961 (2) (2003) 255–260.

[80] J. St-Pierre, J. Lin, S. Krauss, P.T. Tarr, R. Yang, C.B. Newgard, et al., Bioenergetic analysis of peroxisome proliferator-activated receptor gamma coactivators 1alpha and 1beta (PGC-1alpha and PGC-1beta) in muscle cells, J. Biol. Chem. 278 (29) (2003) 26597–26603.

[81] I. Valle, A. Alvarez-Barrientos, E. Arza, S. Lamas, M. Monsalve, PGC-1alpha regulates the mitochondrial antioxidant defense system in vascular endothelial cells, Cardiovasc. Res. 66 (3) (2005) 562–573.

[82] P. Zhang, C. Liu, C. Zhang, Y. Zhang, P. Shen, J. Zhang, et al., Free fatty acids increase PGC-1 alpha expression in isolated rat islets, FEBS Lett. 579 (6) (2005) 1446–1452.

[83] J.C. Yoon, G. Xu, J.T. Deeney, S.N. Yang, J. Rhee, P. Puigserver, et al., Suppression of beta cell energy metabolism and insulin release by PGC-1alpha, Dev. Cell 5 (1) (2003) 73–83.

[84] C. Handschin, J. Lin, J. Rhee, A.K. Peyer, S. Chin, P.H. Wu, et al., Nutritional regulation of hepatic heme biosynthesis and porphyria through PGC-1alpha, Cell 122 (4) (2005) 505–515.

[85] S. Jacob, J. Machann, K. Rett, K. Brechtel, A. Volk, W. Renn, et al., Association of increased intramyocellular lipid content with insulin resistance in lean nondiabetic offspring of type 2 diabetic subjects, Diabetes 48 (5) (1999) 1113–1119.

[86] J.D. Browning, J.D. Horton, Molecular mediators of hepatic steatosis and liver injury, J. Clin. Invest. 114 (2) (2004) 147–152.

[87] J.D. McGarry, R.L. Dobbins, Fatty acids, lipotoxicity and insulin secretion, Diabetologia 42 (2) (1999) 128–138.

[88] J.A. Simoneau, D.E. Kelley, Altered glycolytic and oxidative capacities of skeletal muscle contribute to insulin resistance in NIDDM, J. Appl. Physiol. 83 (1) (1997) 166–171.

[89] D.E. Kelley, J. He, E.V. Menshikova, V.B. Ritov, Dysfunction of mitochondria in human skeletal muscle in type 2 diabetes, Diabetes 51 (10) (2002) 2944–2950.

[90] J. Song, J.Y. Oh, Y.A. Sung, Y.K. Pak, K.S. Park, H.K. Lee, Peripheral blood mitochondrial DNA content is related to insulin sensitivity in offspring of type 2 diabetic patients, Diabetes Care 24 (5) (2001) 865–869.

[91] K.F. Petersen, S. Dufour, D. Befroy, R. Garcia, G.I. Shulman, Impaired mitochondrial activity in the insulin-resistant offspring of patients with type 2 diabetes, N Engl. J. Med. 350 (7) (2004) 664–671.

[92] K.F. Petersen, S. Dufour, G.I. Shulman, Decreased insulin-stimulated ATP synthesis and phosphate transport in muscle of insulin-resistant offspring of type 2 diabetic parents, PLoS Med. 2 (9) (2005) e233.

[93] M.E. Patti, A.J. Butte, S. Crunkhorn, K. Cusi, R. Berria, S. Kashyap, et al., Coordinated reduction of genes of oxidative metabolism in humans with insulin resistance and diabetes: potential role of PGC1 and NRF1, Proc. Natl. Acad. Sci. USA 100 (14) (2003) 8466–8471.

[94] V.K. Mootha, C.M. Lindgren, K.F. Eriksson, A. Subramanian, S. Sihag, J. Lehar, et al., PGC-1 alpha-responsive genes involved in oxidative phosphorylation are coordinately downregulated in human diabetes, Nat. Genet. 34 (3) (2003) 267–273.

[95] R. Sreekumar, P. Halvatsiotis, J.C. Schimke, K.S. Nair, Gene expression profile in skeletal muscle of type 2 diabetes and the effect of insulin treatment, Diabetes 51 (6) (2002) 1913–1920.

[96] V.K. Yechoor, M.E. Patti, R. Saccone, C.R. Kahn, Coordinated patterns of gene expression for substrate and energy metabolism in skeletal muscle of diabetic mice, Proc. Natl. Acad. Sci. USA 99 (16) (2002) 10587–10592.

[97] V.K. Yechoor, M.E. Patti, K. Ueki, P.G. Laustsen, R. Saccone, R. Rauniyar, et al., Distinct pathways of insulin-regulated versus diabetes-regulated gene expression: an *in vivo* analysis in MIRKO mice, Proc. Natl. Acad. Sci. USA 101 (47) (2004) 16525–16530.

[98] D. Larrouy, H. Vidal, F. Andreelli, M. Laville, D. Langin, Cloning and mRNA tissue distribution of human PPARgamma coactivator-1, Int. J. Obes. Relat. Metab. Disord. 23 (12) (1999) 1327–1332.

[99] C. Ling, P. Poulsen, E. Carlsson, M. Ridderstrale, P. Almgren, J. Wojtaszewski, et al., Multiple environmental and genetic factors influence skeletal muscle PGC-1alpha and PGC-1beta gene expression in twins, J. Clin. Invest. 114 (10) (2004) 1518–1526.

[100] K. Hara, K. Tobe, T. Okada, H. Kadowaki, Y. Akanuma, C. Ito, et al., A genetic variation in the PGC-1 gene could confer insulin resistance and susceptibility to Type II diabetes, Diabetologia 45 (5) (2002) 740–743.

[101] H. Oberkofler, V. Linnemayr, R. Weitgasser, K. Klein, M. Xie, B. Iglseder, et al., Complex haplotypes of the PGC-1alpha gene are associated with carbohydrate metabolism and type 2 diabetes, Diabetes 53 (5) (2004) 1385–1393.

[102] J. Pihlajamaki, M. Kinnunen, E. Ruotsalainen, U. Salmenniemi, I. Vauhkonen, T. Kuulasmaa, et al., Haplotypes of PPARGC1A are associated with glucose tolerance, body mass index and insulin sensitivity in offspring of patients with type 2 Diabetes, Diabetologia 48 (7) (2005) 1331–1334.

[103] H. Esterbauer, H. Oberkofler, V. Linnemayr, B. Iglseder, M. Hedegger, P. Wolfsgruber, et al., Peroxisome Proliferator-Activated Receptor-{gamma} Coactivator-1 gene locus: associations with obesity indices in middle-aged women diabetes, 51 (4) (2002) 1281–1286.

[104] J. Ek, G. Andersen, S.A. Urhammer, P.H. Gaede, T. Drivsholm, K. Borch-Johnsen, et al., Mutation analysis of peroxisome proliferator-activated receptor-gamma coactivator-1 (PGC-1) and relationships of identified amino acid polymorphisms to Type II diabetes mellitus, Diabetologia 44 (12) (2001) 2220–2226.

[105] J.H. Kim, H.D. Shin, B.L. Park, Y.M. Cho, S.Y. Kim, H.K. Lee, et al., Peroxisome proliferator-activated receptor gamma coactivator 1 alpha promoter polymorphisms are associated with early onset type 2 diabetes mellitus in the Korean population, Diabetologia 48 (7) (2005) 1323–1330.

[106] Y.L. Muller, C. Bogardus, O. Pedersen, L.A. Baier, Gly482Ser missense mutation in the peroxisome proliferator-activated receptor gamma coactivator-1 is associated with altered lipid oxidation and early insulin secretion in Pima Indians, Diabetes 52 (3) (2003) 895–898.

[107] L. Al-Khalili, M. Forsgren, K. Kannisto, J.R. Zierath, F. Lonnqvist, A. Krook, Enhanced insulin-stimulated glycogen synthesis in response to insulin, metformin or rosiglitazone is associated with increased mRNA expression of GLUT4 and peroxisomal proliferator activator receptor gamma coactivator 1, Diabetologia 48 (6) (2005) 1173–1179.

[108] C. Tiraby, D. Langin, Conversion from white to brown adipocytes: a strategy for the control of fat mass? Trends Endocrinol. Metab. 14 (10) (2003) 439–441.

[109] A. Hammarstedt, P.A. Jansson, C. Wesslau, X. Yang, U. Smith, Reduced expression of PGC-1 and insulin-signaling molecules in adipose tissue is associated with insulin resistance, Biochem. Biophys. Res. Commun. 301 (2) (2003) 578–852.

[110] X. Yang, S. Enerback, U. Smith, Reduced expression of FOXC2 and brown adipogenic genes in human subjects with insulin resistance, Obes. Res. 11 (10) (2003) 1182–1191.

[111] R.K. Semple, V.C. Crowley, C.P. Sewter, M. Laudes, C. Christodoulides, R.V. Considine, et al., Expression of the thermogenic nuclear hormone receptor coactivator PGC-1alpha is reduced in the adipose tissue of morbidly obese subjects, Int. J. Obes. Relat. Metab. Disord. 28 (1) (2004) 176–179.

[112] S. Kashyap, R. Belfort, A. Gastaldelli, T. Pratipanawatr, R. Berria, W. Pratipanawatr, et al., A sustained increase in plasma free fatty acids impairs insulin secretion in nondiabetic subjects genetically predisposed to develop type 2 diabetes, Diabetes 52 (10) (2003) 2461–2474.

[113] C.T. De Souza, E.P. Araujo, P.O. Prada, M.J. Saad, A.C. Boschero, L.A. Velloso, Short-term inhibition of peroxisome proliferator-activated receptor-gamma coactivator-1alpha expression reverses diet-induced diabetes mellitus and hepatic steatosis in mice, Diabetologia 48 (9) (2005) 1860–1871.

[114] M. Lefevre, C.M. Champagne, R.T. Tulley, J.C. Rood, M.M. Most, Individual variability in cardiovascular disease risk factor responses to low-fat and low-saturated-fat diets in men: body mass index, adiposity, and insulin resistance predict changes in LDL cholesterol, Am. J. Clin. Nutr. 82 (5) (2005) 957–963 quiz 1145–1146.

[115] M. Uusitupa, Gene-diet interaction in relation to the prevention of obesity and type 2 diabetes: evidence from the Finnish Diabetes Prevention Study, Nutr. Metab. Cardiovasc. Dis. 15 (3) (2005) 225–233.

[116] H. Esterbauer, H. Oberkofler, F. Krempler, W. Patsch, Human peroxisome proliferator activated receptor gamma coactivator 1 (PPARGC1) gene: cDNA sequence, genomic organization, chromosomal localization, and tissue expression, Genomics 62 (1) (1999) 98–102.

[117] R. Pratley, D. Thompson, M. Prochazka, L. Baier, D. Mott, E. Ravussin, et al., An autosomal genomic scan for loci linked to prediabetic phenotypes in Pima Indians, J. Clin. Invest. 101 (8) (1998) 1757–1764.

[118] S. Stone, V. Abkevich, S.C. Hunt, A. Gutin, D.L. Russell, C.D. Neff, et al., A major predisposition locus for severe obesity, at 4p15-p14, Am. J. Hum. Genet. 70 (6) (2002) 1459–1468.

[119] R. Arya, R. Duggirala, C.P. Jenkinson, L. Almasy, J. Blangero, P. O'Connell, et al., Evidence of a novel quantitative-trait locus for obesity on chromosome 4p in Mexican Americans, Am. J. Hum. Genet. 74 (2) (2004) 272–282.

[120] C. Lacquemant, M. Chikri, P. Boutin, C. Samson, P. Froguel, No association between the G482S polymorphism of the proliferator-activated receptor-gamma coactivator-1 (PGC-1) gene and Type II diabetes in French Caucasians, Diabetologia 45 (4) (2002) 602–603. author reply 604.

[121] I. Barroso, J. Luan, R.P. Middelberg, A.H. Harding, P.W. Franks, R.W. Jakes, et al., Candidate gene association study in type 2 diabetes indicates a role for genes involved in beta-cell function as well as insulin action, PloS Biol. 1 (1) (2003) E20.

[122] M. Stumvoll, A. Fritsche, L.M. t'Hart, J. Machann, C. Thamer, O. Tschritter, et al., The Gly482Ser variant in the peroxisome proliferator-activated receptor gamma coactivator-1 is not associated with diabetes-related traits in non-diabetic German and Dutch populations, Exp. Clin. Endocrinol. Diabetes 112 (5) (2004) 253–257.

[123] M. Ridderstrale, H. Parikh, L. Groop, Calpain 10 and type 2 diabetes: are we getting closer to an explanation?, Curr. Opin. Clin. Nutr. Metab. Care 8 (4) (2005) 361–366.

[124] J.C. Florez, N. Burtt, P.I. de Bakker, P. Almgren, T. Tuomi, I. Holmkvist, et al., Haplotype structure and genotype-phenotype correlations of the sulfonylurea receptor and the islet ATP-sensitive potassium channel gene region, Diabetes 53 (5) (2004) 1360–1368.

[125] D. Altshuler, J.N. Hirschhorn, M. Klannemark, C.M. Lindgren, M.C. Vohl, J. Nemesh, et al., The common PPARgamma Pro12Ala polymorphism is associated with decreased risk of type 2 diabetes, Nat. Genet. 26 (1) (2000) 76–80.

[126] P.W. Franks, I. Barroso, J. Luan, U. Ekelund, V.E. Crowley, S. Brage, et al., PGC-1alpha genotype modifies the association of volitional energy expenditure with [OV0312]O2max, Med. Sci. Sports Exerc. 35 (12) (1999) 1998–2004.

[127] J. Tuomilehto, J. Lindstrom, J.G. Eriksson, T.T. Valle, H. Hamalainen, P. Ilanne-Parikka, et al., Prevention of type 2 diabetes mellitus by changes in lifestyle among subjects with impaired glucose tolerance, N Engl. J. Med. 344 (18) (2001) 1343–1350.

[128] V.I. Lindi, M.I. Uusitupa, J. Lindstrom, A. Louheranta, J.G. Eriksson, T.T. Valle, et al., Association of the Pro12Ala polymorphism in the PPAR-gamma2 gene with 3-year incidence of type 2 diabetes and body weight change in the Finnish Diabetes Prevention Study, Diabetes 51 (8) (2002) 2581–2586.

[129] O. Laukkanen, J. Pihlajamaki, J. Lindstrom, J. Eriksson, T.T. Valle, H. Hamalainen, et al., Polymorphisms of the SUR1 (ABCC8) and Kir6.2 (KCNJ11) genes predict the conversion from impaired glucose tolerance to type 2 diabetes. The Finnish Diabetes Prevention Study, J. Clin. Endocrinol. Metab. 89 (12) (2004) 6286–6290.

[130] O. Laukkanen, J. Pihlajamaki, J. Lindstrom, J. Eriksson, T.T. Valle, H. Hamalainen, et al., Common polymorphisms in the genes regulating the early insulin signalling pathway: effects on weight change and the conversion from impaired glucose tolerance to Type 2 diabetes. The Finnish Diabetes Prevention Study, Diabetologia 47 (5) (2004) 871–877.

[131] A. Kubaszek, J. Pihlajamaki, V. Komarovski, V. Lindi, J. Lindstrom, J. Eriksson, et al., Promoter polymorphisms of the TNF-alpha (G-308A) and IL-6 (C-174G) genes predict the conversion from impaired glucose tolerance to type 2 diabetes: the Finnish Diabetes Prevention Study, Diabetes 52 (7) (2003) 1872–1876.

[132] W.C. Knowler, E. Barrett-Connor, S.E. Fowler, R.F. Hamman, J.M. Lachin, E.A. Walker, et al., Reduction in the incidence of type 2 diabetes with lifestyle intervention or metformin, N. Engl. J. Med. 346 (6) (2002) 393–403.

[133] G. Andersen, L. Wegner, K. Yanagisawa, C.S. Rose, J. Lin, C. Glumer, et al., Evidence of an association between genetic variation of the coactivator PGC-1beta and obesity, J. Med. Genet. 42 (5) (2005) 402–407.

[134] L. Andrulionyte, J. Zacharova, J. L. Chiasson, M. Laakso, Common polymorphisms of the PPAR-gamma2 (Pro12Ala) and PGC-1alpha (Gly482Ser) genes are associated with the conversion from impaired glucose tolerance to type 2 diabetes in the STOP-NIDDM trial, Diabetologia 2004.

[135] K. Yamagata, H. Furuta, N. Oda, P.J. Kaisaki, S. Menzel, N.J. Cox, et al., Mutations in the hepatocyte nuclear factor-4alpha gene in maturity-onset diabetes of the young (MODY1), Nature 384 (6608) (1996) 458–460.

[136] L. Ji, M. Malecki, J. Warram, Y. Yang, S. Rich, A. Krolewski, New susceptibility locus for NIDDM is localized to human chromosome 20q, Diabetes 46 (5) (1997) 876–881.

[137] E. Hani, L. Suaud, P. Boutin, J. Chevre, E. Durand, A. Philippi, et al., A missense mutation in hepatocyte nuclear factor-4 alpha, resulting in a reduced transactivation activity, in human late-onset non-insulin-dependent diabetes mellitus, J. Clin. Invest. 101 (3) (1998) 521–526.

[138] K. Sakurai, N. Seki, R. Fujii, K. Yagui, Y. Tokuyama, F. Shimada, et al., Mutations in the hepatocyte nuclear factor-4alpha gene in Japanese with non-insulin-dependent diabetes: a nucleotide substitution in the polypyrimidine tract of intron 1b, Horm. Metab. Res. 32 (8) (2000) 316–320.

[139] Q. Yang, K. Yamagata, K. Yamamoto, Y. Cao, J. Miyagawa, A. Fukamizu, et al., R127W-HNF-4alpha is a loss of function mutation but not a rare polymorphism and causes Type II diabetes in a Japanese family with MODY1, Diabetologia 43 (4) (2000) 520–524.

[140] L.D. Love-Gregory, J. Wasson, J. Ma, C.H. Jin, B. Glaser, B.K. Suarez, et al., A common polymorphism in the upstream promoter region of the hepatocyte nuclear factor-4 alpha gene on chromosome 20q is associated with type 2 diabetes and appears to contribute to the evidence for linkage in an ashkenazi jewish population, Diabetes 53 (4) (2004) 1134–1140.

[141] J. Ek, C.S. Rose, D.P. Jensen, C. Glumer, K. Borch-Johnsen, T. Jorgensen, et al., The functional Thr130Ile and Val255Met polymorphisms of the hepatocyte nuclear factor-4alpha (HNF4A): gene associations with type 2 diabetes or altered beta-cell function among Danes, J. Clin. Endocrinol. Metab. 90 (5) (2005) 3054–3059.

[142] Y.B. Lombardo, A. G. Chicco, Effects of dietary polyunsaturated n-3 fatty acids on dyslipidemia and insulin resistance in rodents and humans. A review, J. Nutr. Biochem. (2005).

[143] H. Sampath, J.M. Ntambi, Polyunsaturated fatty acid regulation of gene expression, Nutr. Rev. 62 (9) (2004) 333–339.

[144] R.J. Southgate, C.R. Bruce, A.L. Carey, G.R. Steinberg, K. Walder, R. Monks, M.J. Watt, J.A. Hawley, M.J. Birnbaum, M. Febbraio, PGC-1α gene expression is down-regulated by Akt-mediated phosphorylation and nuclear exclusion of FoxO1 in insulin-stimulated skeletal muscle, FASEB J 19 (14) (2005) 2072–2074.

Chapter 13

Hepatic CCAAT/enhancer binding protein β (C/EBPβ): engineer of diabetes, obesity, and inflammatory disease processes

Jill M. Schroeder-Gloeckler[1], Shaikh Mizanoor Rahman[2], Jacob E. Friedman[2]

[1]*Current address: Medical University of Ohio at Toledo, 3035-Arlington Avenue, Block Health Science Bldg, Room 270, Toledo, OH 43614-5804, USA;*
[2]*Department of Pediatrics, Biochemistry & Molecular Genetics, University of Colorado at Denver and Health Sciences Center, Mail Stop 8106, P.O. Box 6511, Aurora, CO 80045, USA*

1. Introduction

The C/EBP family of transcription factors includes C/EBP α, β, γ, δ, ε, ς, and are encoded by separate genes located on different chromosomes. They have been implicated in such diverse cellular functions as differentiation, proliferation, inflammation, and the response to endoplasmic reticulum (ER) stress. Two of these gene family members, C/EBPα and C/EBPβ are central regulators of important integrative metabolic processes in the liver, particularly gluconeogenesis. In addition to gluconeogenic genes, C/EBP binding motifs also exist in many lipogenic gene promoters. Based on gene knockout studies, C/EBPα and C/EBPβ appear to not only to affect gluconeogenesis, but also hepatic lipogenesis as well. Gene inactivation studies also suggest that C/EBPs while overlapping to some degree, have unique metabolic roles and are not at all redundant in function. In this chapter we will outline how C/EBP, particularly C/EBPα and C/EBPβ are involved in the control of gluconeogenesis in the context of other known transcription factors using the PEPCK gene as a model promoter. In addition, we will outline the emerging role for C/EBPβ as a factor in regulation of hepatic lipogenesis, and its important role in integrating the response to ER stress and inflammatory disease processes.

ADVANCES IN MOLECULAR AND CELLULAR ENDOCRINOLOGY
VOLUME 5 ISSN 1569-2566/DOI 10.1016/S1569-2566(06)05013-7

2. Transcriptional control of gluconeogenesis: PEPCK as a model target

The liver plays a critical role in blood glucose homeostasis by maintaining a balance between the uptake and storage of glucose via glycogenesis and the release of glucose via glycogenolysis and gluconeogenesis [1,2]. During periods of fasting, the liver can produce glucose by breaking down glycogen and by *de novo* synthesis of glucose from precursors lactate, pyruvate, glycerol, and alanine. The rate of gluconeogenesis is controlled principally by the availability of substrates and activities of several key enzymes in the pathway, primarily the cytosolic form of phosphoenolpyruvate carboxykinase (PEPCK-c), fructose-1,6-bisphosphatase, and glucose-6-phosphatase [1,2]. The genes encoding these enzymes are tightly controlled at the transcriptional level by hormones, particularly insulin in the feeding state, and glucagon (via cAMP) and glucocorticoids during fasting.

In both type 1 and type 2 diabetes, excessive hepatic gluconeogenesis is a major contributor to both fasting hyperglycemia and exaggerated postprandial hyperglycemia [3–5]. In transgenic animals, just a two-fold overexpression of the PEPCK gene resulted in increased hepatic glucose production and disruption of glucose homeostasis [6,7]. The level of PEPCK in liver is controlled by a wide variety of physiological stimuli including dietary carbohydrate, hormones, and cellular intermediates [8]. PEPCK expression in mammalian liver is induced by starvation and reduced by a high carbohydrate diet [9]. Hormones that control synthesis of PEPCK include glucagon (acting via cAMP), glucocorticoids, and thyroid hormone, all of which increase PEPCK gene expression, and insulin, which acutely inhibits PEPCK synthesis. The major regulatory axis for PEPCK involves the opposing effects of cAMP and insulin [8]. The regulation of PEPCK expression is primarily at the level of gene transcription. Studies of the PEPCK gene promoter have revealed an overlapping set of hormone response units, each one consisting of a specific hormone response element associated with transcription factor binding (Fig. 1).

2.1. *Glucocorticoids and cAMP*

Glucocorticoids induce PEPCK gene transcription through the glucocorticoid response unit (GRU). The GRU is comprised of two glucocorticoid regulatory elements (GRE), three glucocorticoid accessory factor binding sites (AF1-3), and a cAMP response element (CRE) [8,10,11]. Responding to glucocorticoid stimulation, the glucocorticoid receptor binds to the GRE and cooperates with other factors, like hepatic nuclear factor 4α (HNF4α), Foxo1, and C/EBPβ, which binds the CRE, to increase PEPCK gene transcription [12–14]. Likewise, cAMP stimulates PEPCK gene transcription through a cAMP response unit (CRU), which is comprised of a CRE, two C/EBP binding sites, and an AP1 binding site [15].

2.2. *C/EBPs and liver transcriptional control*

Despite a wealth of literature over the last several years characterizing the molecular details of the regulation of gluconeogenic enzymes through hormones and transcription

Model for Insulin Interaction with the PEPCK Transcriptome

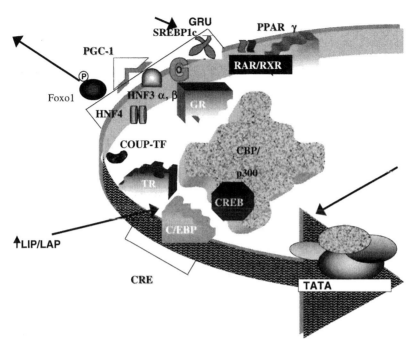

Fig. 1. Model of transcription factor and coactivator binding to the PEPCK promoter. The abbreviations for the factors and binding elements are: CRE, cAMP regulatory element; GRU, glucocorticoid regulatory unit; G, glucocorticoid; SREBP1c, sterol response element binding protein 1c; CREB, CRE binding protein; C/EBP, CCAAT/enhancer binding protein; Foxo1, forkhead transcription factor; HNF-4α, hepatic nuclear factor-4α; TR, thyroid hormone receptor; GR, glucocorticoid receptor; PPARγ, peroxisome proliferator-activated receptor γ; RAR, retinoic acid receptor; RXR, retinoid X receptor; CBP, CREB binding protein; PGC-1, PPARγ coactivator 1; COUP-TF, chicken ovalbumin upstream promoter transcription factor. See Plate 12 in Colour Plate Section.

factors, much less has been incorporated into our understanding of how these factors regulate *one another* in the control of gluconeogenesis. PEPCK is the first committed step in gluconeogenesis in hepatic and renal cells. CCAAT/enhancer binding protein (C/EBP) is a sequence-specific DNA-binding protein that was first identified in crude nuclear extracts from adult rat liver [16,17]. Six different members of this family have been isolated and characterized, including C/EBP α, β, γ, δ, ε, and ζ [18]. The genes encoding these family members give rise to various isoforms that fulfill different metabolic functions. C/EBPα, C/EBPβ, and C/EBPδ are highly expressed in liver, adipose tissue, lung, and intestinal tissue ([19,20], reviewed in [21]). C/EBPα is also expressed in adrenal gland, peripheral blood mononuclear cells, and placenta (reviewed in [21]). C/EBPβ is also expressed in the kidney, heart, spleen, reproductive tract, and mammary gland ([19,20]; reviewed in [21]). C/EBPβ is also found in the hippocampus, pituitary cells, and the hypothalamus where it may play a role in regulation of genes, like propiomelanocortin (POMC) that regulates energy balance ([22–24], unpublished

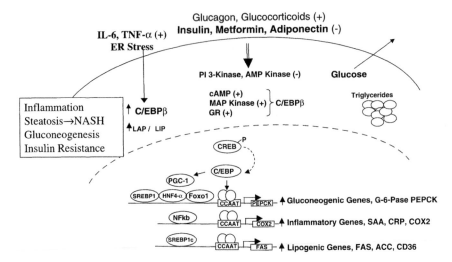

Fig. 2. Hepatic C/EBPβ and its role in gluconeogenesis, steatosis, and inflammatory processes.

data Friedman and Schwartz lab, see Fig. 2). C/EBPγ is expressed ubiquitously with increased expression in non-differentiated progenitor cells. C/EBPε is expressed in myeloid and lymphoid cells. Finally, C/EBPζ is ubiquitously expressed and induced by DNA damage (reviewed in [21]).

Accumulating data strongly indicate that both C/EBP α and β are important regulators of integrative processes that control glucose homeostasis. C/EBPβ gene transcription, like hepatic glucose production is acutely upregulated by cAMP [25,26] and glucocorticoids in hepatoma cells [27] and in primary rat hepatocytes [28]. In the livers of normal mice, C/EBPβ protein increases up to 10-fold within 90 min after injection of $N^6,O^{2'}$-dibutyryladenosine (Bt$_2$)-cAMP [29], suggesting that C/EBPβ is under rapid post-translational control. During streptozotocin-diabetes, C/EBPβ protein accumulates up to three-fold in liver nuclei, while C/EBPα is decreased [30]. This change is reversed by insulin treatment, suggesting that C/EBPβ may be responsible for regulating PEPCK gene transcription in response to cAMP, glucocorticoids, and possibly insulin.

2.2.1. C/EBPβ regulation

C/EBPβ can be regulated at a functional level by phosphorylation, at the level of transcription by cAMP or insulin, or by alternative translation of the protein into its long form LAP (Liver Activating Protein) or truncated form lacking the transactivation domain LIP (Liver Inhibitory Protein) [31,32]. C/EBPβ is an intronless gene, which may account for its rapid appearance in response to cAMP stimulation. There are two CRE-like sites in the C/EBPβ promoter region, which mediate the cAMP response of the gene via protein kinase A (PKA) and the CREB transcription factor pathway [25,29,33,34]. Most recently, two independent studies demonstrated that insulin increases C/EBPβ protein expression in both differentiated 3T3-L1 adipocytes and H4IIE hepatic cells, in favor of an increase in the LIP isoform [25,35].

Insulin also phosphorylates CBP (CREB binding protein) at Ser1834, which disrupts its interactions with C/EBPβ and PEPCK gene transcription [36]. Thus, insulin treatment reduces the LAP/LIP ratio, which may be responsible for the inhibition by insulin on PEPCK gene transcription [25]. However, the mechanisms whereby insulin increases LIP have not been studied. Mice lacking C/EBPβ show fasting hypoglycemia and reduced responsiveness to glucagon-stimulated hepatic glucose production [37], suggesting that C/EBPβ is essential for maintenance of normal glucose homeostasis.

2.2.2. C/EBPβ structural features

The members of the C/EBP family of transcription factors all have a highly conserved basic region-leucine zipper motif (bZIP) in the C-terminal domain. The basic amino acid rich region of this motif binds specifically to the DNA, while the leucine zipper acts to dimerize two C/EBP proteins (reviewed in [38]). Since this region is highly conserved C/EBP proteins can heterodimerize as well as homodimerize to produce a wide variety of responses to stimuli (reviewed in [39]).

Unlike the C-terminal domains, the N-terminal domains are very divergent in their identity. The N-terminal domain usually contains the transactivation domain of the protein. It is this domain, or lack of the domain (in the case of LIP), which supplies the proteins with their individual mechanisms of either positive or negative regulation (reviewed in [38]). There are three alternative C/EBPβ translation products from a single C/EBPβ mRNA: the 38- and 34-kDa forms of C/EBPβ, also known as LAP, and the 20-kDa form of C/EBPβ, known as LIP (reviewed in [38]). LIP lacks the N-terminal activation domain and possesses only DNA-binding and leucine zipper dimerization domains and therefore acts as a dominant-negative inhibitor of C/EBPβ-mediated transcription. Heterodimerization of LIP with full-length LAP attenuates transcriptional activity indicating that the LAP/LIP ratio is important for C/EBPβ-mediated transcription. Wheelhouse et al. showed that a selective increase in LIP relative to LAP induces growth hormone- and amino acid-mediated control of insulin-like growth factor-1 (IGF-1) gene expression in ovine hepatocytes [40]. The LIP/LAP ratio has been reported to change with inflammation [41] during liver development [42] and in liver regeneration [43]. In all of these cases, LIP levels increase transiently, resulting in an increase in the LIP/LAP ratio.

Insulin represses glucocorticoid-induced PEPCK expression within 30 min by increasing LIP expression, which disrupts the association of CBP and pol II with the PEPCK promoter [25]. Other examples of the regulation of the LAP/LIP ration include the following: Epimorphin (EPM), a protein expressed on the surface of myoepithelial and fibroblast cells of the mammary gland, has been shown to mediate luminal morphogenesis of mammary epithelial cells *in vitro* by control of expression of LAP and LIP [44]. Zahnow et al. found elevated levels of LIP in human breast cancer [45]. Recently, Shao et al. [46] showed that treatment of FAO cells with high glucose (20 mM) increases glucose production and PEPCK gene expression and increases the LAP/LIP ratio despite decreases in C/EBPβ expression. These results indicate the crucial role of the LAP/LIP ratio in hyperglycemia-induced hepatic glucose production and PEPCK gene expression.

2.2.3. *Knockout mice: Effects on hepatic gluconeogenesis and lipid storage*
C/EBPα and C/EBPβ are required for mouse embryogenesis. These proteins are coexpressed starting at embryonic day 9.5 (E9.5). When C/EBPα and C/EBPβ are deleted from the embryo, it dies between E10 and E11. A single copy of either of these genes is sufficient for complete development of the embryos. However, a single copy of C/EBPα is not sufficient for the survival of a newborn mouse [47]. This illustrates that C/EBPs are essential for murine development and have some, but not all redundant functions.

The use of gene knockouts has provided important information about the physiological functions of C/EBPs *in vivo*. Mice with a homozygous deletion of the C/EBPα gene are phenotypically normal at birth; however, they die within a few hours after birth. These mice have no hepatic glycogen stores due to decreased expression of glycogen synthase and uncoupling protein genes. C/EBPα knockout mice cannot initiate gluconeogenesis due to the absence of expression of the gluconeogenic genes, PEPCK, glucose-6-phosphatase (G-6-Pase), and Tyrosine Aminotransferase (TAT) during the first 1–2 h after birth. However, PEPCK and G-6-Pase mRNA return to their normal levels 7 h after the birth of these mice, if kept alive via glucose gavage. The lack of glycogen and the delayed expression of gluconeogenic genes lead to a fatal hypoglycemia in C/EBPα knockout mice. The delayed expression of the gluconeogenic genes also suggests that C/EBPα is necessary to activate transcription of these genes during the perinatal period, but this activation is later controlled by other regulatory factors such as C/EBPβ ([48], reviewed in [49]).

C/EBPα knockout mice are also defective in adipose tissue accumulation. The levels of lipid accumulation in brown adipose tissue are abnormally low after birth. The brown adipose tissue expresses no uncoupling protein shortly after birth and its levels do not rise above 5% during the perinatal period compared to normal mice. In addition, the accumulation of lipid in inguinal white adipose tissue during the perinatal period is undetectable ([48], reviewed in [49]). Studies in which a global knockdown of C/EBPα has been accomplished in adult mice are discussed below.

Homozygous deletion of the C/EBPβ gene generates two phenotypes of C/EBPβ -/- mice [50]. Similar to C/EBPα gene knockout mice, phenotype B mice die within 1–2 h after birth of neonatal hypoglycemia, which is caused by a lack of or a delay in initiation of PEPCK gene transcription and mobilization of hepatic glycogen [48,50]. Phenotype A mice survive, but the females are reproductively sterile and both sexes are susceptible to infection due to immunological problems [51,52]. In addition to impairment of hepatic acute-phase response protein expression [52,53] and preadipocyte differentiation [18,54], adult C/EBPβ-/- mice display fasting hypoglycemia and impaired hepatic glucose production [37,55]. These animals also have lower blood lipids and adipose tissue lipolysis when stimulated by epinephrine and/or glucagon [37,55]. These effects may have been influenced by significantly reduced levels of hepatic cAMP, which can be rescued by injection of the mice with (Bt₂)-cAMP [53]. A follow-up paper shows that C/EBPβ is involved in cAMP metabolism through its effect on phosphodiesterase activity and expression [56].

2.2.4. *Replacement of C/EBPα with C/EBPβ*

Normal liver function and hepatic PEPCK mRNA levels are restored in C/EBPα knockout mice when C/EBPβ replaces C/EBPα at its gene locus (*C/ebpα^{β/β}* mice). The increased expression of the C/EBPβ gene compensates for the loss of C/EBPα in the liver. The normal levels of endogenous C/EBPβ mRNA are insufficient for the correction of the lethal C/EBPα-/- phenotype, but when expressed from the C/EBPα locus, C/EBPβ is sufficient to rescue C/EBPα mice from death [57]. Fat storage and adipsin and leptin levels in *C/ebpα^{β/β}* mice are significantly reduced in the white adipose tissue of these mice indicating that C/EBPα is essential, but not sufficient for adipogenesis *in vivo* [57]. These findings indicate that C/EBPβ and C/EBPα have some redundant functions in the liver, for example, C/EBPα is more important for the transition from *in utero* to birth while C/EBPβ is more important in glucose homeostasis in the adult.

2.2.5. *Floxed mice: Role in gluconeogenesis and fatty liver*

Recently the role of C/EBPα in the control of both hepatic lipogenesis and hepatosteatosis became evident from the studies in the Gonzalez laboratory [58,59]. Matsusue et al. produced a C/EBPα-liver null mouse on an ob/ob background (ob/ob-C/EBPα/Cr+) using a *floxed* C/EBP α allele and Cre recombinase under the control of an albumin promoter (AlbCre). They found a significant decrease of triglycerides in C/EBPα-deficient liver in ob/ob mice compared to mice lacking the AlbCre transgene (ob/ob-C/EBPα/Cre⁻). This reduction of triglycerides in ob/ob-C/EBPα/Cre+ mice was accompanied with dramatic reduction in the expression of key lipogenic genes: fatty acid synthase, acetyl-CoA carboxylase, stearoyl-CoA desaturase 1, and ATP-citrate lyase. These results clearly indicate that C/EBP α is a key mediator in the induction of lipogenic genes. To further ascertain the role of C/EBP α in lipogenesis, Inoue et al. fed mice a high carbohydrate (HC) diet for 12 days. The HC feeding resulted increased expression of lipogenic genes, fatty liver, increased liver size, hepatic triglyceride, and cholesterol content in ob/ob-C/EBPα/Cre⁻ mice, but not in ob/ob-C/EBPα/Cr+ mice [58]. Adult C/EBPα null mice were also produced using a floxed C/EBPα allele and the albumin-cre transgene. Interestingly, the 6- and 12-month-old KO mice exhibited steatotic livers compared to 2-week- and 2-month-old KO mice. Oil red O staining showed increased lipid accumulation in the liver of the older mice. Hepatic triglycerides and cholesterol levels were higher in 6- and 12-month-old KO mice compared to floxed mice. The increased level of hepatic lipid in aged KO mice was accompanied by increased expression of lipoprotein lipase and reduced expression of microsomal triglyceride transfer protein, apolipoprotein B100, and A-IV. These results demonstrate the critical role of C/EBPα in hepatic lipid homeostasis in adult mice [59]. Why the aged hepatic C/EBPα knockdown animal has excess hepatic lipid deposition, whereas C/EBPα deletion in the liver of ob/ob mice provides protection from fatty livers is unclear.

A conditional global C/EBPα knockout mouse was recently created, in which C/EBPα is ablated upon the administration of poly I:C, to study the effects of the C/EBPα knockout in adult mice. These mice developed hypophagia and severe weight loss 16 days after the knockout injection, despite total ablation of C/EBPα by day 4, and survived until 1 month post-injection. These animals also showed hypoglycemia, hypoinsulinemia, and depletion of hepatic glycogen as well as decreased plasma-free fatty acids, triglycerides, and cholesterol, and decreased triglycerides in white adipose tissue, though not brown adipose tissue, and they also developed a fatty liver. The mRNAs for the gluconeogenic enzymes PEPCK and G-6-Pase were decreased; however, the levels of these mRNAs were rescued by injection of Bt2-cAMP [60]. These results, combined with the previously mentioned C/EBPβ replacement studies [57], may suggest that C/EBPβ plays a role in the recovery of gluconeogenic expression. These striking results on appetite also suggest that C/EBPα could play a role in feeding behavior, or other metabolic processes that regulate appetite.

2.3. CREB and PEPCK gene expression

The transcription factor CREB can stimulate C/EBPβ and PEPCK expression. The Ser133 phosphorylated form of CREB activates C/EBPβ in a cAMP-responsive manner by binding to two CRE-like C/EBPβ promoter elements [29,33,34]. PEPCK expression can be increased in response to cAMP by the binding of CREB, C/EBPβ, and/or C/EBPα to the five cis elements of the PEPCK cAMP response unit (CRU); one CRE, one AP-1 binding site, and three C/EBP binding sites [61]. All three transcription factors can bind to the PEPCK CRE which causes the promoter to be responsive to cAMP; C/EBPβ or α binding to the distal C/EBP binding sites causes a cAMP-responsive effect on PEPCK transcription [15]. These data indicate that both CREB and C/EBPβ can participate in the cAMP response of the PEPCK promoter and that CREB can also act to activate C/EBPβ expression. It is interesting to note that C/EBPβ acts as an accessory factor in the GRU when it is bound to the CRE [14]. Recently, TORC2 (transducer of regulated CREB) has been suggested to create the differential effects of glucagon and insulin on CREB-mediated gene expression in the liver. Glucagon suppresses TORC2 Ser171 phosphorylation causing nuclear localization of TORC2 in the liver; whereas insulin increases Ser171 phosphorylation which promotes TORC2 cytoplasmic localization [62]. TORC2 interactions with CREB stabilize the interaction between CREB and $TAF_{II}130$ thus enhancing the transcriptional activity of CREB [63]. The CREB–TORC2 interaction also stimulates insulin receptor substrate 2 (IRS2) expression and thus increase insulin signaling in the liver [64]. TORC2, through its effect on CREB may also play a role in other transcription factors that regulate PEPCK. For example, since C/EBPβ is controlled by CREB, and C/EBPβ knockout mice have fasting hypoglycemia, it suggests that CREB via TORC2 may require C/EBPβ in the hierarchy of regulatory factors that control cAMP mediated PEPCK transcription and gluconeogenesis.

2.4. PGC-1α and regulation of PEPCK

PGC-1α was originally identified as a transcriptional coactivator of the nuclear receptor PPARγ. Recent studies of PGC-1α indicate that it acts as an accessory factor involved in the control of blood glucose levels by amplifying transcription of PEPCK in the liver [12,65,66]. The initial observation of increased PGC-1α mRNA in the

PEPCK expression is reduced by treatment with glitazones in cultured rat hepatocytes or streptozotocin-treated rats [85,86]. Later studies illustrated that PPARγ agonists reduce the levels of PEPCK, G-6-Pase, and Pyruvate Carboxylase in the liver as well as decreasing fatty acid oxidation gene expression and increasing the expression of lipogenic genes [87]. This data indicates that PPARγ may play a role in decreasing hepatic glucose production; however, this effect could be amplified by the flux of fatty acids away from the liver [87] *in vivo*. Recently, Cassuto et al. [88] demonstrated that glucocorticoids enhanced the binding of FOXO1 and PPAR-α to the AF2 and site within the glucocorticoid unit and a distant site (−1365) on the PEPCK promoter as well as enhancing the binding of HNF4α. Insulin inhibited the binding of these factors to their respective sites suggesting an extended GRU may include control via interaction with HNF4α and PPARα in the liver to control PEPCK gene transcription.

3. Insulin, glucose, adiponectin, and resistin and PEPCK gene transcription

3.1. *Insulin*

Insulin regulates the expression of more than a hundred genes [89] and plays an essential role in the regulation of glucose homeostasis by inhibiting PEPCK gene transcription, which ultimately decreases the output of glucose from liver [90]. It is known that insulin binds to the insulin receptor, which phosphorylates insulin receptor substrates and activates PI3-kinase. Two of the commercially available inhibitors of PI3-kinase, wortmanin and LY 294002, abolish insulin's suppression of basal and cAMP and dexamethasone-induced PEPCK and G-6-Pase gene expression [91–93]. Adenoviral overexpression of the dominant-negative mutant of the PI-3 kinase regulatory subunit p85α, which lacks a binding site for the catalytic subunit, increases PEPCK and G-6-Pase gene expression as well as hepatic glucose production *in vivo* [94]. Hepatic overexpression of a constitutively active Akt, which mimics the effects of insulin on Akt, in mice leads to hypoglycemia and a decrease in the PEPCK and G-6-Pase expression, however, the mechanism for Akt's effect is still unknown [95]. In addition, one study suggests insulin can act through liver X-activated receptor (LXR) activators to decrease gluconeogenesis by suppressing PEPCK and G-6-Pase [96].

In addition to increasing the concentration of the inhibitory C/EBP isoform LIP [25], insulin also has been shown to regulate gluconeogenesis through transcriptional components forkhead transcription factor 1 (FOXO1) and peroxisome proliferative activated receptor-γ coactivator 1 (PGC-1α). PGC-1α binds to FOXO1 to coactivate gluconeogenic gene expression [13]. This interaction is also vital for insulin induced suppression of FOXO1, via Akt-mediated phosphorylation. Phosphorylation of FOXO1 disrupts it's interaction with PGC-1α, in part by causing FOXO1 to exit from the nucleus, and thus reduces the interactions amplifying effects on gluconeogenesis [13,97]. SREBP-1c, as well as SREBP-1a and SREBP-2, inhibit transcription of the gene encoding the cytosolic form of phosphoenolpyruvate carboxykinase

(GTP) (PEPCK-C). There are two SREBP regulatory elements (SREs) in the PEPCK gene promoter (−322 to −313 and −590 to −581). The SRE at −590 overlaps a Sp1 site on the opposite strand of the DNA. These SREs bound SREBP-1a and SREBP-1c with low affinity but the addition of purified upstream stimulatory activity enhanced the binding of SREBP-1 to both of these sites. Insulin represses transcription of the gene for PEPCK-C by inducing SREBP-1c production in the liver, which interferes with the stimulatory effect of Sp1 at −590 of the PEPCK-C gene promoter [74].

3.2. *Glucose*

Glucose is known to repress PEPCK gene expression in both FAO cells and primary hepatocytes [98,99], requiring metabolism through glucokinase. It is thought that xylulose-5-phosphate might be the metabolite responsible for glucose-induced inhibition of PEPCK gene expression [100] though controversy exists on this point [101]. In cultured hepatocytes, a high glucose concentration induces lipogenesis and at the same time represses PEPCK expression, but does not induce a detectable increase in xylulose-5-phosphate. In HL1C rat hepatoma cells, which do not express GK, 2-deoxyglucose is able to repress PEPCK expression [102]. Based on the results from several experiments it is reasonable to assume that glucose-6-phosphate might be the activating factor for the activating effects of glucose on PEPCK and therefore on gluconeogenesis ([101], reviewed in [103]).

3.3. *Adiponectin*

Adiponectin, also known as Acrp30, or adipoQ, is a 30 kDa adipose tissue-derived hormone that plays an essential role in energy homeostasis and glucose and lipid metabolism. Intraperitoneal injection of adiponectin lowers blood glucose levels in mice within 2–4 h after injection indicating a role in glucose homeostasis [104,105]. The mechanism involved might be either increased glucose uptake or regulation of glucose output [104]. Furthermore, ectopic expression of the adiponectin transgene modulates hepatic gluconeogenesis as demonstrated by reduction of key hepatic genes such as PEPCK [106]. Adiponectin, like resistin, stimulates glucose utilization by activating AMPK, a master switch controlling lipid and glucose metabolism. It is therefore possible that adiponectin regulates PEPCK gene expression by activating AMPK [106,107].

3.4. *Resistin*

The hormone resistin is a 12.5 kDa protein secreted by adipose tissue and plays an important role in glucose homeostasis [108]. Serum levels of resistin are elevated in rodent models of obesity and diabetes [108]. Acute administration of resistin in C57BL/6J mice impairs glucose homeostasis and insulin action [108]. Infusion of resistin protein into Sprague–Dawley rats worsens glucose homeostasis by increasing blood glucose and hepatic glucose production [109] suggesting an acute increase of resistin in rodents may impair glucose homeostasis. Similarly, transgenic mice over-expressing the resistin gene show higher blood glucose, impaired glucose tolerance, and increased glucose production compared to their non-transgenic littermates, consistent with increased hepatic expression of PEPCK [110]. Administration of pyruvate, a gluconeogenic substrate, to mice lacking the resistin gene show decreased blood glucose and reduced liver glucose-6-phosphatase (G-6-Pase) and PEPCK gene expression compared to wild type mice [111]. These findings clearly suggest a modulatory role of resistin in gluconeogenesis.

4. Role of C/EBPs in inflammation and ER stress response

The ER is an organelle that synthesizes various secretory and membrane proteins. These proteins are correctly folded and assembled by chaperones in the ER. During stressful conditions, such as nutrient excess, an increase in the misfolded protein levels can occur, the chaperones become overloaded and the ER fails to fold and export newly synthesized proteins, leading to ER stress [112,113]. Recently ER stress has been linked to activation of Jun Kinase-1 (JNK-1). JNK-1 is increased obesity and its reversal can improve insulin action, and type 2 diabetes [114]. It has been demonstrated that obesity overloads the functional capacity of the ER and that this ER-stress leads to the activation of inflammatory signaling pathways and thus contributes to insulin resistance ([115,116]). Additionally, increased glucose metabolism can lead to a rise in mitochondrial production of reactive oxygen species (ROS) and stress inducible JNK that can increase the ER stress. While it is clear that inhibition of insulin receptor signaling pathways is a central mechanism through which inflammatory and stress responses mediate insulin resistance, it is likely that other relevant pathways, molecules, and alternative mechanisms involved in this interaction have yet to be uncovered. C/EBP's regulate the development and function of the liver and other tissues, however evidence has revealed a remarkable array of additional metabolic regulatory functions, including inflammation, ER stress, and other disease mechanisms that impact diabetes and obesity pathophysiology. Some specific examples of these processes are outlined below.

4.1. C/EBPβ and COX2-mediated inflammation

Cyclooxygenase (COX) is the rate-limiting enzyme in prostaglandin (PG) synthesis, catalyzing the conversion of arachidonic acid to PGH_2 [117]. Two distinct COX isoforms have been characterized so far: COX1, which is present in most cells and is responsible for constitutive PG formation, and COX2, which is induced in response to stress [117]. COX2 exerts diverse action on cell function, including proliferation, migration and DNA damage. Enhanced expression of COX2 is assumed to be protective however; uncontrolled or excessive expression is harmful, causing inflammation, atheromatous plaque instability and intimal hyperplasia. Reports have been published showing a deleterious role of COX2 in myocardial infarction [118,119]. C/EBPβ is thought to be a key transactivator for COX2 expression induced by proinflammatory mediators like interleukinβ (IL-β) and lipopolysaccharides (LPS) [120]. It has been shown that aspirin and salicylate suppress COX2 expression by blocking C/EBPβ activation [120]. Given recent studies suggesting that COX inhibitors (salicylates) may be important in the treatment of insulin resistance [121], this suggests that by inhibiting the proinflammatory genes, C/EBPβ may be an important factor in suppressing inflammation and quite possibly reducing an important pathway for insulin resistance [122]. Saunders et al. [123] demonstrated that sodium salicylate at a therapeutic concentration suppressed COX-2 gene transcription induced by phorbol 12-myristate 13-acetate and interleukin 1 by inhibiting the binding of C/EBPβ binding to its promoter region of COX-2. By contrast, salicylate did not inhibit nuclear factor B-dependent COX-2 induction by tumor necrosis factor. These findings indicate that contrary to the current view that salicylate acts via inhibition of nuclear factor B the pharmacological actions of aspirin and salicylates may be mediated by inhibiting C/EBPβ binding and transactivation. These findings could have a major impact on the conceptual understanding of the mechanism of action of salicylates and on new drug discovery and design.

4.2. C/EBP and vascular inflammation

Vascular inflammation plays an important role in both initiation and progression of atherosclerosis, a key diabetic complication (see chapter on CREB, this volume). It has been shown that increased expression of C/EBPδ in response to inflammation positively regulated transcription and protein expression of PPARγ in vascular smooth muscle cells. PPARγ ligands have been found to suppress C/EBPδ expression through transactivation of PPARγ [124]. These results suggest that C/EBP-δ is negatively autoregulated via transactivation of PPAR-γ. The ultimate molecular event is the downregulation of the transcription of inflammatory cytokines and acute phase proteins and therefore may modulate inflammatory responses in the early phase of atherosclerosis.

4.3. C/EBPs in nitric oxide induced inflammation

NO (nitric oxide) produced by inducible nitric oxide synthase (iNOS) plays a key role in the induction of variety of diseases and inflammation ([125–127]. Expression of the iNOS gene is regulated at different levels including transcriptional, translational, and posttranslational steps [128]. The mouse iNOS promoter contains an enhancer and basal promoter site. It has been shown that NFkB and C/EBPs regulate NO production by binding to promoter site of the iNOS gene [129,131]. The essential role of C/EBPβ in the regulation of NO production was shown by the work of Kim et al. [131]. These authors have shown that 8-hydroxyquinolein (8HQ), a lipophilic metal chelator, inhibited LPS induced NO-production and iNOS expression in Raw 246.7 cells through inhibition of NFkB and C/EBPβ binding to the iNOS promoter and thereby affecting iNOS induction.

4.4. *Role of C/EBPs in endoplasmic reticulum stress response*

The ER, plays a critical role in protein folding, and diseases such as Parkinson's, Alzheimers, Huntington's disease, and obesity are linked to misfolded proteins [114]. Various chemical and biological stressors also induce ER stress, resulting in the unfolded protein response, which both activates and deactivates gene/protein expression to restore the cell to homeostasis ([130,132]). Activation of the ER stress signaling pathway known as the unfolded protein response (UPR) is characterized by (a) upregulation of the genes encoding ER chaperone proteins including Bip/GRP78 and GRP94, which increase protein-folding activity and prevent aggregation (b) attenuation of protein biosynthesis mediated acutely by PERK (PKR-like ER kinase) through phosphorylation of translation initiation factor 2 (eIF2), (c) degradation of misfolded proteins in the ER, which is called ER associated degradation, and (d) apoptosis which occurs when functions of the ER are severely impaired to protect the organism by eliminating the damaged cells [132,133].

The human C/EBPβ gene is activated by ER stress through an unfolded protein response element downstream of the protein coding sequence ([134]). Accumulated data provide evidence that CHOP, a C/EBP homologous protein, also known as growth arrest and DNA damage-inducible gene 153 (GADD 153) is actively involved in ER stress-induced apoptotic pathways [135]. Fawcett et al. [136] showed that in response to oxidative stress, the expression of both C/EBPβ and CHOP is induced and that they interact *in vivo*, unlike other C/EBPs. These authors further proposed that C/EBP transactivates CHOP expression through a C/EBP-ATF composite site in the CHOP promoter. The increased CHOP to C/EBP protein ratio may lead to the heterodimerization of CHOP with C/EBP, and consequently, given the dominant-negative effect of CHOP [136], this heterodimerization could block the transactivation effect of C/EBP on numerous genes. Since the accumulation of unfolded proteins in the ER increases the levels of C/EBPβ in cells, this raises questions about the mechanism of sensing cell stress that ultimately leads to activation of target genes. C/EBPβ may therefore be a switch that links ER stress to changes in apoptosis or genes meant to relieve ER stress.

4.5. *C/EBP and non-alcoholic steatohepatitis (NASH)*

Non-alcoholic steatohepatitis (NASH) is a metabolic liver disease and commonly associated with obesity, type 2 diabetes, and the metabolic syndrome [137–139]. A two-hit model has been proposed in the pathogenesis of NASH. The first hit is hepatic steatosis or fatty liver and is associated with accumulation of triglycerides in liver. The second hit consists of inflammation, cell death and fibrosis [137,140,141]. A large majority of obese subjects have fatty liver and it has been suggested that 30% have NASH [142,143]. The pathophysiological mechanism leading to the progression from steatosis to NASH remains obscure. A methionine-choline-deficient (MCD) diet is being extensively used to produce a dietary model of NASH in animals. Accumulated data reveal that this model produces steatohepatitis and liver fibrosis that is histologically similar to human NASH [144–146]. Studies from our laboratory have shown increased C/EBPβ expression in the livers from MCD fed mice along with increased level of triglycerides and NFkKβ (unpublished observations). Moreover, biochemical markers of NASH are also upregulated in this model along with the induction of ER stress marker proteins. In support of the hypothesis that C/EBPβ contributes to the NASH phenotype, injection of an adenovirus containing the LAP form of C/EBPβ into mice results in an identical phenomena as observed in MCD fed mice. These results suggest that C/EBPβ might be involved in NASH though further studies will be required. Studies examining the independent effects of a high fat or the MCD diet on the NASH phenotype in C/EBPβ deficient mice are currently underway.

Further evidence for a role of C/EBPβ in NASH has come from mice bred for double recessive $Lepr^{db/db}$ + CEBP$\beta^{-/-}$ double knockout (DKO) mice that exhibit partial amelioration of weight gain and reversal of diabetes. This might be expected, since extinguishing the CEBPβ gene blocks differentiation of preadipocytes to adipocytes and reduces gluconeogenesis. Surprisingly however, hepatic triglycerides were normalized in the DKO mice as well, even though serum and muscle triglycerides remain elevated. C/EBPβ deletion normalized the activity of the liver lipogenic enzymes fatty acid synthase (FAS) and ATP-citrate lyase (CL) independent of SREBP1c expression. This important observation suggests C/EBPβ may potentially regulate hepatic lipogenesis as well as gluconeogenesis by mechanisms distinct from or parallel to SREBP1c (Cell^{Metabolism} in review).

5. Summary and future perspective

The basic molecular mechanisms underlying the regulation of hepatic glucose and lipid homeostasis by C/EBPs are complex and involve interaction with other transcription factors. A gene deletion in C/EBPβ affects gluconeogenesis, hepatic lipid storage, and possibly inflammation resulting in hypoglycemia and protection from hepatic steatosis when challenged by overfeeding. Evidence suggests that nutrients, hormones, and cytokines affect the pattern of expression of C/EBPβ, which in turn, regulates key genes that control metabolic processes including lipogenesis and gluconeogenesis. It is very likely that C/EBPβ, like many other transcription factors, represents a funnel through which several extracellular signaling pathways are potentially channeled to generate transcriptional patterns resulting in coordinate regulation of fuel metabolism. Characterization of key tissue-specific functions of the C/EBPβ pathway will lead to a greater understanding of the integration of molecular control over both glucose and lipid metabolism. In addition, further understanding of how external signaling pathways (adiponectin, or ER stressors for example) can control C/EBPβ expression and its gene targets may provide important new insights into potential molecular mechanisms that underlie diabetes, obesity, inflammation, and fatty liver disease.

References

[1] R.C. Nordlie, J.D. Foster, A.J. Lange, Regulation of glucose production by the liver, Annu. Rev. Nutr. 19 (1999) 379–406.

[2] A. Vidal-Puig, S. O'Rahilly, Metabolism. Controlling the glucose factory, Nature 413 (6852) (2001) 125–126.

[3] R.A. DeFronzo, D. Simonson, E. Ferrannini, Hepatic and peripheral insulin resistance: a common feature of type 2 (non-insulin-dependent) and type 1 (insulin-dependent) diabetes mellitus, Diabetologia 23 (4) (1982) 313–319.

[4] C. Bogardus, S. Lillioja, B.V. Howard, G. Reaven, D. Mott, Relationships between insulin secretion, insulin action, and fasting plasma glucose concentration in nondiabetic and noninsulin-dependent diabetic subjects, J. Clin. Invest. 74 (4) (1984) 1238–1246.

[5] R.A. DeFronzo, Lilly lecture 1987, The triumvirate: beta-cell, muscle, liver. A collusion responsible for NIDDM, Diabetes 37 (6) (1988) 667–687.

[6] A. Valera, A. Pujol, M. Pelegrin, F. Bosch, Transgenic mice overexpressing phosphoenolpyruvate carboxykinase develop non-insulin-dependent diabetes mellitus, Proc. Natl. Acad. Sci. USA 91 (19) (1994) 9151–9154.

[7] Y. Sun, S. Liu, S. Ferguson, L. Wang, P. Klepcyk, J.S. Yun, J.E. Friedman, Phosphoenolpyruvate carboxykinase overexpression selectively attenuates insulin signaling and hepatic insulin sensitivity in transgenic mice, J. Biol. Chem. 277 (2002) 23301–23307.

[8] R.W. Hanson, L. Reshef, Regulation of phosphoenolpyruvate carboxykinase (GTP) gene expression, Annu. Rev. Biochem. 66 (1997) 581–611.

[9] S.M. Tilghman, R.W. Hanson, L. Reshef, M.F. Hopgood, F.J. Ballard, Rapid loss of translatable messenger RNA of phosphoenolpyruvate carboxykinase during glucose repression in liver, Proc. Natl. Acad. Sci. USA 71 (4) (1974) 1304–1308.

[10] C. Croniger, P. Leahy, L. Reshef, R.W. Hanson, C/EBP and the control of phosphoenolpyruvate carboxykinase gene transcription in the liver, J. Biol. Chem. 273 (48) (1998) 31629–31632.

[11] T. Sugiyama, D.K. Scott, J.C. Wang, D.K. Granner, Structural requirements of the glucocorticoid and retinoic acid response units in the phosphoenolpyruvate carboxykinase gene promoter, Mol. Endocrinol. 12 (10) (1998) 1487–1498.

[12] J.C. Yoon, P. Puigserve, G. Chen, J. Donovan, Z. Wu, J. Rhee, G. Adelmant, J. Stafford, C.R. Kahn, D.K. Granner, C.B. Newgard, B.M. Spiegelman, Control of hepatic gluconeogenesis through the transcriptional coactivator PGC-1, Nature 413 (6852) (2001) 131–138.

[13] P. Puigserver, J. Rhee, J. Donovan, C.J. Walkey, J.C. Yoon, F. Oriente, Y. Kitamura, J. Altomonte, H. Dong, D. Accili, B.M. Spiegelman, Insulin-regulated hepatic gluconeogenesis through FOXO1-PGC-1alpha interaction, Nature 423 (6939) (2003) 550–555.

[14] K. Yamada, D.T. Duong, D.K. Scott, J.-C. Wang, D.K. Granner, CCAAT/enhancer-binding protein beta is an accessory factor for the glucocorticoid response from the camp response element in the rat phosphoenolpyruvate carboxykinase gene promoter, J. Biol. Chem. 274 (9) (1999) 5880–5887.

[15] W.J. Roesler, What is a cAMP response unit? Mol. Cell Endocrinol. 162 (1–2) (2000) 1–7.

[16] P.F. Johnson, W.H. Landschulz, B.J. Graves, S.L. McKnight, Identification of a rat liver nuclear protein that binds to the enhancer core element of three animal viruses, Genes Dev. 1 (2) (1987) 133–146.

[17] B.J. Graves, P.F. Johnson, S.L. McKnight, Homologous recognition of a promoter domain common to the MSV LTR and the HSV tk gene, Cell 44 (4) (1986) 565–576.

[18] Z. Cao, R.M. Umek, S.L. McKnight, Regulated expression of three C/EBP isoforms during adipose conversion of 3T3-L1 cells, Genes Dev. 5 (9) (1991) 1538–1552.

[19] V. Poli, F.P. Mancini, R. Cortese, IL-6DBP, a nuclear protein involved in interleukin-6 signal transduction, defines a new family of leucine zipper proteins related to C/EBP, Cell 63 (3) (1990) 643–653.

[20] P. Descombes, M. Chojkier, S. Lichtsteiner, E. Falvey, U. Schibler, LAP, a novel member of the C/EBP gene family, encodes a liver-enriched transcriptional activator protein, Genes Dev. 4 (9) (1990) 1541–1551.

[21] J. Lekstrom-Himes, K.G. Xanthopoulos, Biological role of the CCAAT/Enhancer-binding protein family of transcription factors, (Minireview) J. Biol. Chem. 273 (44) (1998) 28545–28548.

[22] S.M. Taubenfeld, K.A. Wiig, B. Monti, B. Dolan, G. Pollonini, C.M. Alberini, Fornix-dependent induction of hippocampal CCAAT enhancer-binding protein β and δ colocalizes with phosphorylated cAMP response element-binding protein and accompanies long-term memory consolidation, J. Neurosci. 21 (1) (2001) 84–91.

[23] J. Chen, S.S. Newton, L. Zeng, D.H. Adams, A.L. Dow, T.M. Madse, E.J. Nestler, R.S. Duman, Downregulation of the CCAAT-enhancer binding protein beta in deltaFosB transgenic mice and by electroconvulsive seizures, Neuropsychopharmacology 29 (1) (2004) 23–31.

[24] R.A. Abbud, R. Kelleher, S. Melmed, Cell-specific pituitary gene expression profiles after treatment with leukemia inhibitory factor reveal novel modulators for proopiomelanocortin expression, Endocrinology 145 (2) (2004) 867–880.

[25] D.T. Duong, M.E. Waltner-Law, R. Sears, L. Sealy, D.K. Granner, Insulin inhibits hepatocellular glucose production by utilizing liver- enriched transcriptional inhibitory protein to disrupt the association of creb-binding protein and rna polymerase II with the phosphoenolpyruvate carboxykinase gene promoter, J. Biol. Chem. 277 (35) (2002) 32234–32242.

[26] E.A. Park, W.J. Roesler, J. Liu, D.J. Klemm, A.L. Gurney, J.D. Thatcher, J. Shuman, A. Friedman, R.W. Hanson, The role of the CCAAT/enhancer-binding protein in the transcriptional regulation of the gene for phosphoenolpyruvate carboxykinase (GTP), Mol. Cell Biol. 10 (12) (1990) 6264–6272.

[27] T. Gotoh, S. Chowdhury, M. Takiguchi, M. Mori, The glucocorticoid-responsive gene cascade, Activation of the rat arginase gene through induction of C/EBPbeta, J. Biol. Chem. 272 (6) (1997) 3694–3698.

[28] F. Matsuno, S. Chowdhury, T. Gotoh, K. Iwase, H. Matsuzaki, K. Takatsuki, M. Mori, M. Takiguchi, Induction of the C/EBP beta gene by dexamethasone and glucagon in primary-cultured rat hepatocytes, J. Biochem. (Tokyo). 119 (3) (1996) 524–532.

[29] S.E. Nizielski, C. Arizmendi, A.R. Shteyngarts, C.J. Farrell, J.E. Friedman, Involvement of transcription factor C/EBP-beta in stimulation of PEPCK gene expression during exercise, Am. J. Physiol. 270 (5 Pt 2) (1996) R1005–R1012.

[30] F. Bosch, J. Sabater, A. Valera, Insulin inhibits liver expression of the CCAAT/Enhancer-binding protein β, Diabetes 44 (3) (1995) 267–271.

[31] G. Piwien-Pilipuk, O. MacDougald, J. Schwartz, Dual regulation of phosphorylation and dephosphorylation of C/EBPbeta modulate its transcriptional activation and DNA binding in response to growth hormone, J. Biol. Chem. 277 (46) (2002) 44557–44565.

[32] C.F. Calkhoven, C. Muller, A. Leutz, Translational control of C/EBPalpha and C/EBPbeta isoform expression, Genes Dev. 14 (15) (2000) 1920–1932.

[33] M. Niehof, M.P. Manns, C. Trautwein, CREB controls LAP/C/EBP beta transcription, Mol. Cell Biol. 17 (7) (1997) 3600–3613.

[34] M. Niehof, S. Kubicka, L. Zender, M.P. Manns, C. Trautwein, Autoregulation enables different pathways to control CCAAT/enhancer binding protein beta (C/EBP beta) transcription, J. Mol. Biol. 309 (4) (2001) 855–868.

[35] S.L. Lay, I. Lefrere, C. Trautwein, I. Dugail, S. Krief, Insulin and Sterol-regulatory Element-binding Protein-1c (SREBP-1C) Regulation of Gene Expression in 3T3-L1 Adipocytes. Identification Of CCAAT/Enhancer-Binding Protein beta As An SREBP-1C Target, J. Biol. Chem. 277 (38) (2002) 35625–35634.

[36] S. Guo, S.B. Cichy, X. He, Q. Yang, M. Ragland, A.K. Ghosh, P.F. Johnson, T.G. Unterman, Insulin suppresses transactivation by CAAT/enhancer-binding proteins beta (C/EBPbeta). Signaling to p300/CREB-binding protein by protein kinase B disrupts interaction with the major activation domain of C/EBPbeta, J. Biol. Chem. 276 (11) (2001) 8516–8523.

[37] S. Liu, C. Croniger, C. Arizmendi, M. Harada-Shiba, J. Ren, V. Poli, R.W. Hanson, J.E. Friedman, Hypoglycemia and impaired hepatic glucose production in mice with a deletion of the C/EBPbeta gene, J. Clin. Invest. 103 (2) (1999) 207–213.

[38] D.P. Ramji, P. Foka, CCAAT/enhancer-binding proteins: structure, function and regulation, Review, Biochem. J. 365 (2002) 561–575.

[39] W.J. Roesler, The role of C/EBP in nutrient and hormonal regulation of gene expression, Review, Annu. Rev. Nutr. 21 (2001) 41–165.

[40] N.M. Wheelhouse, A.K. Stubbs, M.A. Lomax, J.C. MacRae, D.G. Hazlerigg, Growth Hormone and amino acid supply interact synergistically to control insulin-like growth factor-I production and gene expression in cultured ovine hepatocytes, J. Endocrinol. 163 (2) (1999) 353–361.

[41] M.R. An, C.C. Hsieh, P.D. Reisner, J.P. Rabek, S.G. Scott, D.T. Kuninger, J. Papaconstantinou, Evidence for posttranscriptional regulation of C/EBPalphaC/EBPbeta isoform expression during the lipopolysaccharide-mediated acute-phase response, Mol. Cell. Biol. 16 (5) (1996) 2295–2306.

[42] A.M. Diehl, P. Michaelson, S.T. Yang, Selective induction of CCAAT/enhancer binding protein isoforms occurs during rat liver development, Gastroenterology 106 (6) (1994) 1625–1637.

[43] N.A. Timchenko, M. Wilde, K.L. Kosai, A. Heydari, T.A. Bilyeu, M.J. Finegold, K. Mohamedali, A. Richardson, G.J. Darlington, Regenerating livers of old rats contain high levels of C/EBPalpha that correlate with altered expression of cell cycle associated proteins, Nucl. Acids Res. 26 (13) (1998) 3293–3299.

[44] Y. Hirai, D. Radisky, R. Boudreau, M. Simian, M.E. Stevens, Y. Oka, K. Takebe, S. Niwa, M.J. Bissell, Epimorphin mediates mammary luminal morphogenesis through control of C/EBPbeta, J. Cell Biol. 153 (4) (2001) 785–794.

[45] C.A. Zahnow, P. Younes, R. Laucirica, J.M. Rosen, Overexpression of C/EBPbeta-LIP, a naturally occurring, dominant-negative transcription factor, in human breast cancer, J. Natl. Cancer Inst. 89 (24) (1997) 1887–1891.

[46] J. Shao, L. Qiao, R.C. Janssen, M. Pagliassotti, J.E. Friedman, Chronic hyperglycemia enhances PEPCK gene expression and hepatocellular glucose production via elevated liver activating protein/ liver inhibitory protein ratio, Diabetes 54 (4) (2005) 976–984.

[47] V. Begay, J. Smink, A. Leutz, Essential requirement of CCAAT/enhancer binding proteins in embryogenesis, Mol. Cell Biol. 24 (22) (2004) 9744–9751.

[48] N.D. Wang, M.J. Finegold, A. Bradley, C.N. Ou, S.V. Abdelsayed, M.D. Wilde, L.R. Taylor, D.R. Wilson, G.J. Darlington, Impaired energy homeostasis in C/EBP alpha knockout mice, Science 269 (5227) (1995) 1108–1112.

[49] G.J. Darlington, N. Wang, R.W. Hanson, C/EBPα: a critical regulator of genes governing integrative metabolic processes, Curr. Opin. Genet. Dev. 5 (1995) 565–570.

[50] C. Croniger, M. Trus, K. Lysek-Stupp, H. Cohen, Y. Liu, G.J. Darlington, V. Poli, R.W. Hanson, L. Reshef, Role of the isoforms of CCAAT/enhancer-binding protein in the initiation of phosphoenolpyruvate carboxykinase (GTP) gene transcription at birth, J. Biol. Chem. 272 (42) (1997) 26306–26312.

[51] E. Sterneck, L. Tessarollo, P.F. Johnson, An essential role for C/EBPβ in female reproduction, Genes Dev 11 (1997) 2153–2162.

[52] T. Tanaka, S. Akira, K. Yoshida, M. Umemoto, Y. Yoneda, N. Shirafuji, H. Fujiwara, S. Suematsu, N. Yoshida, T. Kishimoto, Targeted disruption of the NF-IL6 gene discloses its essential role in bacteria killing and tumor cytotoxicity by macrophages, Cell 80 (2) (1995) 353–361.

[53] I. Screpanti, P. Musiani, D. Bellavia, M. Cappelletti, F.B. Aiello, M. Maroder, L. Frati, A. Modesti, A. Gulino, V. Poli, Inactivation of the IL-6 gene prevents development of multicentric Castleman's disease in C/EBP beta-deficient mice, J. Exp. Med. 184 (4) (1996) 1561–1566.

[54] R. Herrera, H.S. Ro, G.S. Robinson, K.G. Xanthopoulos, B.M. Spiegelman, A direct role for C/EBP and the AP-I-binding site in gene expression linked to adipocyte differentiation, Mol. Cell Biol. 9 (12) (1989) 5331–5339.

[55] L. Wang, J. Shao, P. Muhlenkamp, S. Liu, P. Klepcyk, J. Ren, J.E. Friedman, Increased insulin receptor substrate-1 and enhanced skeletal muscle insulin sensitivity in mice lacking CCAAT/ enhancer-binding protein beta, J. Biol. Chem. 275 (19) (2000) 14173–14181.

[56] C.M. Croniger, C. Millward, J. Yang, Y. Kawai, I.J. Arinze, S. Liu, M. Harada-Shiba, K. Chakravarty, J.E. Friedman, V. Poli, R.W. Hanson, Mice with a deletion in the gene for

CCAAT/enhancer-binding protein beta have an attenuated response to cAMP and impaired carbohydrate metabolism, J. Biol. Chem. 276 (1) (2001) 629–638.

[57] S.S. Chen, J.-F. Chen, P.F. Johnson, V. Muppala, Y.-H. Lee, C/EBPβ, when expressed from the C/ebpα gene locus, can functionally replace C/EBPα in liver but not in adipose tissue, Mol. Cell Biol. 20 (19) (2000) 7292–7299.

[58] K. Matsusue, O. Gavrilova, G. Lambert, H.B. Brewer Jr., J.M. Ward, Y. Inoue, D. LeRoith, F.J. Gonzalez, Hepatic CCAAT/enhancer binding protein alpha mediates induction of lipogenesis and regulation of glucose homeostasis in leptin-deficient mice, Mol. Endocrinol. 18 (11) (2004) 2751–2764.

[59] Y. Inoue, J. Inoue, G. Lambert, S.H. Yim, F.J. Gonzalez, Disruption of hepatic C/EBPalpha results in impaired glucose tolerance and age-dependent hepatosteatosis, J. Biol. Chem. 279 (43) (2004) 44740–44748.

[60] J. Yang, C.M. Croniger, J. Lekstrom-Himes, P. Zhang, M. Fenyus, D.G. Tenen, G.J. Darlington, R.W. Hanson, Metabolic response of mice to a postnatal ablation of CCAAT/enhancer-binding protein alpha, J. Biol. Chem. 280 (46) (2005) 38689–38699.

[61] J.S. Liu, E.A. Park, A.L. Gurney, W.J. Roesler, R.W. Hanson, Cyclic AMP induction of phosphoenolpyruvate carboxykinase (GTP) gene transcription is mediated by multiple promoter elements, J. Biol. Chem. 266 (28) (1991) 19095–19102.

[62] S.H. Koo, L. Flechner, L. Qi, X. Zhang, R.A. Screaton, S. Jeffries, S. Hedrick, W. Xu, F. Boussouar, P. Brindle, H. Takemori, M. Montminy, The CREB coactivator TORC2 is a key regulator of fasting glucose metabolism, Nature 437 (7062) (2005) 1109–1111.

[63] M.D. Conkright, M. Montminy, CREB: the unindicted cancer co-conspirator, Trends Cell Biol. 15 (9) (2005) 457–459.

[64] G. Canettieri, S.H. Koo, R. Berdeaux, J. Heredia, S. Hedrick, X. Zhang, M. Montminy, Dual role of the coactivator TORC2 in modulating hepatic glucose output and insulin signaling, Cell Metab. 2 (5) (2005) 331–338.

[65] S. Herzig, F. Long, U.S. Jhala, S. Hedrick, R. Quinn, A. Bauer, D. Rudolph, G. Schutz, C. Yoon, P. Puigserver, B. Spiegelman, M. Montminy, CREB regulates hepatic gluconeogenesis through the coactivator PGC-1, Nature 413 (6852) (2001) 179–183.

[66] B. Herzog, R.K. Hall, X.L. Wang, M. Waltner-Law, D.K. Granner, Peroxisome proliferator-activated receptor gamma coactivator-1alpha, as a transcription amplifier, is not essential for basal and hormone-induced phosphoenolpyruvate carboxykinase gene expression, Mol. Endocrinol. 18 (4) (2004) 807–819.

[67] J. Lin, P.H. Wu, P.T. Tarr, K.S. Lindenberg, J. St-Pierre, C.Y. Zhang, V.K. Mootha, S. Jager, C.R. Vianna, R.M. Reznick, L. Cui, M. Manieri, M.X. Donovan, Z. Wu, M.P. Cooper, M.C. Fan, L.M. Rohas, A.M. Zavacki, S. Cinti, G.I. Shulman, B.B. Lowell, D. Krainc, B.M. Spiegelman, Defects in adaptive energy metabolism with CNS-linked hyperactivity in PGC-1alpha null mice, Cell 119 (1) (2004) 121–135.

[68] M. Montminy, S.H. Koo, Diabetes: outfoxing insulin resistance?, Nature 432 (7020) (2004) 958–959.

[69] C. Wolfrum, E. Asilmaz, E. Luca, J.M. Friedman, M. Stoffel, Foxa2 regulates lipid metabolism and ketogenesis in the liver during fasting and in diabetes, Nature 432 (7020) (2004) 1027–1032.

[70] D. Frescas, L. Valenti, D. Accili, Nuclear trapping of the forkhead transcription factor FoxO1 via Sirt-dependent deacetylation promotes expression of glucogenetic genes, J. Biol. Chem. 280 (21) (2005) 20589–20595.

[71] J. Altomonte, A. Richter, S. Harbaran, J. Suriawinata, J. Nakae, S.N. Thung, M. Meseck, D. Accili, H. Dong, Inhibition of Foxo1 function is associated with improved fasting glycemia in diabetic mice, Am. J. Physiol. Endocrinol. Metab. 285 (4) (2003) E718–E728.

[72] R.K. Hall, F.M. Sladek, D.K. Granner, The orphan receptors COUP-TF and HNF-4 serve as accessory factors required for induction of phosphoenolpyruvate carboxykinase gene transcription by glucocorticoids, Proc. Natl. Acad. Sci. USA 92 (2) (1995) 412–416.

[73] T. Yamamoto, H. Shimano, Y. Nakagawa, T. Ide, N. Yahagi, T. Matsuzaka, M. Nakakuki, A. Takahashi, H. Suzuki, H. Sone, H. Toyoshima, R. Sato, N. Yamada, SREBP-1 interacts with

hepatocyte nuclear factor-4 alpha and interferes with PGC-1 recruitment to suppress hepatic gluconeogenic genes, J. Biol. Chem. 279 (13) (2004) 12027–12035.

[74] K. Chakravarty, S.Y. Wu, C.M. Chiang, D. Samols, R.W. Hanson, SREBP-1c and Sp1 interact to regulate transcription of the gene for phosphoenolpyruvate carboxykinase (GTP) in the liver, J. Biol. Chem. 279 (15) (2004) 15385–15395.

[75] J.D. Horton, Y. Bashmakov, I. Shimomura, H. Shimano, Regulation of sterol regulatory element binding proteins in livers of fasted and refed mice, Proc. Natl. Acad. Sci. USA 95 (11) (1998) 5987–5992.

[76] N. Yahagi, H. Shimano, A.H. Hasty, M. Amemiya-Kudo, H. Okazaki, Y. Tamura, Y. Iizuka, F. Shionoiri, K. Ohashi, J. Osuga, K. Harada, T. Gotoda, R. Nagai, S. Ishibashi, N. Yamada, A crucial role of sterol regulatory element-binding protein-1 in the regulation of lipogenic gene expression by polyunsaturated fatty acids, J. Biol. Chem. 274 (50) (1999) 35840–35844.

[77] T. Yoshikawa, H. Shimano, N. Yahagi, T. Ide, M. Amemiya-Kudo, T. Matsuzaka, M. Nakakuki, S. Tomita, H. Okazaki, Y. Tamura, Y. Iizuka, K. Ohashi, A. Takahashi, H. Sone, J. Osuga Ji, T. Gotoda, S. Ishibashi, N. Yamada, Polyunsaturated fatty acids suppress sterol regulatory element-binding protein 1c promoter activity by inhibition of liver X receptor (LXR) binding to LXR response elements, J. Biol. Chem. 277 (3) (2002) 1705–1711.

[78] A.H. Hasty, H. Shimano, N. Yahagi, M. Amemiya-Kudo, S. Perrey, T. Yoshikawa, J. Osuga, H. Okazaki, Y. Tamura, Y. Iizuka, F. Shionoiri, K. Ohashi, K. Harada, T. Gotoda, R. Nagai, S. Ishibashi, N. Yamada, Sterol regulatory element-binding protein-1 is regulated by glucose at the transcriptional level, J. Biol. Chem. 275 (40) (2000) 31069–31077.

[79] I. Shimomura, Y. Bashmakov, S. Ikemoto, J.D. Horton, M.S. Brown, J.L. Goldstein, Insulin selectively increases SREBP-1c mRNA in the livers of rats with streptozotocin-induced diabetes, Proc. Natl. Acad. Sci. USA 96 (24) (1999) 13656–13661.

[80] B.M. Spiegelman, PPAR-gamma: adipogenic regulator and thiazolidinedione receptor, Diabetes 47 (4) (1998) 507–514.

[81] C.L. Eisenberger, H. Nechushtan, H. Cohen, M. Shani, L. Reshef, Differential regulation of the rat phosphoenolpyruvate carboxykinase gene expression in several tissues of transgenic mice, Mol. Cell Biol. 12 (3) (1992) 1396–1403.

[82] M.M. McGrane, J.S. Yun, A.F. Moorman, W.H. Lamers, G.K. Hendrick, B.M. Arafah, E.A. Park, T.E. Wagner, R.W. Hanson, Metabolic effects of developmental, tissue-, and cell-specific expression of a chimeric phosphoenolpyruvate carboxykinase (GTP)/bovine growth hormone gene in transgenic mice, J. Biol. Chem. 265 (36) (1990) 22371–22379.

[83] J. Mitchell, E. Noisin, R. Hall, R. O'Brien, E. Imai, D. Granner, Integration of multiple signals through a complex hormone response unit in the phosphoenolpyruvate carboxykinase gene promoter, Mol. Endocrinol. 8 (5) (1994) 585–594.

[84] P. Tontonoz, E. Hu, J. Devine, E.G. Beale, B.M. Spiegelman, PPAR gamma 2 regulates adipose expression of the phosphoenolpyruvate carboxykinase gene, Mol. Cell Biol. 15 (1) (1995) 351–357.

[85] G.F. Davies, R.L. Khandelwal, W.J. Roesler, Troglitazone inhibits expression of the phosphoenolpyruvate carboxykinase gene by an insulin-independent mechanism, Biochim. Biophys. Acta 1451 (1) (1999) 122–131.

[86] C. Hofmann, K. Lorenz, D. Williams, B.J. Palazuk, J.R. Colca, Insulin sensitization in diabetic rat liver by an antihyperglycemic agent, Metabolism 44 (3) (1995) 384–389.

[87] J.M. Way, W.W. Harrington, K.K. Brown, W.K. Gottschalk, S.S. Sundseth, T.A. Mansfield, R.K. Ramachandran, T.M. Willson, S.A. Kliewer, Comprehensive messenger ribonucleic acid profiling reveals that peroxisome proliferator-activated receptor gamma activation has coordinate effects on gene expression in multiple insulin-sensitive tissues, Endocrinology 142 (3) (2001) 1269–1277.

[88] H. Cassuto, K. Kochan, K. Chakravarty, H. Cohen, B. Blum, Y. Olswang, P. Hakimi, C. Xu, D. Massillon, R.W. Hanson, L. Reshef, Glucocorticoids regulate transcription of the gene for phosphoenolpyruvate carboxykinase in the liver via an extended glucocorticoid regulatory unit, J. Biol. Chem. 280 (40) (2005) 33873–33884.

[89] R.M. O'Brien, D.K. Granner, Regulation of gene expression by insulin, Physiol. Rev. 76 (4) (1996) 1109–1161.

[90] D.K. Granner, R.M. O'Brien, Molecular physiology and genetics of NIDDM, Importance of metabolic staging, Diabetes Care 15 (3) (1992) 369–395.

[91] J.M. Agati, D. Yeagley, P.G. Quinn, Assessment of the roles of mitogen-activated protein kinase, phosphatidylinositol 3-kinase, protein kinase B, and protein kinase C in insulin inhibition of cAMP-induced phosphoenolpyruvate carboxykinase gene transcription, J Biol. Chem. 273 (30) (1998) 18751–18759.

[92] M. Dickens, C.A. Svitek, A.A. Culbert, R.M. O'Brien, J.M. Tavare, Central role for phosphatidylinositide 3-kinase in the repression of glucose-6-phosphatase gene transcription by insulin, J. Biol. Chem. 273 (32) (1998) 20144–20149.

[93] C. Sutherland, R.M. O'Brien, D.K. Granner, Phosphatidylinositol 3-kinase, but not p70/p85 ribosomal S6 protein kinase, is required for the regulation of phosphoenolpyruvate carboxykinase (PEPCK) gene expression by insulin. Dissociation of signaling pathways for insulin and phorbol ester regulation of PEPCK gene expression, J. Biol. Chem. 270 (26) (1995) 15501–15506.

[94] K. Miyake, W. Ogawa, M. Matsumoto, T. Nakamura, H. Sakaue, M. Kasuga, Hyperinsulinemia, glucose intolerance, and dyslipidemia induced by acute inhibition of phosphoinositide 3-kinase signaling in the liver, J. Clin. Invest. 110 (10) (2002) 1483–1491.

[95] H. Ono, H. Shimano, H. Katagiri, N. Yahagi, H. Sakoda, Y. Onishi, M. Anai, T. Ogihara, M. Fujishiro, A.Y. Viana, Y. Fukushima, M. Abe, N. Shojima, M. Kikuchi, N. Yamada, Y. Oka, T. Asano, Hepatic Akt activation induces marked hypoglycemia, hepatomegaly, and hypertriglyceridemia with sterol regulatory element binding protein involvement, Diabetes 52 (12) (2003) 2905–2913.

[96] G. Cao, Y. Liang, C.L. Broderick, B.A. Oldham, T.P. Beyer, R.J. Schmidt, Y. Zhang, K.R. Stayrook, C. Suen, K.A. Otto, A.R. Miller, J. Dai, P. Foxworthy, H. Gao, T.P. Ryan, X.C. Jiang, T.P. Burris, P.I. Eacho, G.J. Etgen, Antidiabetic action of a liver x receptor agonist mediated by inhibition of hepatic gluconeogenesis, J. Biol. Chem. 278 (2) (2003) 1131–1136.

[97] A. Brunet, A. Bonni, M.J. Zigmond, M.Z. Lin, P. Juo, L.S. Hu, M.J. Anderson, K.C. Arden, J. Blenis, M.E. Greenberg, Akt promotes cell survival by phosphorylating and inhibiting a Forkhead transcription factor, Cell 96 (6) (1999) 857–868.

[98] C.R. Kahn, V. Lauris, S. Koch, M. Crettaz, D.K. Granner, Acute and chronic regulation of phosphoenolpyruvate carboxykinase mRNA by insulin and glucose, Mol. Endocrinol. 3 (5) (1989) 840–845.

[99] F. Cournarie, D. Azzout-Marniche, M. Foretz, C. Guichard, P. Ferre, F. Foufelle, The inhibitory effect of glucose on phosphoenolpyruvate carboxykinase gene expression in cultured hepatocytes is transcriptional and requires glucose metabolism, FEBS Lett. 460 (3) (1999) 527–532.

[100] D. Massillon, W. Chen, N. Barzilai, D. Prus-Wertheimer, M. Hawkins, R. Liu, R. Taub, L. Rossetti, Carbon flux via the pentose phosphate pathway regulates the hepatic expression of the glucose-6-phosphatase and phosphoenolpyruvate carboxykinase genes in conscious rats, J. Biol. Chem. 273 (1) (1998) 228–234.   ,

[101] F. Mourrieras, F. Foufelle, M. Foretz, J. Morin, S. Bouche, P. Ferre, Induction of fatty acid synthase and S14 gene expression by glucose, xylitol and dihydroxyacetone in cultured rat hepatocytes is closely correlated with glucose 6-phosphate concentrations, Biochem. J. 326 (Pt 2) (1997) 345–349.

[102] D.K. Scott, R.M. O'Doherty, J.M. Stafford, C.B. Newgard, D.K. Granner, The repression of hormone-activated PEPCK gene expression by glucose is insulin-independent but requires glucose metabolism, J. Biol. Chem. 273 (37) (1998) 24145–24151.

[103] J. Girard, P. Ferre, F. Foufelle, Mechanisms by which carbohydrates regulate expression of genes for glycolytic and lipogenic enzymes, Annu. Rev. Nutr. 17 (1997) 325–352.

[104] A.H. Berg, T.P. Combs, X. Du, M. Brownlee, P.E. Scherer, The adipocyte-secreted protein Acrp30 enhances hepatic insulin action, Nat. Med. 7 (8) (2001) 947–953.

[105] J. Fruebis, T.S. Tsao, S. Javorschi, D. Ebbets-Reed, M.R. Erickson, F.T. Yen, B.E. Bihain, H.F. Lodish, Proteolytic cleavage product of 30-kDa adipocyte complement-related protein increases fatty acid oxidation in muscle and causes weight loss in mice, Proc. Natl. Acad. Sci. USA 98 (4) (2001) 2005–2010.

[106] S. Shklyaev, G. Aslanidi, M. Tennant, V. Prima, E. Kohlbrenner, V. Kroutov, M. Campbell-Thompson, J. Crawford, E.W. Shek, P.J. Scarpace, S. Zolotukhin, Sustained peripheral expression of transgene adiponectin offsets the development of diet-induced obesity in rats, Proc. Natl. Acad. Sci. USA 100 (24) (2003) 14217–14222.

[107] T. Yamauchi, J. Kamon, Y. Minokoshi, Y. Ito, H. Waki, S. Uchida, S. Yamashita, M. Noda, S. Kita, K. Ueki, K. Eto, Y. Akanuma, P. Froguel, F. Foufelle, P. Ferre, D. Carling, S. Kimura, R. Nagai, B.B. Kahn, T. Kadowaki, Adiponectin stimulates glucose utilization and fatty-acid oxidation by activating AMP-activated protein kinase, Nat. Med. 8 (11) (2002) 1288–1295.

[108] C.M. Steppan, S.T. Bailey, S. Bhat, E.J. Brown, R.R. Banerjee, C.M. Wright, H.R. Patel, R.S. Ahima, M.A. Lazar, The hormone resistin links obesity to diabetes, Nature 409 (6818) (2001) 307–312.

[109] M.W. Rajala, S. Obici, P.E. Scherer, L. Rossetti, Adipose-derived resistin and gut-derived resistin-like molecule-beta selectively impair insulin action on glucose production, J. Clin. Invest. 111 (2) (2003) 225–230.

[110] S.M. Rangwala, A.S. Rich, B. Rhoades, J.S. Shapiro, S. Obici, L. Rossetti, M.A. Lazar, Abnormal glucose homeostasis due to chronic hyperresistinemia, Diabetes 53 (8) (2004) 1937–1941.

[111] R.R. Banerjee, S.M. Rangwala, J.S. Shapiro, A.S. Rich, B. Rhoades, Y. Qi, J. Wang, M.W. Rajala, A. Pocai, P.E. Scherer, C.M. Steppan, R.S. Ahima, S. Obici, L. Rossetti, M.A. Lazar, Regulation of fasted blood glucose by resistin, Science 303 (5661) (2004) 1195–1198.

[112] M. Aridor, W.E. Balch, Integration of endoplasmic reticulum signaling in health and disease, Nat. Med. 5 (7) (1999) 745–751.

[113] H.P. Harding, Y. Zhang, D. Ron, Protein translation and folding are coupled by an endoplasmic-reticulum-resident kinase, Nature 397 (6716) (1999) 271–274.

[114] U. Ozcan, Q. Cao, E. Yilmaz, A.H. Lee, N.N. Iwakoshi, E. Ozdelen, G. Tuncman, C. Gorgun, L.H. Glimcher, G.S. Hotamisligil, Endoplasmic reticulum stress links obesity, insulin action, and type 2 diabetes, Science 306 (5695) (2004) 457–461.

[115] Y. Nakatani, H. Kaneto, D. Kawamori, K. Yoshiuchi, M. Hatazaki, T.A. Matsuoka, K. Ozawa, S. Ogawa, M. Hori, Y. Yamasaki, M. Matsuhisa, Involvement of endoplasmic reticulum stress in insulin resistance and diabetes, J. Biol. Chem. 280 (1) (2005) 847–851.

[116] K. Ozaeua, M. Miyazaki, M. Matsuhisa, Y. Nakatani, M. Hatazaki, T. Tamatani, K. Yamagata, J. Miyagawa, Y. Kitao, O. Hori, Y. Yamasaki, S. Ozawa, The endoplasmic reticulum chaperone improves insulin resistance in type 2 diabetes, Diabetes 54 (3) (2005) 657–663.

[117] W.L. Smith, R.M. Garavito, D.L. DeWitt, Prostaglandin endoperoxide H synthases (cyclooxygenases)-1 and -2, J. Biol. Chem. 271 (52) (1996) 33157–33160.

[118] K. Shinmura, X.L. Tang, Y. Wang, Y.T. Xuan, S.Q. Liu, H. Takano, A. Bhatnagar, R. Bolli, Cyclooxygenase-2 mediates the cardioprotective effects of the late phase of ischemic preconditioning in conscious rabbits, Proc. Natl. Acad. Sci. USA 97 (18) (2000) 10197–10202.

[119] N.P. Dowd, M. Scully, S.R. Adderley, A.J. Cunningham, D.J. Fitzgerald, Inhibition of cyclooxygenase-2 aggravates doxorubicin-mediated cardiac injury *in vivo*, J. Clin. Invest. 108 (4) (2001) 585–590.

[120] K.A. Cieslik, Y. Zhu, M. Shtivelband, K.K. Wu, Inhibition of p90 ribosomal S6 kinase-mediated CCAAT/enhancer-binding protein beta activation and cyclooxygenase-2 expression by salicylate, J. Biol. Chem. 280 (18) (2005) 18411–18417.

[121] S.E. Shoelson, J. Lee, M. Yuan, Inflammation and the IKK/IB/NF-B axis in obesity- and diet-induced insulin resistance, Int. J. Obesity 27 (2003) S49–S52.

[122] R.S. Hundal, K.F. Petersen, A.B. Mayerson, P.S. Randhawa, S. Inzucchi, S.E. Shoelson, G.I. Shulman, Mechanism by which high-dose aspirin improves glucose metabolism in type 2 diabetes, J. Clin. Invest. 109 (10) (2002) 1321–1326.

[123] M.A. Saunders, L.S. Garcia, G.W. Gilroy, K.K. Wu, Selective suppression of CCAAT/enhancer-binding protein binding and cyclooxygenase-2 promoter activity by sodium salicylate in quiescent human fibroblasts, J. Biol. Chem. 276 (22) (2001) 18897–18904.

[124] Y. Takata, Y. Kitami, Z.H. Yang, M. Nakamura, T. Okura, K. Hiwada, Vascular inflammation is negatively autoregulated by interaction between CCAAT/enhancer-binding protein-delta and peroxisome proliferator-activated receptor-gamma, Circ. Res. 91 (5) (2002) 427–433.

[125] S. Moncada, R.M. Palmer, E.A. Higgs, Nitric oxide: physiology, pathophysiology, and pharmacology, Pharmacol. Rev. 43 (2) (1991) 109–142.

[126] J. MacMicking, Q.W. Xie, C. Nathan, Nitric oxide and macrophage function, Annu. Rev. Immunol. 15 (1997) 323–350.

[127] W.K. Alderton, C.E. Cooper, R.G. Knowles, Nitric oxide synthases: structure, function and inhibition, Biochem. J. 357 (Pt 3) (2001) 593–615.

[128] Y. Vodovotz, M.S. Lucia, K.C. Flanders, L. Chesler, Q.W. Xie, T.W. Smith, J. Weidner, R. Mumford, R. Webber, C. Nathan, A.B. Roberts, C.F. Lippa, M.B. Sporn, Inducible nitric oxide synthase in tangle-bearing neurons of patients with Alzheimer's disease, J. Exp. Med. 184 (4) (1996) 1425–1433.

[129] Q.W. Xie, Y. Kashiwabara, C. Nathan, Role of transcription factor NF-kappa B/Rel in induction of nitric oxide synthase, J. Biol. Chem. 269 (7) (1994) 4705–4708.

[130] A.K. Lee, S.H. Sung, Y.C. Kim, S.G. Kim, Inhibition of lipopolysaccharide-inducible nitric oxide synthase, TNF-alpha and COX-2 expression by sauchinone effects on I-kappaBalpha phosphorylation, C/EBP and AP-1 activation, Br. J. Pharmacol. 139 (1) (2003) 11–20.

[131] Y.H. Kim, K.J. Woo, J.H. Lim, S. Kim, T.J. Lee, E.M. Jung, J.M. Lee, J.M. Park, T.K. Kwon, 8-Hydroxyquinoline inhibits iNOS expression and nitric oxide production by down-regulating LPS-induced activity of NF-kappaB and C/EBPbeta in Raw 264.7 cells, Biochem. Biophys. Res. Commun. 329 (2) (2005) 591–597.

[132] D. Ron, Translational control in the endoplasmic reticulum stress response, J. Clin. Invest. 110 (10) (2002) 1383–1388.

[133] R.J. Kaufman, Orchestrating the unfolded protein response in health and disease, J. Clin. Invest. 110 (10) (2002) 1389–1398.

[134] C. Chen, E.E. Dudenhausen, Y.X. Pan, C. Zhong, M.S. Kilberg, Human CCAAT/enhancer-binding protein beta gene expression is activated by endoplasmic reticulum stress through an unfolded protein response element downstream of the protein coding sequence, J. Biol. Chem. 279 (27) (2004) 27948–27956.

[135] K.D. McCullough, J.L. Martindale, L.-O. Klotz, T.Y. Aw, N.J. Holbrook, Gadd153 Sensitizes Cells to Endoplasmic Reticulum Stress by Down-Regulating Bcl2 and Perturbing the Cellular Redox State, Mol. Cell. Biol. 21 (4) (2001) 1249–1259.

[136] T.W. Fawcett, H.B. Eastman, J.L. Martindale, N.J. Holbrook, Physical and functional association between GADD153 and CCAAT/Enhancer-binding protein during cellular stress, J. Biol. Chem. 271 (1996) 14285–14289.

[137] P. Angulo, Non-alcoholic fatty liver disease, N. Engl. J. Med. 346 (2002) 1221–1231.

[138] G. Pagano, G. Pacini, G. Musso, R. Gambino, F. Mecca, N. Depetris, M. Cassader, E. David, P. Cavallo-Perin, M. Rizzetto, Nonalcoholic steatohepatitis, insulin resistance, and metabolic syndrome: further evidence for an etiologic association, Hepatology 35 (2) (2002) 497–499.

[139] J. Choudhury, A.J. Sanyal, Insulin resistance in NASH, Front. Biosci. (10) (2005) 1520–1533.

[140] C.P. Day, O.F. James, Steatohepatitis: a tale of two "hits"?, Gastroenterology 114 (4) (1998) 842–845.

[141] A.E. Reid, Nonalcoholic steatohepatitis, Gastroenterology 121 (3) (2001) 710–723.

[142] D. Festi, A. Colecchia, T. Sacco, M. Bondi, E. Roda, G. Marchesini, Hepatic steatosis in obese patients: clinical aspects and prognostic significance, Obes. Rev. 5 (1) (2004) 27–42.

[143] L.S. Szczepaniak, P. Nurenberg, D. Leonard, J.D. Browning, J.S. Reingold, S. Grundy, H.H. Hobbs, R.L. Dobbins, Magnetic resonance spectroscopy to measure hepatic triglyceride content: prevalence of hepatic steatosis in the general population, Am. J. Physiol. Endocrinol. Metab. 288 (2) (2005) E462–E468.

[144] E. Ip, G.C. Farrell, G. Robertson, P. Hall, R. Kirsch, I. Leclercq, Central role of PPARalpha-dependent hepatic lipid turnover in dietary steatohepatitis in mice, Hepatology 38 (1) (2003) 14–17.

[145] R. Kirsch, V. Clarkson, E.G. Shephard, D.A. Marais, M.A. Jaffer, V.E. Woodburne, R.E. Kirsch, P.L. Hall, Rodent nutritional model of non-alcoholic steatohepatitis: species, strain and sex difference studies, J. Gastroenterol. Hepatol. 18 (11) (2003) 1272–1282.

[146] I.A. Leclercq, G.C. Farrell, J. Field, D.R. Bell, F.J. Gonzalez, G.R. Robertson, CYP2E1 and CYP4A as microsomal catalysts of lipid peroxides in murine nonalcoholic steatohepatitis, J. Clin. Invest. 105 (8) (2000) 1067–1075.

Chapter 14

Insulin resistance, inflammation, and the IKK/IκB/NF-κB pathway

Bankim A. Bhatt[1], Robert M. O'Doherty[1,2]

[1]*Department of Medicine, Division of Endocrinology/Metabolism, University of Pittsburgh, Pittsburgh, PA 15261, USA;*
[2]*Department of Molecular Genetics and Biochemistry, University of Pittsburgh, Pittsburgh, PA 15261, USA*

Overview

Insulin resistance is a characteristic of human obesity, and a primary risk factor for the development of type II diabetes (T2DM). However, despite tremendous effort and great progress in a number of areas of research, the biochemical mechanisms underlying the pathogenesis of insulin resistance in obesity remain poorly understood. In short, defects in insulin signaling, alterations in the expression and/or activity of a variety of adipokines and cytokines, dyslipidemia/dysregulated lipid metabolism, and most recently, increased intracellular stress and activation of inflammatory pathways have each been implicated as important contributory mechanisms in insulin resistance. In all likelihood it is the interplay of these factors, combined with genetic predisposition and environmental influences that results in the full metabolic manifestation of insulin resistance. This chapter accentuates a bias and recent progress in one area of research that implicates increased activity of the pro-inflammatory IKK/IκB/NF-κB (NF-κB) pathway in the pathogenesis of insulin resistance. The purpose of the chapter is to (i) review seminal studies addressing the potential role of increased activity of the NF-κB pathway in decreasing insulin action; (ii) discuss the potential relevance of these studies to human obesity; (iii) address putative mechanisms of activation of the NF-κB pathway in obesity and how activation of the NF-κB activity may reduce insulin action; and (iv) briefly discuss the potential of targeting activity of the NF-κB pathway in the treatment of insulin resistance. Because of the narrow focus of the subject matter in this chapter, the reader is referred to a number of other excellent studies that address the potential detrimental effects on insulin action of activity of other inflammatory pathways [1], endoplasmic reticulum (ER) stress [2], and mitochondrial dysfunction [3,4].

ADVANCES IN MOLECULAR AND CELLULAR ENDOCRINOLOGY
VOLUME 5 ISSN 1569-2566/DOI 10.1016/S1569-2566(06)05014-9

1. The obesity/T2DM epidemic

The prevalence of obesity and T2DM has reached epidemic proportions in Western societies, with concomitant increases in health-care costs. It has been estimated that ~30% of adults are obese in the USA, and more worryingly, childhood obesity is increasing rapidly [5,6]. Obesity is also recognized as the single greatest risk factor for the development of T2DM [5,6], and direct health-care costs associated with obesity are estimated to be > $100 billion/year in the USA alone [5,6]. Because of the health and cost consequences of obesity/T2DM, or the so-called diabesity, it is vital that the pathogenesis of the metabolic abnormalities of these conditions be understood if effective, rational treatments are to be developed.

2. Insulin resistance in obesity

Insulin resistance is a hallmark of obesity, and predisposes to the development of T2DM. However, the biochemical and molecular mechanisms that may mediate the detrimental effects of obesity on insulin action remain poorly understood. Defects in insulin signaling (increased serine phosphorylation of IRS-1, decreased responsiveness of PI3-kinase) have been identified in a number of insulin-resistant states, and they likely contribute to the principal metabolic manifestations of insulin resistance in obesity (decreased stimulation of glucose uptake and glycogen synthesis (skeletal muscle), impaired suppression of gluconeogenesis (liver), decreased suppression of lipolysis (adipose tissue), and fatty acid oxidation (skeletal muscle)). Indeed, elegant experiments using targeted mutagenesis and transgenic approaches in mice have emphasized the absolute requirement for components of the insulin-signaling pathway in mediating the metabolic actions of insulin [7].

One obvious candidate mechanism for the development of insulin resistance is the hyperlipidemia, dysregulated lipid metabolism, and increased adiposity associated with obesity. Supporting the hypothesis that dyslipidemia has direct or indirect roles in the pathogenesis of insulin resistance are observations that (i) acute hyperlipidemia induces insulin resistance [8–12]; (ii) plasma and tissue lipid levels are inversely correlated with insulin sensitivity [13,14]; and (iii) decreasing/increasing the metabolic availability of lipids *in vivo* increases/decreases insulin sensitivity [15–17]. Further insight comes from observations that changes in the expression or actions of factors such as leptin [18–22], adiponectin [23–27], resistin [28–32], IL-6 [33,34], TNFα [35–39], and PAI-1 [40], which are associated with increased adiposity have each been implicated in altering insulin sensitivity. Most recently, a body of opinion has begun to coalesce around the hypothesis that stress/inflammatory responses, involving activation of the innate immune system [41–43], increased activity of pro-inflammatory signaling pathways in peripheral tissues [1,43–48], ER stress [2], and possibly mitochondrion dysfunction [3,4] contribute to the decrease in insulin sensitivity observed in obesity. The current chapter will focus on one aspect of the inflammatory/stress response, namely activation of the pro-inflammatory IKK/IκB/ NF-κB pathway.

3. The IKK/IκB/NF-κB pathway

Cell responses to inflammatory and stress signals are mediated by a number of ubiquitously expressed signaling cascades. Of these, the NF-κB and mitogen-activated protein kinase (MAPK) pathways, specifically c-Jun N-terminal kinase (JNK) and p38 MAPK, are best described. Altered activity of each of these pathways has been implicated in changing insulin action. However, of central relevance to this chapter are a number of studies demonstrating a role for elevated activity of the IKK/IκB/NF-κB pathway [49–51] in the pathogenesis of insulin resistance [43–48,52,53]. NF-κBs (nuclear factor kappa B) are a family of structurally similar transcription factors (NF-κB1 (p50), p65/RelA, c-Rel, RelB, and NF-κB2 (p52)) containing Rel homology, DNA binding, nuclear localization, and dimerization domains. Described first by Sen and Baltimore [54,55] as a transcription factor that bound to an enhancer element in the gene for the Igκ light chain, and believed to be B cell-specific, NF-κB is now known to be expressed ubiquitously. NF-κBs function as homo- or heterodimers, which are activated in response to a variety of stimuli, notably stress and inflammatory signals. Indeed, the NF-κB pathway is considered to be one of the central pathways mediating the inflammatory response [51]. NF-κB regulates the expression of numerous pro-inflammatory, immunomodulatory, and anti-apoptotic genes, functioning predominantly as the p65/p50 heterodimer [49–51]. In the inactive state, NF-κBs are normally confined to the cytoplasm (Fig. 1), and are bound to one of the family inhibitory proteins, termed inhibitors of κb (IκB). There are seven mammalian IκBs (IκBα, IκBβ, IκBε, IκBγ, Bcl-3, and the precursor Rel

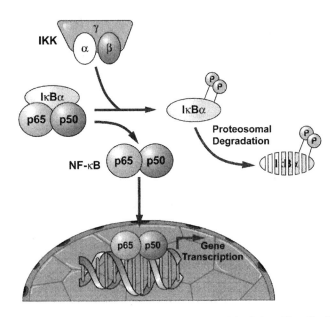

Fig. 1. The IKK/IκB /NF-κB pathway. See Plate 13 in Colour Plate Section.

proteins p100 and p105). Of these, the function and regulation of IκBα and IκBβ are best understood. Activation of NF-κB occurs when IκB is serine-phosphorylated, an event that releases the NF-κB dimer and targets IκB for ubquitination and proteosomal degradation. Serine phosphorylation of IκB is catalyzed by the IκB kinase (IKK), a protein complex comprised of two catalytic subunits, IKKα and IKKβ, and a regulatory subunit IKKγ, also known as NEMO (NF-κB essential modulator). Data indicate that activation of IKKβ, rather then IKKα, participates in the primary pathway by which pro-inflammatory stimuli induce NF-κB function [51]. The release of the NF-κB dimer from IκB allows NF-κB to translocate to the nucleus and activate gene transcription by binding to a consensus DNA sequence in the promoter region of target genes, including cytokine, chemokine, and cell adhesion molecule genes, which are involved in the inflammatory cascade. As one might expect of such an important signaling pathway, the regulation of the activity of NF-κB pathway is highly complex, and the brief overview given here only touches on this complexity. The reader is directed to a number of excellent reviews that address in greater detail the regulation and details of NF-κB action [49–51].

4. Making the connection: The IKK/IκB/NF-κB pathway and insulin resistance

A potential role for altered activity of the NF-κB pathway in the determination of insulin action was not suspected prior to the 2001 study of Yuan et al. [44]. The intellectual foundations of this study were built on two salient, but initially unconnected, observations. The first was studies dating back to the early 20th century demonstrating the capacity of high doses of aspirin (salicylates) to lower blood glucose levels in diabetics [56,57]. These observations, interesting in themselves, came into sharper focus when a 1998 study identified salicylates as inhibitors of IKKβ activity [58], raising the possibility that the effects of salicylates on blood glucose levels and IKK activity were connected. This hypothesis was addressed in the subsequent study of Yuan et al. [44], which demonstrated that suppressing activity of IKK improves insulin action in insulin-resistant states in cell culture and rodent models. The authors first studied the effects of aspirin on insulin sensitivity in two genetic models of obesity-induced diabetes, the *fa/fa* rats and *ob/ob* mouse. A continuous 3–4-week aspirin infusion improved insulin sensitivity as measured by glucose and insulin tolerance tests compared to controls in both models. These metabolic improvements were accompanied by increased responsiveness of skeletal muscle and liver insulin receptor, and AKT to insulin-stimulated tyrosine phosphorylation in the *fa/fa* rat. In follow-up studies, the authors investigated *in vivo* the effects of a whole-body heterozygous deficiency of IKKβ (IKK$^{+/-}$) on readouts of insulin action in response to aging and obesity. Age- and obesity-related increases in plasma insulin concentration were reduced in IKK$^{+/-}$ mice, while *ob/ob* mice crossed onto an IKK$^{+/-}$ background, and IKK$^{+/-}$ mice on a high-fat diet displayed improved glucose tolerance compared to controls. Taken together with confirmatory *in vitro* data the authors concluded that reduced IKKβ activity improves insulin sensitivity in obesity.

5. Tissue specificity: Insights from targeted manipulations of the IKK/IκB/NF-κB pathway *in vivo*

Although informative, the Yuan study design (salicylates and whole-body hetero-zygous knockout of IKK*β*) gave no insight into the specific tissues that may play a role in conferring beneficial effects of salicylate and decreased activity of IKK*β* on insulin action in obesity. This issue has been addressed in a number of recent studies that have examined the effects of manipulation of activity of the NF-κB pathway in liver, skeletal muscle, or monocytes.

5.1. *Liver*

Two studies [43,48] have addressed the effects of liver-specific manipulation of IKK*β* activity on hepatic and whole-body insulin action. In the first study [43], a liver-specific deletion of IKK*β* in mice decreased hepatic insulin resistance induced by a high-fat diet, obesity (*ob/ob* genetic background), or aging. However, systemic insulin resist-ance, i.e., skeletal muscle and adipose tissue insulin resistance, developed to the same extent as controls, suggesting that liver-specific decreases in activity of the NF-κB pathway are not sufficient to protect against the development of whole-body insulin resistance. Improvements in hepatic insulin responsiveness in IKK*β*-deficient mice presented as an increased capacity of insulin to suppress gluconeogenesis and activate PI3-kinase and Akt, and decreased gluconeogenic (PEPCK and G6Pase) gene ex-pression. In the second study [48], an opposing strategy of liver-specific transgenic overexpression of IKK*β* was used (LIKK). This intervention increased IKK*β* activity by ~two-fold, similar to that observed in the liver of obese animals, and was sufficient to induce not only hepatic insulin resistance, but also systemic (skeletal muscle) insulin resistance. Thus, insulin was unable to suppress hepatic glucose production, hepatic glycogen synthesis was decreased, as was insulin-stimulated activation of PI3-kinase and Akt, expression of PEPCK and G6Pase was elevated, and skeletal muscle glucose uptake and glycogen synthesis were decreased. In follow-up studies, the authors demonstrated a reversal of insulin resistance in LIKK mice upon treatment with salicylates or by crossing LIKK mice with mice expressing an IκBα super-repressor (an IκBα mutant lacking the serine 32 and 36 phosphorylation sites), an intervention that would be expected to decrease the activity of NF-κB. Taken together, these studies demonstrate that manipulation of IKK*β* activity, specifically in liver, alters hepatic insulin action, and suggests that increased hepatic IKK activity can induce systemic insulin resistance. However, the demonstration that deletion of liver IKK*β* cannot protect against the development of systemic insulin resistance in *ob/ob* mice or mice on a high-fat diet suggests caution when considering a role for the liver NF-κB pathway in mediating whole-body insulin resistance induced by obesity.

5.2. *Skeletal muscle*

Skeletal muscle is the largest insulin sensitive tissue by mass in the body, and is insulin resistant in obesity and T2DM. As such it is an obvious candidate for manipulation of activity of the NF-κB pathway to determine effects on insulin action. Two studies have directly manipulated NF-κB pathway activity in skeletal muscle while leaving activity of the pathway intact in other tissues [59,60]. Similar to the complete knockout of IKKβ in liver, Rohl et al. [60] generated a mouse with a targeted knockout of skeletal muscle IKKβ. These mice, together with wild-type controls, were subjected to an injection of gold thioglucose (GTG), an intervention that induces hyperphagia and obesity or were placed on a high-fat diet (diet-induced obesity). Glucose tolerance tests were then performed. Glucose tolerances were similar in wild type and skeletal muscle IKKβ-deficient GTG-treated mice. Furthermore, tyrosine phosphorylation of the skeletal muscle insulin receptor in response to an insulin bolus was decreased in obese (GTG-treated) wild type and IKKβ-deficient animals to a similar extent compared to lean (non-GTG treated) controls. Glucose tolerance was also similar in high-fat-fed wild type compared to high-fat-fed skeletal muscle IKKβ-deficient mice. The authors conclude that knockout of skeletal muscle IKKβ does not alter whole-body insulin sensitivity in GTG-treated or high-fat-fed mice. However, having generated these mice, it is unfortunate that a more in-depth metabolic and biochemical analysis was not undertaken. Glucose tolerance tests are not strictly a method for the assessment of insulin sensitivity, due to the potentially confounding issues of insulin secretion and hepatic glucose output. The authors state that insulin tolerance tests indicated similar insulin sensitivity of GTG-treated wild-type and GTG-treated skeletal muscle IKKβ knockout animals, but do not report the data, and insulin tolerance tests were not performed on high-fat-fed animals. Furthermore, since the authors also report that the whole-body heterozygous deletion of IKKβ did not protect against the effects of obesity on insulin action, an opposite finding to that reported by Yuan et al. [44], the potential role of the skeletal muscle NF-κB pathway in the development of insulin resistance in obesity remained unresolved by this study. Similar to their study in liver, a second study from the Shoelson group [59] addressed the physiological effects of transgenic overexpression of IKKβ (MIKK) or the IκBα super-repressor (MISR) in mouse skeletal muscle. The central conclusion from the MIKK intervention was that activation of the skeletal muscle NF-κB pathway causes severe muscle wasting (~50% reduction in muscle mass compared to wild-type controls), and body weight at 20 weeks of age is decreased by ~30% compared to wild-type controls. However, the authors also report that increased skeletal muscle IKKβ activity does not decrease skeletal muscle insulin sensitivity and that the expression of the IκBα super-repressor is not sufficient to protect against the detrimental effects of a high-fat diet on skeletal muscle insulin sensitivity. Three caveats should be appended to these conclusions. First, direct *in vivo* measurements of insulin sensitivity were not made. Rather, fasting insulin and glucose concentrations and glucose tolerance tests were used to estimate insulin sensitivity in both MISR and MIKK mice. Second, differences in body weight may be a confounding factor. Third, in MIKK mice *ex vivo* glucose uptake in isolated EDL muscles was also measured and was reported as not different from wild-type controls. However, since the EDL muscle from a wild-type mouse weighs ~2 × that of an EDL muscle from a MIKK mouse, it is unclear if (or how) insulin action is comparable in these two muscles. Regardless of these issues, it can be stated that both this study and that of Rohl et al. [60] support the view that activation of the NF-κB pathway in skeletal muscle may not be required for the development of insulin resistance in obesity. However, this raises a further issue of explaining data from studies [47,53,61,62] that have implicated activation of the muscle NF-κB pathway as a mechanism of lipid-induced insulin resistance [8–12] in skeletal muscle. Of particular note, IKKβ-deficient mice and salicylate-infused mice are resistant to the detrimental effects of acute (5 h) hyperlipidemia on skeletal muscle insulin action [47], suggesting that activation of the NF-κB pathway in skeletal muscle can induce insulin resistance.

5.3. *Myeloid cells*

Notwithstanding the importance and novelty of the foregoing data, perhaps the most intriguing study is that of Arkan et al. [43], which addressed the effects of a myeloid cell-specific deletion of IKKβ on insulin action. The importance of the Arkan study is that it is the first to establish a mechanistic bridge between NF-κB activity in an integral element of the innate immune system (myeloid cells) and whole-body insulin sensitivity. Deletion of the IKKβ gene from myeloid cells resulted in an absence of IKKβ in macrophages and neutrophils [63]. Whole-body insulin sensitivity in these animals, as measured by insulin suppression of hepatic glucose production and stimulation of glucose disposal under euglycemic conditions, was greater on a high-fat diet compared to control animals on a similar diet. Thus, the authors conclude that activation of the NF-κB pathway in a myeloid lineage contributes to the development of insulin resistance in diet-induced obesity. This study is not the first to implicate activation of the innate immune system, and specifically macrophages, as a contributing mechanism to the development of insulin resistance. Indeed, the Arkan study builds on previous seminal observations that have established that obese and insulin-resistant states are associated with macrophage infiltration of adipose tissue [41,42]. Thus, two studies have independently demonstrated increased expression of macrophage markers and elevated numbers of macrophages in the adipose tissue of a number of mouse obesity models (diet-induced, *ob/ob*, *agouti*, *db/db*, *tubby*) compared to lean controls [41,42]. These increases are also evident in adipose tissue from obese humans, displaying a positive correlation with BMI [42]. Interestingly, in diet-induced obesity, the extent of macrophage infiltration is dependent on the length of diet and precedes a substantial increase in plasma insulin concentration [41], possibly indicating a mechanistic relationship between infiltration and insulin resistance, although this hypothesis was not addressed directly. Furthermore, Weisberg et al. [42] demonstrate that adipose tissue macrophages are bone marrow-derived, and are absent in the adipose tissue of macrophage-deficient *Csf1$^{op/op}$* mice, suggesting a stimulated activation and recruitment of macrophages into adipose tissue as obesity develops. Finally, the insulin-sensitizer rosiglitazone, which is proposed to have substantial effects on adipose tissue, decreases the expression of putative macrophage markers in adipose tissue of *ob/ob* mice [41].

5.4. *Adipose tissue, β cells, and the central nervous system*

Adipose tissue, the β-cell of the islet of Langerhans, and as has been described recently, the central nervous system, each play important roles in the regulation of whole-body glucose homeostasis and insulin action. However, there are no published *in vivo* studies addressing the metabolic effects of tissue-specific manipulation of activity of the NF-κB pathway in these tissues. A preliminary report [64] from the Shoelson group suggests that inhibition of activation of adipose tissue NK-κB protects against the development of diet-induced insulin resistance. Also, a recent study [65] demonstrates the activation of the NF-κB pathway and a pro-inflammatory response in the CNS of rats fed a high-fat diet. Thus, further investigation of the contributions of NF-κB in these tissues to the metabolic abnormalities of obesity is warranted.

6. Of mice and men: Relevance of rodent studies to human obesity/T2DM

The studies discussed above categorically implicate activation of the NF-κB pathway in the pathogenesis of insulin resistance in genetic and environmental models of obesity in mice. However, can data from these studies be applied to our understanding of the pathogenesis of insulin resistance in human obesity and/or T2DM? Obesity and T2DM are complex polygenic diseases, whose development is strongly influenced by the environment. Furthermore, the endocrine/metabolic derangements of these diseases are numerous, with insulin resistance being just one, albeit vitally important, defect. For both of these reasons, it is unlikely that any single mechanism will explain the pathogenesis of insulin resistance in obesity or T2DM. Rather, it is more likely that a combination of metabolic, biochemical, and genetic defects will contribute to the full manifestation of insulin resistance. To some extent this point is brought home by studies that have genetically manipulated activity of the NF-κB pathway. In studies where animals are protected against the development of obesity-induced insulin resistance, the protection is not complete, i.e., insulin sensitivity is not returned to that observed in lean animals. With these caveats in mind, what is it possible to say regarding the potential contribution of elevated activity of the NF-κB pathway to decreased insulin sensitivity in humans? First, a series of reports have demonstrated increased levels of inflammatory markers in obesity, and an association between elevated inflammatory status, insulin resistance and increased risk for the development of T2DM [66–77]. Second, the nature of the inflammatory response observed in human obesity implies a role for NF-κB in its manifestation, since expression of many of the acute phase reactants and cytokines that have been reported to be elevated in human obesity are regulated by NF-κB, and the NF-κB pathway plays a vital role in macrophage activation and recruitment [49,51,78]. Third, there is evidence to suggest that altering the activity of the NF-κB pathway in human effects insulin sensitivity. Thus, classic studies [56,57] addressing the beneficial effects of high-dose aspirin on blood glucose levels in diabetics suggest that inhibition of IKK improves glycemic control, but these studies did not directly assess aspirin effects on insulin sensitivity. More recently, Hundal et al. [46] addressed the effects of a 2-week regime of high-dose aspirin ($\sim$7 g per day) on insulin sensitivity in T2DM. The data demonstrate that aspirin reduces fasting glucose, triglycerides, C-reactive protein (an acute phase reactant) concentrations, and the basal rate of hepatic glucose production ($\sim$20%), and improves ($\sim$20%) insulin-stimulated peripheral glucose uptake. The authors conclude that these data support the hypothesis that inhibition of IKK improves insulin sensitivity in T2DM. Finally, it has been shown that one effect of thiazolidinediones (TZDs), a class of insulin-sensitizers, is to inhibit NF-κB activity [79], an indirect action mediated through TZD effects on peroxisome proliferator-activated receptor-gamma (PPARγ). It has also become apparent that TZDs have anti-inflammatory effects [80], with direct actions of these drugs on macrophages being one mechanism of action. While none of these examples are conclusive in and of themselves, and effects on insulin action described for salicylates and TZDs may be explained by actions that do not involve inhibition of the NF-κB pathway, the hypothesis that activation of the NF-κB pathway contributes to the development of insulin resistance in human obesity/T2DM deserves extensive consideration and testing.

7. Putative mechanisms of insulin resistance arising from activation of the IKK/IκB/ NF-κB pathway

Since activation of the NF-κB pathway induces insulin resistance, and inhibition of the pathway offers protection against the development of insulin resistance, the issue of how the NF-κB pathway contributes to impairments in insulin action arises. Given the relative infancy of this field, the putative mechanisms discussed below are at best informed insights based on a small population of studies. There are currently, in our view, no definitive insights into this issue, and as such the time for establishing paradigms is not yet upon us. Figure 2 illustrates the mechanisms that are discussed below.

7.1. *IKK and IRS serine phosphorylation*

Studies have demonstrated increased serine phosphorylation of IRS-1 in insulin-resistant states [8,81–83]. This phosphorylation event is commonly regarded as being inhibitory for insulin signaling (decreased tyrosine phosphorylation of IRS and decreased PI3-kinase activity) and the metabolic actions of insulin. In particular, the Shulman group has demonstrated a correlation between skeletal muscle insulin resistance induced by acute ($\sim$5 h) hyperlipidemia, and decreased tyrosine phosphorylation and increased serine phosphorylation of IRS-1 [8,84–86]. In more recent studies, this group [47] demonstrated in mice that salicylates prevent the detrimental effects of hyperlipidemia on skeletal muscle insulin-stimulated glucose disposal and insulin signaling. Furthermore, heterozygous-deficient IKKβ mice were protected against the effects of lipids on skeletal muscle insulin action. Clearly then, lipid-induced insulin resistance in skeletal muscle appears to require the activation of

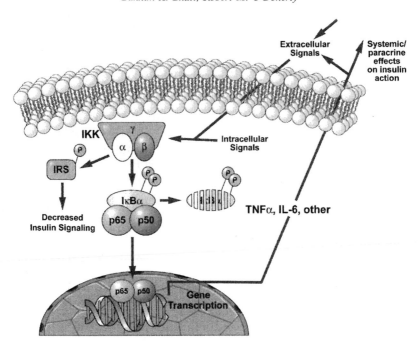

Fig. 2. Potential mechanisms of insulin resistance arising from activation of the NF-κB pathway. See Plate 14 in Colour Plate Section.

IKK, a conclusion supported by recent studies that directly demonstrate the activation of the NF-κB pathway in rodent [61,62] and human skeletal muscle [53] by acute hyperlipidemia, and demonstrate the protective effects of NF-κB inhibitors on fatty acid-induced insulin resistance in isolated myotubes [62]. Given that IKKβ is a serine kinase, one hypothesis arising from these data is that the inhibitory serine phosphorylation of IRS-1 may be mediated directly by IKKβ. Evidence in support of this hypothesis comes from a variety of sources. Thus, in adipocytes, the fatty acid linoleic acid induces insulin resistance, as measured by impaired insulin-stimulated glucose uptake [87], and the reduction in glucose uptake is associated with increased serine 307 phosphorylation and subsequent degradation of IRS-1. The authors demonstrate that this phosphorylation reaction is catalyzed by IKK and JNK, and that the effects of linoleic acid are prevented by inhibitors of IKK and JNK. Similar to 3T3-L1 adipocytes, palmitate-induced decreases in insulin-stimulated IRS-1 tyrosine phosphorylation are prevented by salicylates in L6 myotubes [62]. Furthermore, an inhibitor of NF-κB activation, but not IKK, is unable to prevent the effects of palmitate, lending further weight to the hypothesis that IKK activation, but not NF-κB activation, is required for free fatty acid-induced detriments in insulin signaling. Of interest, both IKK (salicylates and parthenolide) and NF-κB inhibitors (NF-κB SN50) prevent palmitate-induced decreases in insulin stimulation of glucose uptake, demonstrating a divergence of the effects of free fatty acids (FFA) on insulin signaling and metabolism. In neonatal rat myotubes, TNFα increases IKK activity, decreases insulin-stimulated glucose uptake, promotes serine 307 phosphorylation of

IRS-1, and impairs insulin stimulation of insulin receptor, and IRS-1 and IRS-2 tyrosine phosphorylation [88]. Salicylate completely restores insulin signaling, as do the p38 MAPK inhibitors PD169316 or SB203580, but not the JNK inhibitor SP600125. Since in this study the activation of IKKβ by TNFα is dependent on p38 MAPK, the authors conclude that TNFα, through activation of p38 MAPK and IKK, produces insulin resistance through serine phosphorylation of IRS-1. Generally, similar observations have been made of TNFα effects on 3T3-L1 adipocytes and HepG2 s, a hepatocyte cell line [89]. Thus, in both cell types, TNFα promotes serine phosphorylation of IRS-1, and in an informative experiment, this study also demonstrates that the effects of TNFα are reduced in embryo fibroblasts derived from IKK knockout animals. Salicylate treatment again prevents IRS-1 serine phosphorylation and restores insulin-stimulated glucose uptake in 3T3-L1 cells exposed to TNFα. Gao et al. present two lines of evidence that IRS-1 can function as a direct substrate for IKK activity [90]. First, using co-immunoprecipitation assays, interactions between endogenous IRS-1 and IKKβ in HepG2 cells are demonstrated. Second, *in vitro* kinase assays were used to demonstrate that recombinant IRS-1 is serine-phosphorylated by recombinant IKKβ. In summary, there is strong evidence from *in vitro* studies in adipocyte, skeletal muscle, and liver models demonstrating that activation of IKK by lipids or TNFα leads to increased serine 307 phosphorylation of IRS-1, an event that would be expected to and does decrease insulin activation (tyrosine phosphorylation) of IRS-1 and insulin-stimulated glucose uptake. In addition, inhibition of IKK activity reduces IRS-1 serine phosphorylation and restores insulin sensitivity (tyrosine phosphorylation and glucose uptake). *In vivo* evidence of IKK-mediated serine phosphorylation of IRS-1 remains correlative, extending only as far as the observation that lipid-induced skeletal muscle insulin resistance are prevented by salicylates or a deficiency of IKKβ. Evidence that IRS-1 is a direct substrate for IKKβ activity is sparse. One *in vitro* study demonstrates that IKK directly serine phosphorylates IRS-1, but it remains unknown if IRS-1 is a physiological (*in vivo*) substrate for IKKβ activity. Lastly, it should be noted that there remains no definitive demonstration that the IKKβ-mediated serine phosphorylation of IRS proteins is a mechanism of insulin resistance in rodent or human obesity.

7.2. *NF-κB responsive genes*

A primary function of NF-κB is to regulate the expression of genes required for mounting an appropriate physiological response to an inflammatory/stress stimulus, leading to the obvious implication that products of NF-κB responsive genes are involved in the pathogenesis of insulin resistance and the elevated inflammatory status in obesity. A challenge that is faced when addressing this hypothesis is the sheer number of genes that are regulated by NF-κB, numbering upwards of 200, and ranging through genes expressing cytokines/chemokines, immunoreceptors, antigen presentation proteins, acute phase proteins, stress response genes, cell-surface receptors, regulators of apoptosis, growth factors, transcription factors, and enzymes [78]. Notwithstanding this complexity, there are a number of NF-κB target genes that are implicated directly in the pathogenesis of insulin resistance. The cytokines IL-6 and TNFα and the acute-phase reactant PAI-1 are elevated in obesity, their expression are regulated by NF-κB [78,91–98], and each has been implicated in the pathogenesis of insulin resistance. Thus, chronic elevation of IL-6 induces insulin resistance in rodents [33], TNFα exposure induces insulin resistance in a number of models [35,39], while PAI-1 [40] and TNFα [37] deficient mice are protected against the development of obesity-related insulin resistance. However, given that other transcription factors are also involved in the regulation of expression of these factors, more direct evidence for a role of activation of NF-κB in the pathogenesis of insulin resistance is required. As discussed above, mice with a liver-specific increase in IKKβ activity (LIKK) display hepatic and systemic insulin resistance [48]. Furthermore, these mice also have increased expression of a number of NF-κB responsive genes, including IL-6 and TNFα. To demonstrate a direct role of NF-κB in this phenotype, Cai et al. [48] performed three experiments. First, the elevated systemic IL-6 protein concentrations in LIKK mice was neutralized by injection of αIL-6 antibodies, an intervention that normalized the "insulin resistance index" during a glucose tolerance test (glucose concentration × insulin concentration). Second, LIKK mice were crossed to mice (LISR) with a liver-specific expression of a dominant inhibitory IκBα super-repressor, leading to an improvement in the insulin resistance index. Finally, LISR mice were subjected to an obesity-inducing high-fat diet. Compared to control mice on a high-fat diet, the LISR mice had an improved insulin resistance index. Taken together, these data strongly suggest a role for NF-κB activation in the development of insulin resistance that is independent of IKK activity. *In vitro* studies are supportive of this general conclusion. Thus, a 6-h exposure of rat L6 myotubes to the saturated fatty acid palmitate reduces insulin-stimulated glucose uptake, phosphatidylinositol-3-kinase (PI3-kinase) activity, and PKB phosphorylation, and stimulates IκBα degradation and the nuclear translocation of NF-κB [62]. The IKK inhibitors acetylsalicylate and parthenolide prevent palmitate-induced reductions in insulin-stimulated glucose uptake and NF-κB nuclear translocation. Most importantly, NF-κB SN50, a cell-permeable peptide that inhibits NF-κB nuclear translocation downstream of IKK is sufficient to prevent NF-κB activation and palmitate-induced reductions in insulin-stimulated glucose uptake. Similar to L6 cells, exposure of C2C12 myotubes, a mouse skeletal muscle cell line, to palmitate increases NF-κB activity, IL-6 mRNA expression, and IL-6 protein secretion, and reduces insulin-stimulated glucose uptake [96]. Elevated IL-6 expression and secretion in the presence of palmitate are prevented by the NF-κB inhibitor pyrrolidine dithiocarbamate, while an anti-IL-6 antibody prevents reductions in insulin-stimulated glucose uptake induced by palmitate. In a mixed human adipocyte/stromovascular tissue explant, *trans*-10, *cis*-12 conjugated linoleic acid (CLA) increases IL-6 and TNFα expression, and induces insulin resistance as measured by decreased GLUT-4 expression/translocation and insulin stimulation of glucose uptake [97]. The effects of CLA are prevented by inhibition of NF-κB activation or depletion of p65 NF-κB expression by RNA interference.

7.3. *Monocyte activation and recruitment*

As discussed above, Arkan et al. [43] demonstrate that a conditional knockout of IKKβ in monocytes protects against diet-induced insulin resistance and infiltration of macrophages into adipose tissue. Taken together with the studies of Xu et al. [41] and Weisberg et al. [42], which demonstrate adipose tissue macrophage activation and infiltration in mouse and human obesity, these data suggest a third, although not completely separate mechanism from those discussed above, by which activation of the NF-κB pathway may contribute to the development of insulin resistance in obesity. Thus, NF-κB-dependent macrophage activation and infiltration of peripheral tissues may in and of itself have effects on insulin action by as yet unidentified mechanisms. Alternatively, infiltrated macrophages may increase expression of NF-κB-dependent proteins, such as cytokines, that act locally on the adipocyte to induce insulin resistance and/or activate inflammatory pathways. In this respect, the observations that the source of increased expression of TNFα in adipose tissue in obesity appears to be from macrophages is suggestive [42].

8. Potential mechanisms of activation of the IKK/IκB/NF-κB pathway in obesity

A vitally important issue is the identification of potential mediators of activation of the NF-κB pathway, in particular, and the inflammatory response, in general, in obesity and insulin-resistant states. There is no overarching reason to expect *a priori* that obesity would be associated with a chronic, sub-acute inflammatory state, and by extension, activation of the NF-κB pathway. That it has taken the studies demonstrating a mechanistic relationship between inflammation and insulin resistance to generate the recent surge in interest in this area is perhaps indicative of this. What then may be driving the activation of the NF-κB pathway in insulin-resistant states such as obesity? As the excellent review of Pahl [78] documents there are more than 200 described activators of the NF-κB pathway, including classes of bacteria and bacterial products, viruses and viral products, cytokines, physiological, physical, and oxidative stress, environmental hazards, chemical agents, drugs, modified proteins, apoptotic mediators, mitogens, growth factors, hormones, and metabolites. The challenge is to identify possible candidate mechanisms from this group, while also acknowledging that there may be other as yet unidentified mechanisms that may contribute to activation of the NF-κB pathway in insulin-resistant states. One approach to identify the most likely candidates would be to concentrate on those mechanisms that have in common the capacity to activate the NF-κB pathway and a putative role in the pathogenesis of insulin resistance. Figure 3 illustrates the mechanisms discussed below.

8.1. *Cytokines*

As discussed above, obesity is associated with increased levels of cytokines, particularly IL-6 and TNFα, which have been implicated in the pathogenesis of insulin

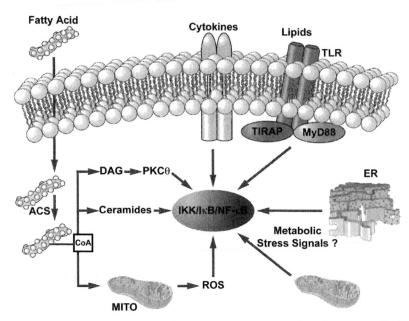

Fig. 3. Potential mechanisms of activation of the NF-κB pathway in insulin-resistant states. See Plate 15 in Colour Plate Section.

resistance and are well-described activators of the NF-κB pathway [78]. As such, they are a strong candidate mechanism for the activation of the NF-κB pathway in insulin-resistant states.

8.2. Lipids

Dyslipidemia is the most common metabolic abnormality associated with obesity, incorporating elevated circulating FFA and triglycerides, an atherogenic lipoprotein profile, accumulation of lipids in peripheral tissues, and altered intracellular lipid metabolism. Lipids and lipid metabolites (notably saturated fatty acids, oxidized lipids, diacylglycerol and ceramide) have been implicated in the activation of the NF-κB pathway [47,62,99–102] and, as discussed previously, there is a growing body of evidence that dyslipidemia plays an important role in the pathogenesis of insulin resistance. In this regard, the capacity of salicylates to protect against the skeletal muscle insulin resistance induced by acute hyperlipidemia, and the failure of acute hyperlipidemia to induce insulin resistance in heterozygous IKKβ knockout mice [47], suggests that lipid activation of the NF-κB pathway plays a role in the development of insulin resistance in this model. Indeed, lipid infusions activates the NF-κB pathway in human [53] and rodent [61] skeletal muscle and in human mononuclear cells [103]. Lipid-induced activation of the NF-κB pathway has also been demonstrated in a number of other cell types, including macrophages [101,102], hepatic Kupffer cells [104], and adipose tissue [97]. Of particular interest are observations in macrophages [101,102], and skeletal muscle [105] that saturated fatty acid-induced activation of the NF-κB pathway is mediated by toll-like receptor-4 (TLR-4), the lipopolysaccaride (LPS) receptor [106]. This observation suggests a link between dyslipidemia and activation of elements of the innate immune system.

8.3. *Other metabolic stress situations: Oxidative stress, ER stress, and mitochondrial dysfunction*

Reactive oxygen species (ROS) are potent activators of the NF-κB pathway [107–109], and increased levels of ROS can result from elevated fatty acid and glucose oxidation [110–112], and potentially impairments of mitochondrial oxidative metabolism. The mechanisms by which ROS activates the NF-κB pathway include modulating transport of NF-κB from the cytoplasm to the nucleus and modulation of IKK activity and other kinases upstream of IKK. ER stress has recently been demonstrated to contribute to the development of insulin resistance in obesity, possibly through the activation of JNK and subsequent serine phosphorylation of IRS-1 [2]. However, ER stress can also result in the activation of the NF-κB pathway [113,114], raising the possibility that obesity induces activation of the NF-κB pathway via ER stress signals. However, this hypothesis is yet to be tested.

In summary, there is ample evidence that a number of mediators (cytokines, lipids and lipid metabolites, ROS, ER stress) that are altered in obesity and implicated in the pathogenesis of insulin resistance can activate the NF-κB pathway. However, it remains to be determined which, if any, of these mechanisms may be important in the activation of this pathway in obesity.

9. Therapeutics

Given the recent upsurge of interest in the potential role of activity of the NF-κB pathway in the pathogenesis of insulin resistance, a brief discussion on potential drug intervention is warranted. As discussed above, aspirin/salicylate improves glycemic control and insulin action in T2DM, most likely by inhibiting IKK activity. In 1901, Williamson reported that sodium salicylate decreases glycosuria in patients with diabetes [56]. Fifty years later, Reid et al. [57] showed that treatment with aspirin leads to a near normal glucose tolerance in a patient with diabetes. Upon further study, they found that aspirin therapy leads to improvement of fasting blood sugar, decreased glycosuria and ketonuria in seven patients with diabetes. Finally, Hundal et al. recently demonstrated improvements in insulin sensitivity in T2DM after a 2-week regime of salicylate [46]. However, a major drawback of aspirin is the effective dose (4–7 g of aspirin per day), which has significant unwanted adverse effects including peptic and duodenal ulcers, gastrointestinal bleeding, and renal failure. Thus, interest has been generated in chemical compounds that may have the same therapeutic value as salicylates, but without the same side effects. In this context salsalate, a dimer of salicylic acid that is hydrolyzed in the small intestine prior to and after systemic absorption, has been used in doses as high as 3 g per day in the treatment of rheumatoid arthritis and osteoarthritis. This dose is well tolerated and has significantly less toxicity compared to salicylic acid, possibly because it has minimal effects on the production of prostaglandins, which are necessary for protecting the mucosal lining of the stomach from gastric acid. The most common side effects include rash, abdominal pain, edema, and tinnitus. Salsalate is currently being evaluated for use in the treatment of insulin-resistant states.

TZDs are currently used in the treatment of diabetes as insulin sensitizers. However, it has recently become clear that TZDs also have anti-inflammatory effects [80]. Although the mechanism of action is not completely understood, there is substantial evidence that activation of the nuclear PPARγ is important for TZD's effects. Activation of these receptors alters gene transcription by (i) transactivation, a DNA-dependent process that involves binding to the PPAR-response element of target genes and (ii) transrepression, a process that interferes with function of other transcription factors in a DNA independent manner. It has been demonstrated that one anti-inflammatory activity of PPARγ involves transrepression of expression of NF-κB responsive genes such as iNOS [79]. Furthermore, in rodent models, rosiglitazone decreases the expression of NF-κB responsive inflammatory genes in macrophages and adipose tissue of *db/db*, *ob/ob* or diet-induced obese animals [41]. In obese non-diabetic or obese diabetic individuals, TZD (troglitazone or rosiglitazone) treatment decreases the plasma levels of C-reactive protein, plasminogen activator inhibitor-1, TNFα, and MCP-1, increases mononuclear IκB levels, decreases activation of mononuclear NF-κB, and decreases generation of ROS in mononuclear cells [115–117]. Taken together, these data suggest that one mechanism of action of TZDs is to dampen NF-κB activity. However, it is not clear if these effects are required for the insulin-sensitizing effects of TZDs. The side effects of these drugs are minimal and include edema, weight gain, headache, myalgia, and anemia.

An alternative strategy to decreasing activity of the NF-κB pathway would be to target products of NF-κB-regulated genes that are implicated in the development of insulin resistance. In this context, it has been proposed that inactivation of TNFα by sequestering the cytokine with an α-TNFα antibody may improve insulin sensitivity in obesity. In obese insulin-resistant humans, a single administration of α-TNFα antibody did not improve insulin-mediated glucose disposal compared to placebo. A weakness of the study design was that only one injection of the antibody was given and the measurement of insulin sensitivity was done 48 h after the injection [118]. However, a separate study in diabetic humans showed similar results [119]. A more recent study suggests long-term use of TNFα antibodies may improve insulin resistance. Thus, Yazdani-Biuki et al. show that treatment with infliximab, an α-TNFα antibody, every 8 weeks improves insulin sensitivity in obese and diabetic humans [120]. Currently, the approved agents available for studies in insulin-resistant states are infliximab and adalimunab (another α-TNFα antibody), which are presently used for the treatment of inflammatory diseases such as rheumatoid arthritis and inflammatory bowel disease. Side effects vary depending on the agent but include injection site reaction, nausea, vomiting, and abdominal pain. Some of the more serious side effects of the drugs are increased susceptibility to infection, demyelinating disease of the CNS, and aplastic anemia.

The importance of increased activity of the NF-κB pathway in diseases such as rheumatoid arthritis and inflammatory bowel disease has generated significant interest in developing strategies for decreasing the activity of the NF-κB pathway in these diseases. There are many agents that have been shown to (i) decrease IKK activation; (ii) inhibit the phosphorylation of IκBα; (iii) inhibit proteosome activity; (iv) inhibit translocation of NF-κB from the cytosol to the nucleus; and (v) inhibit DNA binding of NF-κB [121–123]. However, many of these reagents are used for research purposes only. Some are in the process of being developed for potential human use.

In closing, one important point to make is that chronic systemic inhibition of the NF-κB pathway in humans may have unwanted side effects, due to the vital role of this pathway as a mediator of early responses to infection. A tissue specific or local approach to NF-κB inhibition is an alternative strategy that may be considered if inhibitors of the NF-κB pathway are to be regarded as a potential therapeutic approach to the treatment of insulin resistance.

10. Conclusions

A series of studies in rodents has established that genetic or pharmaceutical interventions that alter the activity of the NF-κB pathway effects insulin action. There is strong evidence to suggest that activation of the pathway in liver induces hepatic, and possibly systemic, insulin resistance, while activation in monocytes causes systemic insulin resistance that may be associated with macrophage infiltration of tissues. There is contradictory evidence in skeletal muscle, with studies providing evidence for and against a role for the NF-κB pathway in the induction of insulin resistance. Currently, there are no studies that directly assess the relationship between NF-κB activity in adipose tissue, β-cells, or the CNS and insulin action. In humans, there is evidence that the NF-κB pathway is activated in insulin-resistant states, but it remains to be clearly established if the NF-κB pathway plays a role in the pathogenesis of insulin resistance in obesity or T2DM. In support of this possibility, treatment of T2DM with salicylate, the IKK inhibitor, improves insulin sensitivity. Mechanisms of activation of the NF-κB pathway of relevance to insulin-resistant states (particularly, cytokines and dyslipidemia but also potentially ER stress and mitochondrial dysfunction) have been proposed and putative mechanisms (IRS-1 serine phosphorylation, TNFα, IL-6) by which activation of the NF-κB pathway induces insulin resistance can be identified. However, a clearer understanding of the potential role and modes of actions of these mechanisms is required. In humans, there are therapeutic interventions that improve insulin action and are proposed to lower activity of the NF-κB pathway (salicylates, TZDs). However, it is not clear if other NF-κB inhibitors currently available have any potential therapeutic value.

Acknowledgments

Studies from the authors group cited in this chapter were supported by the National Institute of Health (NIH RO1 DK58855-01 to ROD and NIH KO8 DK069363-01 to

BB) and the American Diabetes Association (Research Award to ROD). BB was previously supported by NIH T32-DK07052 (Research Training in Diabetes and Endocrinology). Our apologies to the authors of those studies that we may have failed to cite in this chapter. This can be attributed to oversight on our part, space considerations, or the narrow focus of the subject matter.

References

[1] J. Hirosumi, G. Tuncman, L. Chang, C.Z. Gorgun, K.T. Uysal, K. Maeda, M. Karin, G.S. Hotamisligil, A central role for JNK in obesity and insulin resistance, Nature 420 (2002) 333–336.

[2] U. Ozcan, Q. Cao, E. Yilmaz, A.H. Lee, N.N. Iwakoshi, E. Ozdelen, G. Tuncman, C. Gorgun, L.H. Glimcher, G.S. Hotamisligil, Endoplasmic reticulum stress links obesity, insulin action, and type 2 diabetes, Science 306 (2004) 457–461.

[3] V.B. Ritov, E.V. Menshikova, J. He, R.E. Ferrell, B.H. Goodpaster, D.E. Kelley, Deficiency of subsarcolemmal mitochondria in obesity and type 2 diabetes, Diabetes 54 (2005) 8–14.

[4] K.F. Petersen, S. Dufour, D. Befroy, R. Garcia, G.I. Shulman, Impaired mitochondrial activity in the insulin-resistant offspring of patients with type 2 diabetes, N. Engl. J. Med. 350 (2004) 664–671.

[5] Joint WHO/FAO Expert Consultation, WHO Technical Report Series on Diet, nutrition, and the prevention of chronic diseases, 2003.

[6] M. Nestle, M. Jacobson, Halting the obesity epidemic: a public health policy approach, Public Health Rep 115 (2000) 12–24.

[7] A. Nandi, Y. Kitamura, C.R. Kahn, D. Accili, Mouse models of insulin resistance, Physiol. Rev. 84 (2004) 623–647.

[8] C. Yu, Y. Chen, G.W. Cline, D. Zhang, H. Zong, Y. Wang, R. Bergeron, J.K. Kim, S.W. Cushman, G.J. Cooney, B. Atcheson, M.F. White, E.W. Kraegen, G.I. Shulman, Mechanism by which fatty acids inhibit insulin activation of insulin receptor substrate-1 (IRS-1)-associated phosphatidylinositol 3-kinase activity in muscle, J. Biol. Chem. 277 (2002) 50230–50236.

[9] O.P. Bachmann, D.B. Dahl, K. Brechtel, J. Machann, M. Haap, T. Maier, M. Loviscach, M. Stumvoll, C.D. Claussen, F. Schick, H.U. Haring, S. Jacob, Effects of intravenous and dietary lipid challenge on intramyocellular lipid content and the relation with insulin sensitivity in humans, Diabetes 50 (2001) 2579–2584.

[10] G. Boden, B. Lebed, M. Schatz, C. Homko, S. Lemieux, Effects of acute changes of plasma free fatty acids on intramyocellular fat content and insulin resistance in healthy subjects, Diabetes 50 (2001) 1612–1617.

[11] S.M. Chalkley, M. Hettiarachchi, D.J. Chisholm, E.W. Kraegen, Five-hour fatty acid elevation increases muscle lipids and impairs glycogen synthesis in the rat, Metabolism 47 (1998) 1121–1126.

[12] M.E. Griffin, M.J. Marcucci, G.W. Cline, K. Bell, N. Barucci, D. Lee, L.J. Goodyear, E.W. Kraegen, M.F. White, G.I. Shulman, Free fatty acid-induced insulin resistance is associated with activation of protein kinase C theta and alterations in the insulin signaling cascade, Diabetes 48 (1999) 1270–1274.

[13] D.E. Kelley, B.H. Goodpaster, L. Storlien, Muscle triglyceride and insulin resistance, Annu. Rev. Nutr. 22 (2002) 325–346.

[14] B.D. Hegarty, S.M. Furler, J. Ye, G.J. Cooney, E.W. Kraegen, The role of intramuscular lipid in insulin resistance, Acta. Physiol. Scand. 178 (2003) 373–383.

[15] B.A. Swinburn, P.A. Metcalf, S.J. Ley, Long-term (5-year) effects of a reduced-fat diet intervention in individuals with glucose intolerance, Diabetes Care 24 (2001) 619–624.

[16] G. Paolisso, B.V. Howard, Role of non-esterified fatty acids in the pathogenesis of type 2 diabetes mellitus, Diabetes Med. 15 (1998) 360–366.

[17] N.D. Oakes, K.S. Bell, S.M. Furler, S. Camilleri, A.K. Saha, N.B. Ruderman, D.J. Chisholm, E.W. Kraegen, Diet-induced muscle insulin resistance in rats is ameliorated by acute dietary lipid

withdrawal or a single bout of exercise: parallel relationship between insulin stimulation of glucose uptake and suppression of long-chain fatty acyl-CoA, Diabetes 46 (1997) 2022–2028.

[18] R. Buettner, C.B. Newgard, C.J. Rhodes, R.M. O'Doherty, Correction of diet-induced hyperglycemia, hyperinsulinemia, and skeletal muscle insulin resistance by moderate hyperleptinemia, Am. J. Physiol. Endocrinol. Metab. 278 (2000) E563–E569.

[19] K.F. Petersen, E.A. Oral, S. Dufour, D. Befroy, C. Ariyan, C. Yu, G.W. Cline, A.M. DePaoli, S.I. Taylor, P. Gorden, G.I. Shulman, Leptin reverses insulin resistance and hepatic steatosis in patients with severe lipodystrophy, J. Clin. Invest. 109 (2002) 1345–1350.

[20] S. Kamohara, R. Burcelin, J.L. Halaas, J.M. Friedman, M.J. Charron, Acute stimulation of glucose metabolism in mice by leptin treatment, Nature 389 (1997) 374–377.

[21] N. Barzilai, J. Wang, D. Massilon, P. Vuguin, M. Hawkins, L. Rossetti, Leptin selectively decreases visceral adiposity and enhances insulin action, J. Clin. Invest. 100 (1997) 3105–3110.

[22] L. Rossetti, D. Massillon, N. Barzilai, P. Vuguin, W. Chen, M. Hawkins, J. Wu, J. Wang, Short term effects of leptin on hepatic gluconeogenesis and *in vivo* insulin action, J. Biol. Chem. 272 (1997) 27758–27763.

[23] T.P. Combs, A.H. Berg, S. Obici, P.E. Scherer, L. Rossetti, Endogenous glucose production is inhibited by the adipose-derived protein Acrp30, J. Clin. Invest. 108 (2001) 1875–1881.

[24] T. Yamauchi, J. Kamon, H. Waki, Y. Terauchi, N. Kubota, K. Hara, Y. Mori, T. Ide, K. Murakami, N. Tsuboyama-Kasaoka, O. Ezaki, Y. Akanuma, O. Gavrilova, C. Vinson, M.L. Reitman, H. Kagechika, K. Shudo, M. Yoda, Y. Nakano, K. Tobe, R. Nagai, S. Kimura, M. Tomita, P. Froguel, T. Kadowaki, The fat-derived hormone adiponectin reverses insulin resistance associated with both lipoatrophy and obesity, Nat. Med. 7 (2001) 941–946.

[25] A.H. Berg, T.P. Combs, P.E. Scherer, ACRP30/adiponectin: an adipokine regulating glucose and lipid metabolism, Trends Endocrinol. Metab. 13 (2002) 84–89.

[26] J. Fruebis, T.S. Tsao, S. Javorschi, D. Ebbets-Reed, M.R. Erickson, F.T. Yen, B.E. Bihain, H.F. Lodish, Proteolytic cleavage product of 30-kDa adipocyte complement-related protein increases fatty acid oxidation in muscle and causes weight loss in mice, Proc. Natl. Acad. Sci. USA 98 (2001) 2005–2010.

[27] N. Maeda, I. Shimomura, K. Kishida, H. Nishizawa, M. Matsuda, H. Nagaretani, N. Furuyama, H. Kondo, M. Takahashi, Y. Arita, R. Komuro, N. Ouchi, S. Kihara, Y. Tochino, K. Okutomi, M. Horie, S. Takeda, T. Aoyama, T. Funahashi, Y. Matsuzawa, Diet-induced insulin resistance in mice lacking adiponectin/ACRP30, Nat. Med. 8 (2002) 731–737.

[28] C.M. Steppan, S.T. Bailey, S. Bhat, E.J. Brown, R.R. Banerjee, C.M. Wright, H.R. Patel, R.S. Ahima, M.A. Lazar, The hormone resistin links obesity to diabetes, Nature 409 (2001) 307–312.

[29] A. Vidal-Puig, S. O'Rahilly, Resistin: a new link between obesity and insulin resistance?, Clin. Endocrinol. (Oxford) 55 (2001) 437–438.

[30] M. Pravenec, L. Kazdova, V. Landa, V. Zidek, P. Mlejnek, P. Jansa, J. Wang, N. Qi, T.W. Kurtz, Transgenic and recombinant resistin impair skeletal muscle glucose metabolism in the spontaneously hypertensive rat, J. Biol. Chem. 278 (2003) 45209–45215.

[31] C.M. Steppan, M.A. Lazar, Resistin and obesity-associated insulin resistance, Trends Endocrinol. Metab. 13 (2002) 18–23.

[32] H. Satoh, M.T. Nguyen, P.D. Miles, T. Imamura, I. Usui, J.M. Olefsky, Adenovirus-mediated chronic "hyper-resistinemia" leads to *in vivo* insulin resistance in normal rats, J. Clin. Invest. 114 (2004) 224–231.

[33] P.J. Klover, T.A. Zimmers, L.G. Koniaris, R.A. Mooney, Chronic exposure to interleukin-6 causes hepatic insulin resistance in mice, Diabetes 52 (2003) 2784–2789.

[34] P.J. Klover, A.H. Clementi, R.A. Mooney, Interleukin-6 depletion selectively improves hepatic insulin action in obesity, Endocrinology 146 (2005) 3417–3427.

[35] D.E. Moller, Potential role of TNF-alpha in the pathogenesis of insulin resistance and type 2 diabetes, Trends Endocrinol. Metab. 11 (2000) 212–217.

[36] R. Halse, S.L. Pearson, J.G. McCormack, S.J. Yeaman, R. Taylor, Effects of tumor necrosis factor-alpha on insulin action in cultured human muscle cells, Diabetes 50 (2001) 1102–1109.

[37] K.T. Uysal, S.M. Wiesbrock, M.W. Marino, G.S. Hotamisligil, Protection from obesity-induced insulin resistance in mice lacking TNF-alpha function, Nature 389 (1997) 610–614.

[38] P.D. Miles, O.M. Romeo, K. Higo, A. Cohen, K. Rafaat, J.M. Olefsky, TNF-alpha-induced insulin resistance *in vivo* and its prevention by troglitazone, Diabetes 46 (1997) 1678–1683.

[39] G.S. Hotamisligil, Mechanisms of TNF-alpha-induced insulin resistance, Exp. Clin. Endocrinol. Diabetes 107 (1999) 119–125.

[40] L.J. Ma, S.L. Mao, K.L. Taylor, T. Kanjanabuch, Y. Guan, Y. Zhang, N.J. Brown, L.L. Swift, O.P. McGuinness, D.H. Wasserman, D.E. Vaughan, A.B. Fogo, Prevention of obesity and insulin resistance in mice lacking plasminogen activator inhibitor 1, Diabetes 53 (2004) 336–346.

[41] H. Xu, G.T. Barnes, Q. Yang, G. Tan, D. Yang, C.J. Chou, J. Sole, A. Nichols, J.S. Ross, L.A. Tartaglia, H. Chen, Chronic inflammation in fat plays a crucial role in the development of obesity-related insulin resistance, J. Clin. Invest. 112 (2003) 1821–1830.

[42] S.P. Weisberg, D. McCann, M. Desai, M. Rosenbaum, R.L. Leibel, A.W. Ferrante Jr., Obesity is associated with macrophage accumulation in adipose tissue, J. Clin. Invest. 112 (2003) 796–1808.

[43] M.C. Arkan, A.L. Hevener, F.R. Greten, S. Maeda, Z.W. Li, J.M. Long, A. Wynshaw-Boris, G. Poli, J. Olefsky, M. Karin, IKK-beta links inflammation to obesity-induced insulin resistance, Nat. Med. 11 (2005) 191–198.

[44] M. Yuan, N. Konstantopoulos, J. Lee, L. Hansen, Z.W. Li, M. Karin, S.E. Shoelson, Reversal of obesity- and diet-induced insulin resistance with salicylates or targeted disruption of Ikkbeta, Science 293 (2001) 1673–1677.

[45] S.E. Shoelson, J. Lee, M. Yuan, Inflammation and the IKK beta/I kappa B/NF-kappa B axis in obesity- and diet-induced insulin resistance, Int. J. Obes. Relat. Metab. Disord. 27 (Suppl 3) (2003) S49–S52.

[46] R.S. Hundal, K.F. Petersen, A.B. Mayerson, P.S. Randhawa, S. Inzucchi, S.E. Shoelson, G.I. Shulman, Mechanism by which high-dose aspirin improves glucose metabolism in type 2 diabetes, J. Clin. Invest. 109 (2002) 1321–1326.

[47] J.K. Kim, Y.J. Kim, J.J. Fillmore, Y. Chen, I. Moore, J. Lee, M. Yuan, Z.W. Li, M. Karin, P. Perret, S.E. Shoelson, G.I. Shulman, Prevention of fat-induced insulin resistance by salicylate, J. Clin. Invest. 108 (2001) 437–446.

[48] D. Cai, M. Yuan, D.F. Frantz, P.A. Melendez, L. Hansen, J. Lee, S.E. Shoelson, Local and systemic insulin resistance resulting from hepatic activation of IKK-beta and NF-kappaB, Nat. Med. 11 (2005) 183–190.

[49] Q. Li, I.M. Verma, NF-kappaB regulation in the immune system, Nat. Rev. Immunol. 2 (2002) 725–734.

[50] S. Ghosh, M. Karin, Missing pieces in the NF-kappaB puzzle, Cell 109 (Suppl 1) (2002) S81–S96.

[51] P.P. Tak, G.S. Firestein, NF-kappaB: a key role in inflammatory diseases, J. Clin. Invest. 107 (2001) 7–11.

[52] S. Sinha, G. Perdomo, N.F. Brown, R.M. O'Doherty, Fatty acid-induced insulin resistance in L6 myotubes is prevented by inhibition of activation and nuclear localization of NF-κB, J. Biol. Chem. 279 (2004) 41294–41301.

[53] S.I. Itani, N.B. Ruderman, F. Schmieder, G. Boden, Lipid-induced insulin resistance in human muscle is associated with changes in diacylglycerol, protein kinase C, and IkappaB-alpha, Diabetes 51 (2002) 2005–2011.

[54] R. Sen, D. Baltimore, Inducibility of kappa immunoglobulin enhancer-binding protein Nf-kappa B by a posttranslational mechanism, Cell 47 (1986) 921–928.

[55] R. Sen, D. Baltimore, Multiple nuclear factors interact with the immunoglobulin enhancer sequences, Cell 46 (1986) 705–716.

[56] R.T. Williamson, On the treatment of glycosuria and diabetes mellitus with sodium salicylate, Br. Med. J. 1 (1901) 760–761.

[57] J. Reid, A.I. Macdougall, M.M. Andrews, Aspirin and diabetes mellitus, Br. Med. J. 33 (1957) 1071–1074.

[58] M.J. Yin, Y. Yamamoto, R.B. Gaynor, The anti-inflammatory agents aspirin and salicylate inhibit the activity of I(kappa)B kinase-beta, Nature 396 (1998) 77–80.

[59] D. Cai, J.D. Frantz, N.E. Tawa Jr., P.A. Melendez, B.C. Oh, H.G. Lidov, P.O. Hasselgren, W.R. Frontera, J. Lee, D.J. Glass, et al., IKKbeta/NF-kappaB activation causes severe muscle wasting in mice, Cell 119 (2004) 285–298.

[60] M. Rohl, M. Pasparakis, S. Baudler, J. Baumgartl, D. Gautam, M. Huth, R. De Lorenzi, W. Krone, K. Rajewsky, J.C. Bruning, Conditional disruption of IkappaB kinase 2 fails to prevent obesity-induced insulin resistance, J. Clin. Invest. 113 (2004) 474–481.

[61] B.A. Bhatt, J.J. Dube, N. Dedousis, J.A. Reider, R.M. O'Doherty, Diet-induced obesity and acute hyperlipidemia reduce IkappaBalpha levels in rat skeletal muscle in a fiber-type dependent manner, Am. J. Physiol. Regul. Integr. Comp. Physiol. 290 (2006) R233–R240.

[62] S. Sinha, G. Perdomo, N.F. Brown, R.M. O'Doherty, Fatty acid-induced insulin resistance in L6 myotubes is prevented by inhibition of activation and nuclear localization of nuclear factor kappa B, J. Biol. Chem. 279 (2004) 41294–41301.

[63] F.R. Greten, L. Eckmann, T.F. Greten, J.M. Park, Z.W. Li, L.J. Egan, M.F. Kagnoff, M. Karin, IKKbeta links inflammation and tumorigenesis in a mouse model of colitis-associated cancer, Cell 118 (2004) 285–296.

[64] D. Cai, M. Yuan, J. Guo, L. Hansen, J. Lee, Y. Ben-Neriah, S. Shoelson, Prevention of insulin resistance by NF-κB inhibition in fat or liver of transgenic FISR or LISR mice, Diabetes 53 (Suppl 2) (2004) A19.

[65] C.T. De Souza, E.P. Araujo, S. Bordin, R. Ashimine, R.L. Zollner, A.C. Boschero, M.J. Saad, L.A. Velloso, Consumption of a fat-rich diet activates a proinflammatory response and induces insulin resistance in the hypothalamus, Endocrinology 146 (2005) 4192–4199.

[66] B. Vozarova, C. Weyer, K. Hanson, P.A. Tataranni, C. Bogardus, R.E. Pratley, Circulating interleukin-6 in relation to adiposity, insulin action, and insulin secretion, Obes. Res. 9 (2001) 414–417.

[67] T. Wu, J.P. Dorn, R.P. Donahue, C.T. Sempos, M. Trevisan, Associations of serum C-reactive protein with fasting insulin, glucose, and glycosylated hemoglobin: the Third National Health and Nutrition Examination Survey, 1988–1994, Am. J. Epidemiol. 155 (2002) 65–71.

[68] T. Temelkova-Kurktschiev, G. Siegert, S. Bergmann, E. Henkel, C. Koehler, W. Jaross, M. Hanefeld, Subclinical inflammation is strongly related to insulin resistance but not to impaired insulin secretion in a high risk population for diabetes, Metabolism 51 (2002) 743–749.

[69] A. Festa, R. D'Agostino Jr., K. Williams, A.J. Karter, E.J. Mayer-Davis, R.P. Tracy, S.M. Haffner, The relation of body fat mass and distribution to markers of chronic inflammation, Int. J. Obes. Relat. Metab. Disord. 25 (2001) 1407–1415.

[70] J.C. Chambers, S. Eda, P. Bassett, Y. Karim, S.G. Thompson, J.R. Gallimore, M.B. Pepys, J.S. Kooner, C-reactive protein,insulin resistance, central obesity, and coronary heart disease risk in Indian Asians from the United Kingdom compared with European whites, Circulation 104 (2001) 145–150.

[71] N.G. Forouhi, N. Sattar, P.M. McKeigue, Relation of C-reactive protein to body fat distribution and features of the metabolic syndrome in Europeans and South Asians, Int. J. Obes. Relat. Metab. Disord. 25 (2001) 1327–1331.

[72] J.M. Fernandez-Real, B. Lainez, J. Vendrell, M. Rigla, A. Castro, G. Penarroja, M. Broch, A. Perez, C. Richart, P. Engel, et al., Shedding of TNF-alpha receptors, blood pressure, and insulin sensitivity in type 2 diabetes mellitus, Am. J. Physiol. Endocrinol. Metab. 282 (2002) E952–E959.

[73] A.E. Hak, H.A. Pols, C.D. Stehouwer, J. Meijer, A.J. Kiliaan, A. Hofman, M.M. Breteler, J.C. Witteman, Markers of inflammation and cellular adhesion molecules in relation to insulin resistance in nondiabetic elderly: the Rotterdam study, J. Clin. Endocrinol. Metab. 86 (2001) 4398–4405.

[74] N. Pannacciulli, F.P. Cantatore, A. Minenna, M. Bellacicco, R. Giorgino, G. De Pergola, C-reactive protein is independently associated with total body fat, central fat, and insulin resistance in adult women, Int. J. Obes. Relat. Metab. Disord. 25 (2001) 1416–1420.

[75] R.F. Grimble, Inflammatory status and insulin resistance, Curr. Opin. Clin. Nutr. Metab. Care 5 (2002) 551–559.

[76] A. Festa, R. D'Agostino Jr., R.P. Tracy, S.M. Haffner, Elevated levels of acute-phase proteins and plasminogen activator inhibitor-1 predict the development of type 2 diabetes: the insulin resistance atherosclerosis study, Diabetes 51 (2002) 1131–1137.

[77] A.D. Pradhan, J.E. Manson, N. Rifai, J.E. Buring, P.M. Ridker, C-reactive protein, interleukin 6, and risk of developing type 2 diabetes mellitus, Jama 286 (2001) 327–334.

[78] H.L. Pahl, Activators and target genes of Rel/NF-kappaB transcription factors, Oncogene 18 (1999) 6853–6866.

[79] G. Pascual, A.L. Fong, S. Ogawa, A. Gamliel, A.C. Li, V. Perissi, D.W. Rose, T.M. Willson, M.G. Rosenfeld, C.K. Glass, A SUMOylation-dependent pathway mediates transrepression of inflammatory response genes by PPAR-gamma, Nature 437 (2005) 759–763.

[80] A. Consoli, E. Devangelio, Thiazolidinediones and inflammation, Lupus 14 (2005) 794–797.

[81] A. Corbould, Y.B. Kim, J.F. Youngren, C. Pender, B.B. Kahn, A. Lee, A. Dunaif, Insulin resistance in the skeletal muscle of women with PCOS involves intrinsic and acquired defects in insulin signaling, Am. J. Physiol. Endocrinol. Metab. 288 (2005) E1047–E1054.

[82] M. Ueno, J.B. Carvalheira, R.C. Tambascia, R.M. Bezerra, M.E. Amaral, E.M. Carneiro, F. Folli, K.G. Franchini, M.J. Saad, Regulation of insulin signalling by hyperinsulinaemia: role of IRS-1/2 serine phosphorylation and the mTOR/p70 S6 K pathway, Diabetologia 48 (2005) 506–518.

[83] K. Morino, K.F. Petersen, S. Dufour, D. Befroy, J. Frattini, N. Shatzkes, S. Neschen, M.F. White, S. Bilz, S. Sono, M. Pypaert, G.I. Shulman, Reduced mitochondrial density and increased IRS-1 serine phosphorylation in muscle of insulin-resistant offspring of type 2 diabetic parents, J. Clin. Invest. 115 (2005) 3587–3593.

[84] K.F. Petersen, G.I. Shulman, Cellular mechanism of insulin resistance in skeletal muscle, J. R. Soc. Med. 95 (Suppl 42) (2002) 8–13.

[85] K.F. Petersen, G.I. Shulman, Pathogenesis of skeletal muscle insulin resistance in type 2 diabetes mellitus, Am. J. Cardiol. 90 (2002) 11G–18G.

[86] G. Boden, G.I. Shulman, Free fatty acids in obesity and type 2 diabetes: defining their role in the development of insulin resistance and beta-cell dysfunction, Eur. J. Clin. Invest. 32 (Suppl 3) (2002) 14–23.

[87] Z. Gao, X. Zhang, A. Zuberi, D. Hwang, M.J. Quon, M. Lefevre, J. Ye, Inhibition of insulin sensitivity by free fatty acids requires activation of multiple serine kinases in 3T3-L1 adipocytes, Mol. Endocrinol. 18 (2004) 2024–2034.

[88] C. de Alvaro, T. Teruel, R. Hernandez, M. Lorenzo, Tumor necrosis factor alpha produces insulin resistance in skeletal muscle by activation of inhibitor kappaB kinase in a p38 MAPK-dependent manner, J. Biol. Chem. 279 (2004) 17070–17078.

[89] Z. Gao, A. Zuberi, M.J. Quon, Z. Dong, J. Ye, Aspirin inhibits serine phosphorylation of insulin receptor substrate 1 in tumor necrosis factor-treated cells through targeting multiple serine kinases, J. Biol. Chem. 278 (2003) 24944–24950.

[90] Z. Gao, D. Hwang, F. Bataille, M. Lefevre, D. York, M.J. Quon, J. Ye, Serine phosphorylation of insulin receptor substrate 1 by inhibitor kappa B kinase complex, J. Biol. Chem. 277 (2002) 48115–48121.

[91] K. Yamamoto, T. Shimokawa, H. Yi, K. Isobe, T. Kojima, D.J. Loskutoff, H. Saito, Aging accelerates endotoxin-induced thrombosis: increased responses of plasminogen activator inhibitor-1 and lipopolysaccharide signaling with aging, Am. J. Pathol. 161 (2002) 1805–1814.

[92] Q.R. Ruan, W.J. Zhang, P. Hufnagl, C. Kaun, B.R. Binder, J. Wojta, Anisodamine counteracts lipopolysaccharide-induced tissue factor and plasminogen activator inhibitor-1 expression in human endothelial cells: contribution of the NF-kappa b pathway, J. Vasc. Res. 38 (2001) 13–19.

[93] M.A. Collart, P. Baeuerle, P. Vassalli, Regulation of tumor necrosis factor alpha transcription in macrophages: involvement of four kappa B-like motifs and of constitutive and inducible forms of NF-kappa B, Mol. Cell Biol. 10 (1990) 1498–1506.

[94] A.N. Shakhov, M.A. Collart, P. Vassalli, S.A. Nedospasov, C.V. Jongeneel, Kappa B-type enhancers are involved in lipopolysaccharide-mediated transcriptional activation of the tumor necrosis factor alpha gene in primary macrophages, J. Exp. Med. 171 (1990) 35–47.

[95] M. Jove, A. Planavila, R.M. Sanchez, M. Merlos, J.C. Laguna, M. Vazquez-Carrera, Palmitate induces tumor necrosis factor-alpha expression in C2C12 skeletal muscle cells by a mechanism involving protein kinase C and nuclear factor-kappaB activation, Endocrinology 147 (2006) 552–561.

[96] M. Jove, A. Planavila, J.C. Laguna, M. Vazquez-Carrera, Palmitate-induced interleukin 6 production is mediated by protein kinase C and nuclear-factor kappaB activation and leads to glucose transporter 4 down-regulation in skeletal muscle cells, Endocrinology 146 (2005) 3087–3095.

[97] S. Chung, J.M. Brown, J.N. Provo, R. Hopkins, M.K. McIntosh, Conjugated linoleic acid promotes human adipocyte insulin resistance through NFkappaB-dependent cytokine production, J. Biol. Chem. 280 (2005) 38445–38456.

[98] C. Weigert, K. Brodbeck, H. Staiger, C. Kausch, F. Machicao, H.U. Haring, E.D. Schleicher, Palmitate, but not unsaturated fatty acids, induces the expression of interleukin-6 in human myotubes through proteasome-dependent activation of nuclear factor-kappaB, J. Biol. Chem. 279 (2004) 23942–23952.

[99] D. Wu, M. Marko, K. Claycombe, K.E. Paulson, S.N. Meydani, Ceramide-induced and age-associated increase in macrophage COX-2 expression is mediated through up-regulation of NF-kappa B activity, J. Biol. Chem. 278 (2003) 10983–10992.

[100] M.L. Schmitz, S. Bacher, O. Dienz, NF-kappaB activation pathways induced by T cell costimulation, FASEB J. 17 (2003) 2187–2193.

[101] J.Y. Lee, K.H. Sohn, S.H. Rhee, D. Hwang, Saturated fatty acids, but not unsaturated fatty acids, induce the expression of cyclooxygenase-2 mediated through toll-like receptor 4, J. Biol. Chem. 276 (2001) 16683–16689.

[102] J.Y. Lee, J. Ye, Z. Gao, H.S. Youn, W.H. Lee, L. Zhao, N. Sizemore, D.H. Hwang, Reciprocal modulation of toll-like receptor-4 signaling pathways involving MyD88 and phosphatidylinositol 3-kinase/AKT by saturated and polyunsaturated fatty acids, J. Biol. Chem. 278 (2003) 37041–37051.

[103] D. Tripathy, P. Mohanty, S. Dhindsa, T. Syed, H. Ghanim, A. Aljada, P. Dandona, Elevation of free fatty acids induces inflammation and impairs vascular reactivity in healthy subjects, Diabetes 52 (2003) 2882–2887.

[104] I. Rusyn, C.A. Bradham, L. Cohn, R. Schoonhoven, J.A. Swenberg, D.A. Brenner, R.G. Thurman, Corn oil rapidly activates nuclear factor-kappaB in hepatic Kupffer cells by oxidant-dependent mechanisms, Carcinogenesis 20 (1999) 2095–2100.

[105] M. Radin, B.A. Bhatt, R.M. O'Doherty, The lipopolysaccharide receptor, toll-like receptor 4, mediates palmitate-induced activation of the IKK/IkB/NF-kB pathway in L6 myotubes, Diabetes 54 (2005) A59.

[106] B. Beutler, E.T. Rietschel, Innate immune sensing and its roots: the story of endotoxin, Nat. Rev. Immunol. 3 (2003) 169–176.

[107] G. Bonizzi, J. Piette, M.P. Merville, V. Bours, Cell type-specific role for reactive oxygen species in nuclear factor-kappaB activation by interleukin-1, Biochem. Pharmacol. 59 (2000) 7–11.

[108] B. Kaltschmidt, T. Sparna, C. Kaltschmidt, Activation of NF-kappa B by reactive oxygen intermediates in the nervous system, Antioxid. Redox Signal. 1 (1999) 129–144.

[109] J.L. Evans, I.D. Goldfine, B.A. Maddux, G.M. Grodsky, Oxidative stress and stress-activated signaling pathways: a unifying hypothesis of type 2 diabetes, Endocr. Rev. 23 (2002) 599–622.

[110] T. Inoguchi, P. Li, F. Umeda, H.Y. Yu, M. Kakimoto, M. Imamura, T. Aoki, T. Etoh, T. Hashimoto, M. Naruse, H. Sano, H. Utsumi, H. Nawata, High glucose level and free fatty acid stimulate reactive oxygen species production through protein kinase C-dependent activation of NAD(P)H oxidase in cultured vascular cells, Diabetes 49 (2000) 1939–1945.

[111] L.L. Listenberger, D.S. Ory, J.E. Schaffer, Palmitate-induced apoptosis can occur through a ceramide-independent pathway, J. Biol. Chem. 276 (2001) 14890–14895.

[112] A. Cabrero, M. Alegret, R.M. Sanchez, T. Adzet, J.C. Laguna, M.V. Carrera, Increased reactive oxygen species production down-regulates peroxisome proliferator-activated alpha pathway in C2C12 skeletal muscle cells, J. Biol. Chem. 277 (2002) 10100–10107.

[113] H.L. Pahl, P.A. Baeuerle, The ER-overload response: activation of NF-kappa B, Trends Biochem. Sci. 22 (1997) 63–67.

[114] H.L. Pahl, Signal transduction from the endoplasmic reticulum to the cell nucleus, Physiol. Rev. 79 (1999) 683–701.

[115] H. Ghanim, R. Garg, A. Aljada, P. Mohanty, Y. Kumbkarni, E. Assian, W. Hamouda, P. Dandona, Suppression of nuclear factor-kappaB and stimulation of inhibitor kappaB by troglitazone: evidence

for an anti-inflammatory effect and a potential antiatherosclerotic effect in the obese, J. Clin. Endocrinol. Metab. 86 (2001) 1306–1312.

[116] A. Aljada, R. Garg, H. Ghanim, P. Mohanty, W. Hamouda, E. Assian, P. Dandona, Nuclear factor-kappaB suppressive and inhibitor-kappaB stimulatory effects of troglitazone in obese patients with type 2 diabetes: evidence of an antiinflammatory action?, J. Clin. Endocrinol. Metab. 86 (2001) 3250–3256.

[117] P. Mohanty, A. Aljada, H. Ghanim, D. Hofmeyer, D. Tripathy, T. Syed, W. Al-Haddad, S. Dhindsa, P. Dandona, Evidence for a potent antiinflammatory effect of rosiglitazone, J. Clin. Endocrinol. Metab. 89 (2004) 2728–2735.

[118] N. Paquot, M.J. Castillo, P.J. Lefebvre, A.J. Scheen, No increased insulin sensitivity after a single intravenous administration of a recombinant human tumor necrosis factor receptor: Fc fusion protein in obese insulin-resistant patients, J. Clin. Endocrinol. Metab. 85 (2000) 1316–1319.

[119] F. Ofei, S. Hurel, J. Newkirk, M. Sopwith, R. Taylor, Effects of an engineered human anti-TNF-alpha antibody (CDP571) on insulin sensitivity and glycemic control in patients with NIDDM, Diabetes 45 (1996) 881–885.

[120] B. Yazdani-Biuki, H. Stelzl, H.P. Brezinschek, J. Hermann, T. Mueller, P. Krippl, W. Graninger, T.C. Wascher, Improvement of insulin sensitivity in insulin resistant subjects during prolonged treatment with the anti-TNF-alpha antibody infliximab, Eur. J. Clin. Invest. 34 (2004) 641–642.

[121] I.M. Verma, Nuclear factor (NF)-kappaB proteins: therapeutic targets, Ann. Rheum. Dis. 63 (Suppl 2) (2004) ii57–ii61.

[122] V. Pande, M.J. Ramos, NF-kappaB in human disease: current inhibitors and prospects for *de novo* structure based design of inhibitors, Curr. Med. Chem. 12 (2005) 357–374.

[123] J.C. Epinat, T.D. Gilmore, Diverse agents act at multiple levels to inhibit the Rel/NF-kappaB signal transduction pathway, Oncogene 18 (1999) 6896–6909.

Index

Colour Plate Section

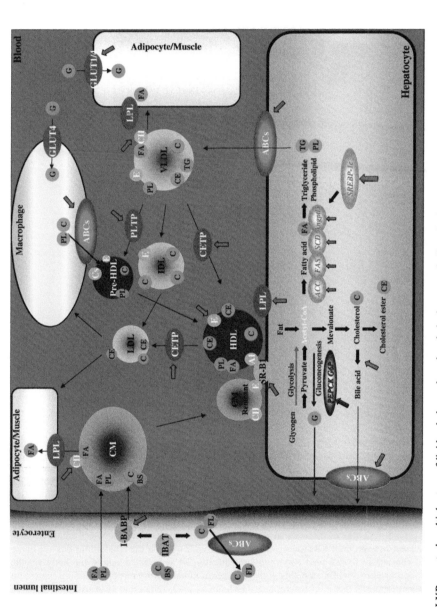

Plate 1. The LXRs control multiple steps of lipid-, cholesterol- and carbohydrate metabolism. Red arrows indicate LXR induced effects while blue arrows indicate LXR repressed effects. C: cholesterol, CE: cholesterol ester, FA: fatty acid, PL: phospspholipid, TG: triglyceride, BS: bile salt, G: glucose, AI: apolipoprotein AI, Cs: apolipoprotein C-I/C-IV/ C-II, E: apolipoprotein E. See text for further details.

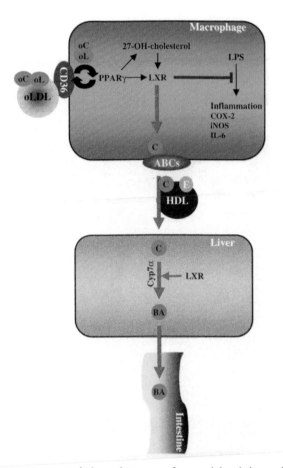

Plate 2. The LXRs promote reverse cholesterol transport from peripheral tissues, including machrophages, to the liver. On machrophages oxidized LDL (oLDL) docks at the CD36 receptor off loading
oxidized cholesterol (oC) and oxidized lipids (oL). OoL activates PPARγ which induces expression of
CD36 further enhancing uptake of oC and oL. This indicates a pro-atherosclerotic effect of PPARγ also
activates. However, PPARγ induces LXRα expression directly via a PPAR response element in the promoter of LXRα. It also activates the LXR by inducing expression of Cyp27 thereby producing the 27-
hydroxycholesterol (27-OH-cholesterol) LXR agonist. Activated LXRs then induce expression of apoE
and ABCA1 promoting efflux of intracellular cholesterol (C) to the HDL particle which transport cholesterol to the liver. In liver, the LXRs induce expression of Cyp7α which is the rate-limiting enzyme in the
conversion of cholesterol to bile acid (BA) and subsequently BA is excreted out of the body via the
intestines. Lipopolysaccharide (LPS), a highly potent inducer of inflammatory responses, induce expression
of inflammatory responsive genes in macrophages including Cox-2, iNOS and IL-6. Activation of the
LXRs suppresses the LPS-induced expression of these inflammatory mediators pointing towards an anti-
inflammatory role of the LXR. Hence, the LXRs are both anti-atherosclerotic and anti-inflammatory
mediators which suggest a positive effect of these receptors in terms of cardiovascular diseases.

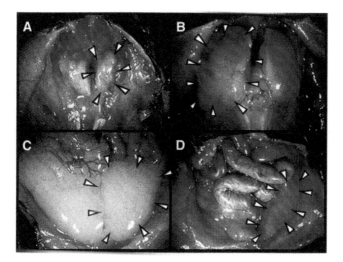

Plate 3. Wild-type mouse (A, C) with normal interscapular BAT depot (A) and intraabdominal WAT depots (C). In aP2 FOXC2, tg mice there is a dramatic increase in BAT depot size (B) and a reduction in intraabdominal WAT depots.

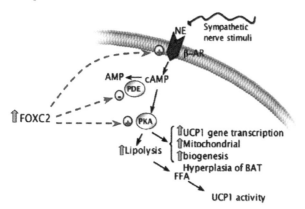

Plate 4. FOXC2 induces increased sensitivity in the β-adrenergic pathway by acting at three different levels.

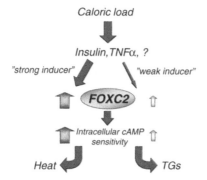

Plate 5. FOXC2 as a regulator of metabolic efficency. According to this hypothesis a strong induction of FOXC2 in response to a caloric load leads to a metabolic situation in which a large portion of the ingested calories would be dissipated as heat, due to increased sensitivity of the β-adrenergic/PKA pathway, whereas a weaker induction induces conservation of the caloric load as triglycerides. (Reproduced with permission from *Cell*, copyright Elsevier Science.)

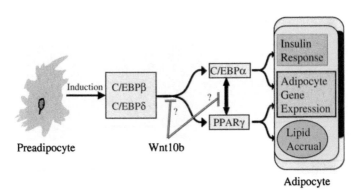

Preadipocyte   Wnt10b

Adipocyte

Plate 6. Program of Adipogenesis. Inducers of preadipocyte differentiation stimulate expression of C/EBPβ and C/EBPδ, which then activate transcription of both C/EBPα and PPARγ. The master adipogenic transcription factors, C/EBPα and PPARγ, enforce each other's expression through a positive feedback loop. During adipogenesis, C/EBPα is required for acquisition of insulin sensitivity, while PPARγ is necessary for accumulation of lipid. Although not fully characterized, both transcription factors play key roles in expression of a subset of adipocyte genes. Together, C/EBPα and PPARγ stimulate the full complement of genes required to create the adipocyte phenotype. Wnt signaling inhibits differentiation by blocking expression of these master adipogenic transcription factors.

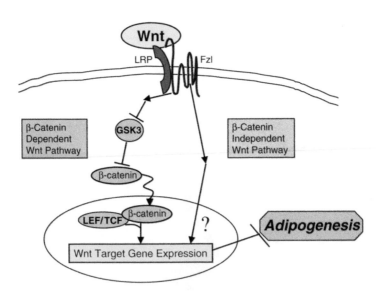

Plate 7. Wnt signaling inhibits adipogenesis through β-catenin dependent and independent pathways. Wnt acts through Frizzled receptors and LRP coreceptors to inhibit activity of glycogen synthase kinase 3, thus resulting in hypophosphorylation and stabilization of β-catenin. After translocation to the nucleus, β-catenin acts through TCF/LEF transcription factors to ultimately inhibit expression of C/EBPα and PPARγ, and thereby block preadipocyte differentiation. In addition, Wnt may inhibit adipocyte conversion through a Wnt signaling pathway independent of β-catenin.

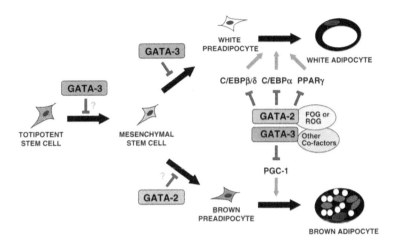

Plate 8. Precursor cells of mesenchymal origin give rise to adipocytes. While it is not clear whether white and brown adipocytes emerge from a common precursor such as a mesenchymal stem cell, many developmental mechanisms are common to both cell types. In this same context, whether GATA factors contribute to lineage development of white and/or brown adipocytes is currently unknown. On the other hand, it is established that both GATA-2 and GATA-3 control the transition from a preadipocyte to adipocyte. To control this critical transition, GATA factors interfere with the activity of at least two key groups of molecules that govern terminal differentiation, the C/EBP family and PPARγ. In the brown adipogenesis, PGC-1 is also targeted by GATA and several transcriptional co-factors are likely contributors to their actions.

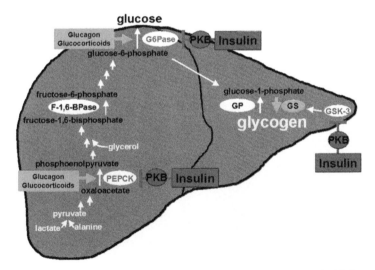

Plate 9. Regulation of hepatic glucose production. *Note*: Glucagon and glucocorticoids increase hepatic gluconeogenesis by inducing the expression of PEPCK and G6 Pase, two key gluconeogenic enzymes (left). In contrast, insulin inhibits hepatic glucose production by inhibiting gluconeogenesis on the level of G6 Pase and PEPCK gene expression and by stimulating glycogen storage via inhibition of GSK-3 (right). Activation of PKB is a central mechanism in the mediation of the metabolic effects of insulin and parts of the effects of PKB on gene expression are mediated by FoxO-transcription factors.

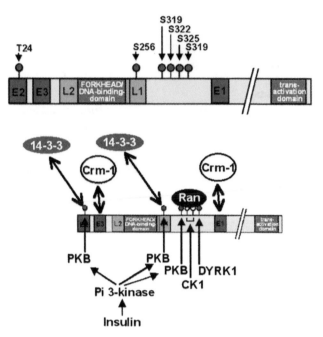

Plate 10. The structure and regulation of FoxO-proteins. *Note*: Upper panel: phosphorylation sites and structural elements involved in the nuclear/cytoplasmic distribution of FoxO1. Lower panel: phosphorylation of FoxO-proteins by PKB, CK1, and DYRK1 results in inactivation and cytoplasmic localization by facilitating the interaction of FoxO-proteins with proteins of the nuclear export machinery like Crm1, 14-3-3, and Ran.

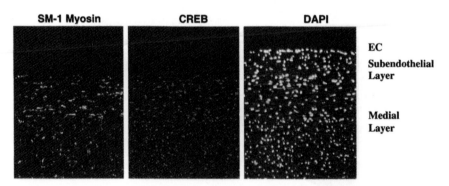

Plate 11. Correlation between CREB content and SMC differentiation markers *in vivo*: fluorescent immunostaining of bovine aorta for cellularity (blue- DAPI), SMC (green-SM Myosin 1) and CREB (red). CREB staining co-localized with medial SMC. For experimental detail, see ref. [1]. *Source:* Adapted figure reproduced with permission ref. [1].

Model for Insulin Interaction with the PEPCK Transcriptome

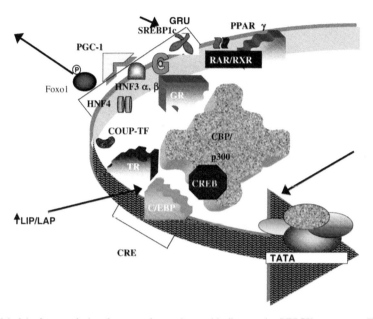

Plate 12. Model of transcription factor and coactivator binding to the PEPCK promoter. The abbreviations for the factors and binding elements are: CRE, cAMP regulatory element; GRU, glucocorticoid regulatory unit; G, glucocorticoid; SREBP1c, sterol response element binding protein 1c; CREB, CRE binding protein; C/EBP, CCAAT/enhancer binding protein; Foxo1, forkhead transcription factor; HNF-4α, hepatic nuclear factor-4α; TR, thyroid hormone receptor; GR, glucocorticoid receptor; PPARγ, peroxisome proliferator-activated receptor γ; RAR, retinoic acid receptor; RXR, retinoid X receptor; CBP, CREB binding protein; PGC-1, PPARγ coactivator 1; COUP-TF, chicken ovalbumin upstream promoter transcription factor.

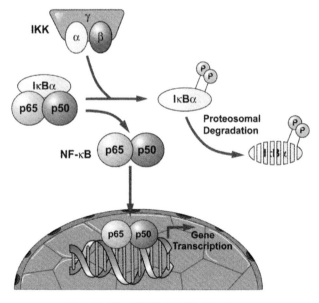

Plate 13. The IKK/IκB /NF-κB pathway.

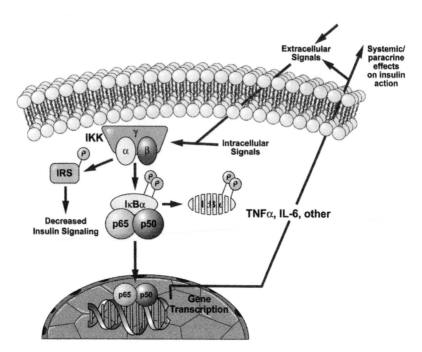

Plate 14. Potential mechanisms of insulin resistance arising from activation of the NF-κB pathway.

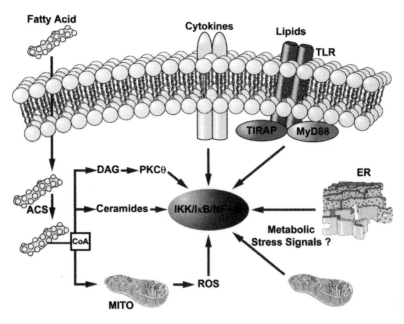

Plate 15. Potential mechanisms of activation of the NF-κB pathway in insulin-resistant states.

Printed and bound by CPI Group (UK) Ltd, Croydon, CR0 4YY

08/05/2025

01865007-0003